Giving Through Teaching

How Nurse Educators Are Changing the World

Giving Through Teaching

How Nurse Educators Are Changing the World

Joyce J. Fitzpatrick, PhD, MBA, RN, FAAN

Cathleen M. Shultz, PhD, RN, CNE, FAAN

Tonia D. Aiken, JD, RN

Editors

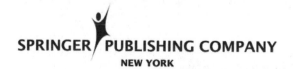

SPRINGER PUBLISHING COMPANY

NEW YORK

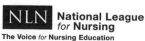

National League
for **Nursing**
The Voice *for* Nursing Education

Springer Publishing Company, LLC
11 West 42nd Street
New York, NY 10036
www.springerpub.com

Acquisitions Editor: Allan Graubard
Production Editor: Gayle Lee
Cover Design: Steve Pisano
Composition: Ashita Shah at Newgen Imaging Systems Ltd.

ISBN: 978–0–8261–1862–2
E-book ISBN: 978–0–8261–1863–9

10 11 12 13/ 5 4 3 2 1

The author and the publisher of this Work have made every effort to use sources believed to be reliable to provide information that is accurate and compatible with the standards generally accepted at the time of publication. Because medical science is continually advancing, our knowledge base continues to expand. Therefore, as new information becomes available, changes in procedures become necessary. We recommend that the reader always consult current research and specific institutional policies before performing any clinical procedure. The author and publisher shall not be liable for any special, consequential, or exemplary damages resulting, in whole or in part, from the readers' use of, or reliance on, the information contained in this book. The publisher has no responsibility for the persistence or accuracy of URLs for external or third-party Internet Web sites referred to in this publication and does not guarantee that any content on such Web sites is, or will remain, accurate or appropriate.

Library of Congress Cataloging-in-Publication Data
Giving through teaching : how nurse educators are changing the world / [edited by] Joyce Fitzpatrick, Cathleen M. Shultz, Tonia D. Aiken.
      p. ; cm.
Includes bibliographical references and index.
ISBN 978-0-8261-1862-2
1. Nursing—Study and teaching—International cooperation. I.
Fitzpatrick, Joyce J., 1944- II. Shultz, Cathleen M. (Cathleen Michaele) III. Aiken, Tonia D.
   [DNLM: 1. Education, Nursing—trends. 2. Faculty, Nursing. 3. Leadership.
4. Nurse's Role—psychology. 5. Power (Psychology) 6.Teaching—trends. WY 18 G539 2010]
   RT73.G58 2010
   610.73071'1—dc22   2010012537

Printed in the United States of America by Hamilton Printing.

Contents

SECTION I: HISTORICAL AND CONTEMPORARY LEGACY NURSE EDUCATORS

Joyce J. Fitzpatrick, Editor

SECTION II: INFLUENTIAL NURSE EDUCATORS IN THE UNITED STATES

Cathleen M. Shultz, Editor

SECTION III: NURSE EDUCATORS WHO CHANGE AND SHAPE HEALTH CARE GLOBALLY
   Cathleen M. Shultz, Editor

SECTION IV: NURSING AMIDST DISASTER
Tonia D. Aiken, Editor

Contributors

Evelyn L. Acheson, PhD, RN, University of Oklahoma College of Nursing, Tulsa, OK

Salpy Akaragian, MN, RN-BC, FIAN, UCLA School of Nursing, Los Angeles, CA

Angela V. Albright, PhD, RN, Samuel Merritt College School of Nursing, Oakland, CA

Patricia Allen, EdD, RN, Texas Tech University Health Sciences Center, Anita Thigpen Perry School of Nursing, Lubbock, TX

Kathleen C. Ashton, PhD, APRN, BC, Thomas Jefferson University School of Nursing, Philadelphia, PA

Brooke Bailey, BSN, RN, University of North Carolina at Chapel Hill School of Nursing, Chapel Hill, NC

Esther G. Bankert, PhD, RN, SUNY Institute of Technology School of Nursing, Utica, NY

Agnes Beachman, PhD, RN, International University of Nursing, St. Kitts

Deborah Bell, MSN, FNP-C, RN, University of Texas at Tyler College of Nursing and Health Sciences, Tyler, TX

Marietta Bell-Scriber, PhD, FNP-BC, Ferris State University School of Nursing, Big Rapids, MI

Lynda Billings, PhD, MFA, Texas Tech University Health Sciences Center, Anita Thigpen Perry School of Nursing, Lubbock, TX

Diane Blanchard, PhD, CNS, RN, Alcorn State University School of Nursing, Natchez, MS

Mary P. Bourke, PhD, MSN, RN, Indiana University Kokomo School of Nursing, Kokomo, IN

Diane M. Breckenridge, PhD, RN, La Salle University School of Nursing and Health Sciences, Philadelphia, PA

Linda M. Brice, PhD, RN, Texas Tech University of Health Sciences Center, Anita Thigpen Perry School of Nursing, Lubbock, TX

Sandra J. Cadena, PhD, ARNP, CNE, University of South Florida College of Nursing, Tampa, FL

Jamie Cash, BSN, RN, University of North Carolina at Chapel Hill School of Nursing, Chapel Hill, NC

Debbie Ciesielka, EdD, CNRP, ANP-BC, Clarion University School of Nursing, Pittsburgh, PA

Rebecca C. Clark, PhD, RN, Carilion Clinic, Roanoke, VA

Pamela Cone, PhD, CNS, RN, Azusa Pacific University School of Nursing, Azusa, CA

Catherine R. Coverston, PhD, RNC, Brigham Young University College of Nursing, Provo, UT

Elissa Crocker, BSN, RN, on behalf of Carole Kenner, DNS, RNC-NIC, FAAN, University of Oklahoma College of Nursing, Tulsa, OK

Deborah L. Curry, APN, BC, DNP, RN, Lurleen B. Wallace College of Nursing and Health Sciences, Jacksonville State University, Jacksonville, FL

Kim Curry, PhD, ARNP, University of Tampa Department of Nursing, Tampa, FL

Sarah Day Dickson, BSN, RN, University of North Carolina at Chapel Hill School of Nursing, Chapel Hill, NC

Jane DeFazio, MS, RN, The Evelyn L. Spiro School of Nursing, Wagner College, Staten Island, NY

Betty Pierce Dennis, DrPH, RN, Dillard University Division of Nursing, New Orleans, LA

Chris DeWilde, RN, Bon Secours Memorial School of Nursing, Richmond, VA

Sharon W. Dowdy, PhD, RN, Belmont University School of Nursing, Nashville, TN

Karen B. Drake, PhD, RNBC, Bethel University Department of Nursing, St. Paul, MN

Elicia Egozcue, BSN, Florida International University College of Nursing and Health Sciences, Miami, FL

Carrie B. Elkins, PHCNS-BC, DHSc, Lurleen B. Wallace College of Nursing and Health Sciences, Jacksonville State University, Jacksonville, FL

Shannon Finley, MSN, RN, University of Arkansas for Medical Sciences College of Nursing, Little Rock, AR

Susan E. Fletcher, EdD, MSN(r), RN, Chamberlain College of Nursing, St. Louis, MO

Sylvia Fox, PhD, CNS, RN, Samuel Merritt College School of Nursing, Oakland, CA

Catherine Garner, DrPH, RN, FAAN, American Sentinel University, Aurora, CO

Ghidey Ghebreyohanes, MSN, RN, Samuel Merritt College School of Nursing, Oakland, CA

Maryann Godshall, PhD(c), CNS, CCRN, CPN, DeSales University Department of Nursing and Health, Center Valley, PA

Jennifer Gray, PhD, RN, The University of Texas at Arlington School of Nursing, Arlington, TX

Michelle Hartman, MSN, PNP, RN, Carilion Clinic, Roanoke, VA

Guanetta Haynes, MSN, APRN, BSN, PHN, RN, University of Phoenix, Phoenix, AZ

Alison Helmink, BSN, RN, University of North Carolina at Chapel Hill School of Nursing, Chapel Hill, NC

Cheryl Herrmann, APN, CCRN, CCNS-CSC/CMC, Methodist Medical Center, Peoria, IL

Katie Horrow, BSN, RN, University of North Carolina at Chapel Hill School of Nursing, Chapel Hill, NC

Sandra L. Hould, MSN, RN, Community Health Systems (CHS), Brandywine Hospital, Coatesville, PA

Faye Hummel, PhD, RN, CTN, University of Northern Colorado School of Nursing, Greeley, CO

Sara L. Jarrett, MS, CNS, EdD, CNE, RN, Regis University School of Nursing, Denver, CO

Joy Jennings, MSN, CNE, RN, University of Arkansas for Medical Sciences College of Nursing, Little Rock, AR

Joanne Joseph, PhD, SUNY Institute of Technology School of Nursing, Utica, NY

Teri Kaul, PhD, APRN-BC, Concordia University Wisconsin Division of Nursing, Mequon, WI

Florence Keane, DNS, MBA, ARNP, NP-C, Florida International University College of Nursing and Health Sciences, Miami, FL

Patricia Kinser, MSN, WHNP, RN, Bon Secours Memorial School of Nursing, Richmond, VA

Rita Knobloch, RN, EMT-B, Sanford Children's Hospital, Sioux Falls, SD

Joanne C. Langan, PhD, RN, Saint Louis University School of Nursing, St. Louis, MO

Kim Larson, PhD, RN, College of Nursing, East Carolina University, Greenville, NC

Kathie Lasater, EdD, RN, Oregon Health Sciences University School of Nursing, Ashland, OR

Mary M. Lebold, EdD, RN, Mercy Hospital and Medical Center, Chicago, IL

Shirleen B. Lewis-Trabeaux, PhD, RN, Nicholls State University College of Nursing and Allied Health, Thibodaux, LA

Huaping Liu, PhD, RN, FAAN, Peking Union Medical College, Beijing, China

James Ludemann, BSN, RN, University of North Carolina at Chapel Hill School of Nursing, Chapel Hill, NC

Karen A. Lumia, MS, RN, Gannon University Villa Maria School of Nursing, Erie, PA

Dawn Michelle Mabry, MSN, RN, University of St. Francis Department of Nursing, Fort Wayne, IN

Andrew J. Mahoney, BSN, SANE-A, RN, Interim LSU Public Hospital, New Orleans, LA

Debbie Mahoney, PhD, ANP-C, RN, University of Texas at Tyler College of Nursing and Health Sciences, Tyler, TX

Erin Maughan, PhD, RN, Brigham Young University College of Nursing, Provo, UT

Kimberly McClane, PhD, RN, International University of Nursing, St. Kitts

Pamela A. Mead, BSN, RN, Erie Home Health Services, Erie, PA

Kay Medlin, BSN, RN, Arkansas Northeastern College Associate Degree Nursing Program, Blytheville, AR

Martha J. Morrow, PhD, FNP-C, Shenandoah University, Department of Nursing, Winchester, VA

Jennifer Morton, DNP, MS, MPH, RN, University of New England Department of Nursing, Biddeford, ME

Carolyn Mosley, PhD, RN, CS, FAAN, College of Health Sciences, University of Arkansas, Fort Smith, AR

Fran Muldoon, MSN, RN, Delaware Technical and Community College Nursing Department, Georgetown, DE

Jemimah Mary Mutabaazi, RM, DipNED, BNS, MCNS, RN, Uganda Christian University Nursing Programme, Mukono, Uganda

Marie Napolitano, PhD, FNP, RN, University of Portland School of Nursing, Portland, OR

Mackie H. Norris, PhD, MN, RN, Africa University, Zimbabwe

Darlene O'Callaghan, MSN, RN, Mercy Hospital and Medical Center, Chicago, IL

Susie Oliver, MSN, NP, RNC, University of Indianapolis School of Nursing, Indianapolis, IN

Jackline Opollo, MSN, MPH, RN, University of Texas at Arlington
School of Nursing, Arlington, TX

Melissa Ott, MS, NP-C, FNP, RN, College of Nursing, East Carolina
University, Greenville, NC

Dorothy A. Otto, EdD, RN, ANEF, University of Texas Health Science
Center at Houston, Houston, TX

Bozena M. Padykula, MSN, RN, AHN-BC, University of Connecticut
School of Nursing, Storrs, CT

Angela Pasco, MSN, RN, Pottsville Hospital School of Nursing,
Drexel University, College of Nursing and Health Professions,
Philadelphia, PA

G. Elaine Patterson, EdD, MA, MdD, FNP-C, Ramapo College of
New Jersey Nursing Program, Mahwah, NJ

Lee A. Perry, JD, MSN, MA, BSN, RN, University of Texas Health
Science Center, Department of Chronic Nursing Care,
San Antonio, TX

Elvira Phelps, EdD, MSN, MAEd, APRN, Denver School of Nursing,
Denver, CO

Nancy Phoenix Bittner, PhD, CCRN, RN, Regis College, School of
Nursing and Health Professions, Weston, MA

Kristen Poe, BSN, RN, University of North Carolina at Chapel Hill
School of Nursing, Chapel Hill, NC

Michele Poradzisz, PhD, RN, Mercy Hospital and Medical Center,
Chicago, IL

Lisa A. Quinn, PhD, CRNP, RNC, Gannon University Villa Maria
School of Nursing, Erie, PA

Paula Reams, PhD, CNE, LMT, RN, Kettering College of Medical Arts
Nursing Program, Dayton, OH

Linda Rickabaugh, MSN, RN, Carilion Clinic, Roanoke, VA

Susan Ritchie, MN, RN, University of Arkansas for Medical Sciences
College of Nursing, Little Rock, AR

Rory Rochelle, PhD(c), MSN, RN, Skagit Valley College Nursing Program, Mount Vernon, WA

Vickie L. Rogers, DNP, RN, University of Southern Mississippi School of Nursing, Hattiesburg, MS

Jan Rooker, MNSc, RNP, University of Arkansas for Medical Sciences College of Nursing, Little Rock, AR

Ecoee Rooney, MSN, SANE-A, RN, Interim LSU Public Hospital, New Orleans, LA

Priscilla Limbo Sagar, PhD, Mount Saint Mary College Nursing Program, Newburgh, NY

Cheryl K. Schmidt, PhD, CNE, RN, ANEF, University of Arkansas for Medical Sciences College of Nursing, Little Rock, AR

Kathleen Sellers, PhD, RN, SUNY Institute of Technology School of Nursing, Utica, NY

Gwen Sherwood, PhD, RN, FAAN, University of North Carolina at Chapel Hill School of Nursing, Chapel Hill, NC

Brenda Simmons, MSN, RN, International University of Nursing, St. Kitts

Eileen M. Smit, MSN, RN, Northern Michigan University Department of Nursing, Marquette, MI

Charlotte Souers, MSN, Ohio University School of Nursing, Athens, OH

Lori Spies, PhD(c), MS, NP-C, RN, University of Texas at Arlington School of Nursing, Arlington, TX

Helena Stanaitis, MS, RN, Saint Anthony College of Nursing, Rockford, IL

Cara Stone, MSN, WHNP-BC, RN, International University of Nursing, St. Kitts

Annette Strickland, MSN, RN, Carilion Clinic, Roanoke, VA

Jane Sumner, PhD, APRN, BC, RN, Louisiana State University Health Sciences Center, New Orleans, LA

Susan C. Taplin, MSN, RN, Belmont University School of Nursing, Nashville, TN

Sharon J. Thompson, PhD, MPH, RN, Gannon University Villa Maria School of Nursing, Erie, PA

Pat Tooker, MSN, FNP, RN, The Evelyn L. Spiro School of Nursing, Wagner College, Staten Island, NY

Amy Toone, PhD, FNP-C, RN, Patty Hanks Shelton School of Nursing, Abilene, TX

Mary Jane Tremethick, PhD, RN, Northern Michigan University Department of Nursing, Marquette, MI

Sarah M. Ware, MSN, RN, Alcorn State University School of Nursing, Natchez, MS

Beth Weaver, RN, World Team, Warrington, PA

Kathleen L. Whitney, MS, ANP, MA, RN, Friendship Bridge Nurses Group, Aurora, CO

Jeana Wilcox, PhD, CNS, RN, Graceland University School of Nursing, Independence, MO

Sarah J. Williams, PhD, RN, BC, University of the Incarnate Word School of Nursing and Health Professions, San Antonio, TX

Marvel L. Williamson, PhD, CNE, RN, ANEF, Kramer School of Nursing at Oklahoma City University, Oklahoma University, OK

Ruth Wittman-Price, PhD, CNS, CNE, RN, DeSales University Department of Nursing and Health, Center Valley, PA

Jenna Woodruff, BSN, RN, University of North Carolina at Chapel Hill School of Nursing, Chapel Hill, NC

Kenneth J. Wysocki, PhD(c), FNP-C, RN, University of Arizona College of Nursing, Phoenix, AZ

Diane Yorke, MSN, MBA, PhD, CPNP, RN, University of North Carolina at Chapel Hill School of Nursing, Chapel Hill, NC

Changrong Yuan, PhD, RN, Second Military Medical University, College of Nursing, Shanghai, China

Patricia E. Zander, PhD, MSN, RN, Viterbo University School of Nursing, La Crosse, WI

Meg Zomorodi, PhD, RN, CNL, University of North Carolina at Chapel Hill School of Nursing, Chapel Hill, NC

Foreword

I am truly writing a "before" word for the book, *Giving Through Teaching: How Nurse Educators Are Changing the World*. The real substance, the word to be received, considered, integrated, and acted upon follows my simple offering. In these pages, you will find many of our heroes. Some of them you will recall from your History of Nursing course if you're my age; or if you are younger, perhaps these names have been required study via Google. Some of the names you and I have never known before. Surprise! These represent the hidden treasures of the nursing profession as it gives with grace, generosity, and brilliance.

I think every nurse educator has a secret wish to make a difference in the world, to change the world. Many of the gift givers described in this book did not realize that their actions, their life journeys, and their heart-felt contributions to society were changing the world. Dr. Joyce Fitzpatrick recalls how she became inspired to write this book. Her inspiration came from President Bill Clinton (whose mother was a nurse) through the pages of his compelling book on giving. We now have a cascade effect. I know that many of you will become inspired to do more from your encounter with the giving work of nurse educators, the giving through teaching so aptly described in this book.

I remember when the call for chapters went out from the NLN. There was an overwhelming response from nurse educators through-out our country. As our NLN president Cathie Shultz, NLN Foundation for Nursing Education trustee Tonia Aiken, and Joyce labored enthu-siastically to bring this lived experience of giving to light, I was regu-larly updated about the impressive stories of nurse educators and their students involved in the practice of giving. And since I have used the term "the practice of giving," the nurse educators and those described in the following chapters are clearly advanced practitioners in giving. The authors' stories are not limited to the United States, but capture nursing's commitment to the world.

It is with great appreciation and respect that I acknowledge the gift that the existence of this book offers to the NLN Foundation for Nursing Education. The royalties generated from the sale of this book will be used to create scholarships for future nursing students. This is quite a remarkable feat: a book on giving by nurse educators that gives back to the treasure of our nursing profession, our students. Finally, let's keep our hands and our hearts open, so the gifts can flow from and through us. You will discover in the following pages that it's no secret that teaching is a beautiful gift.

Beverly Malone, PhD, RN, FAAN

Introduction

In his remarkable book, *Giving: How Each of Us Can Change the World* (2007), former President Bill Clinton presents many types of giving, and provides examples of each. He especially profiles health care and community development, key concepts for nursing education at all levels. Clinton describes gifts of money (e.g., Bill and Melinda Gates, who have given millions of dollars through their foundation, most of which has been targeted to health care globally); gifts of time, including volunteers who provide services to others in need, whether in times of disaster or in areas where there are few services; gifts of things (clothes, books, supplies); gifts of skills, especially education (teaching others how to read, providing health care services); and gifts provided through churches and missions, thus providing new beginnings. Clinton also describes two other important kinds of gifts: gifts of philanthropy (gifts that keep on giving); and gifts to good ideas, funding social entrepreneurs.

As I read the stories profiled by President Clinton, I realized that nursing education held a treasure trove of similar stories. Throughout my career in nursing I have met hundreds of nurse educators who have designed "giving" projects for themselves and their students (Fitzpatrick, 2007). Nurse educators give much of their selves and also encourage their students to give to others. Service learning, a form of meaningful experiential learning that combines classroom activities with community service projects, has become commonplace in nursing curricula at both the basic and graduate levels. While service learning is most often found in community health nursing courses, it also may be woven throughout other educational programs.

In concert with the National League for Nursing (NLN), we have constructed the present book. NLN issued a call for stories from nurse educators about how they and their students give of their time, talents, skills, and resources to make the world a better place. These stories are presented in this book. Stories of legacy nursing educators also are presented to demonstrate that giving is woven throughout our history.

The "giants" of nursing education, then and now, have given much to demonstrate that each of us can make a difference in some small corner of the world, in some project, large or small. Similarly, we expect that the stories of nurse educators presented here will inspire others to do likewise, and to tell their stories as well. We can learn so much from storytelling; it is an educational tool used throughout history and across cultures. As a way to build relationships with others, storytelling is also at the core of nursing, which is built on interpersonal relationships. To close the circle on giving among nurse educators, funds raised through the sales of this book will be used for scholarship support for future nursing students through the NLN Foundation for Nursing Education.

In selecting stories of legacy nurse educators, we used several sources. They are cited as examples only, rather than as an inclusive list. Many of these nurse educators have been honored by their peers, as Living Legends of the American Academy of Nursing, through the International Council of Nurses International Achievement Award, or through Sigma Theta Tau International Founders Awards for nursing education excellence. We also referred to reference works for some background information here, particularly for historical nursing leaders. Contemporary nurse educators were contacted to describe their stories of giving.

The results are inspirational and will serve future generations of nurse educators, encouraging them not only to give to the world, but to tell their stories to others, and continue to weave the rich heritage of nursing education.

Although this book focuses on nurse educators and their students, we are aware that there are many, many nurses in clinical practice, administration, and a myriad of other roles who give of their time, talents, skills, knowledge, and money to make the world a better place. We are all of aware of the remarkable work of Miss Lillian, mother of President Jimmy Carter, who joined the Peace Corps at the age of 68 and used her nursing skills in India. She subsequently established the Lillian Carter Center for International Nursing in continuing support for global nursing. There are many other nurses who have served in the Peace Corps and in AmeriCorps, and many Peace Corps volunteers who, after their years of service, have returned home to attend nursing school. Many of these new nurses have sustained their connections in the countries they came to know during their Peace Corps years. One need only review the alumni magazines of the many schools of nursing to learn of the wonderful work of nurses everywhere.

President Clinton (2007) also has recognized and profiled nurses who are exemplary "givers," including Madonna Coffman, who started "Locks of Love," an organization that provides hairpieces to those who have lost their hair due to health problems, and Greg Mortenson, a nurse who launched an elementary education program through the Central Asia Institute, certainly a model program for giving.

We are convinced that current and future generations of nurses can do much to help achieve the United Nations Millennium Development Goals, for health is at the center of those goals. In 2000, eight United Nations Millennium Development Goals were adopted at the United Nations Millennium Summit by the international community as a framework for development activities in over 190 countries and 10 regions. They have been articulated into over twenty targets and over sixty indicators. The goals speak to global health; their achievement must involve nurses worldwide, as nurses are on the front lines of health care delivery systems in all countries. These United Nations Millennium Development Goals include:

1. Eradicate Extreme Poverty and Hunger
2. Achieve Universal Primary Education
3. Promote Gender Equality and Empower Women
4. Reduce Child Mortality
5. Improve Maternal Health
6. Combat HIV/AIDS, Malaria and Other Diseases
7. Ensure Environmental Sustainability
8. Develop a Global Partnership for Development

There are also countless nurses working for both large and small foundations that are addressing global health issues. These include the Clinton and the Gates Foundations, major foundations that are leading the way for development in global health. The Dreyfus Health Foundation programmatic initiative, Problem Solving for Better Health Nursing stands out for its specific focus on nurses and nursing as a key solution to health challenges. The Dreyfus Health Foundation uses a partnership model between a central foundation and local foundations, nongovernmental organizations, and governmental partners. The model used by the Dreyfus Health Foundation is one of empowering health professionals and communities to identify solutions to problems at the grass roots level, and address the problems locally. Problem Solving for Better Health Nursing is active in fifteen countries around the world; the model has been implemented into the curricula in several nursing schools in several countries, and recently was implemented in curricula in three nursing schools in the United States.

We prepared this book to highlight great stories of giving by nurse educators. We know that we have not been inclusive of all of the work ongoing in the thousands of nursing education programs in the United States and the world. We expect that these stories will lead to hundreds more stories told in countless classrooms by nurse educators and their students. Through the NLN and its Foundation, we will do all that we can to keep alive the storytelling of giving by nurse educators and nurses everywhere.

Joyce J. Fitzpatrick, PhD, MBA, RN, FAAN

REFERENCES

Clinton, B. (2007). *Giving: How each of us can change the world*. NY: Knopf.
Fitzpatrick, J. J. (2007). How nurse educators are changing the world. *Nursing Education Perspectives, 28*(6)305.

Historical and Contemporary Legacy Nurse Educators

Throughout the history of the nursing profession, strong nurse educators around the globe have left lasting impressions through their teaching, writing, and as role models for students. This section includes five chapters that profile the historical contributions of nurse educators and the stellar contributions of contemporary nurse educators. Both the historical and contemporary leaders included in these chapters will serve as inspiration for future generations of nurse educators.

—*Joyce J. Fitzpatrick*

1

A Heritage of Giving
Leading Nurse Educators From Past to Present

Joyce J. Fitzpatrick

FLORENCE NIGHTINGALE (1820–1910)

The "Lady with the Lamp," is the most famous name in nursing history. Although most well known of all of her work, Nightingale's service on the battlefields of the Crimean War was but one of her major contributions. Nightingale also was a health policy activist, a statistician, and a reformer of both nursing practice and education. In 1860, she opened the Nightingale School and Home for Training Nurses in London's St. Thomas Hospital, which paved the way for formalized nurse training throughout the world, and became the precursor for nursing educational programs today. Her book, *Notes on Nursing*, first published in 1859, remains a classic. It is noteworthy that in that same year Nightingale published a second book, *Notes on Hospitals*, in which she advocated the same principles on a system-wide basis (McKown, 1966).

CLARA BARTON (1821–1912)

Clara Barton was a pioneer in nursing and the founder of the American Red Cross. Just as Florence Nightingale is best known for her work in the Crimean War, Barton is remembered for her humanitarian efforts in the American Civil War. She established an agency to minister to the needs of the soldiers and lobbied the military in order to bring her own supplies to the battlefield. In 1865, President Abraham Lincoln placed her in charge of the search for soldiers of the Union Army missing in action. She became known as the "Angel of the Battlefield" for her care of the wounded and the dying. While recuperating from the strenuous years of service to the soldiers in the American Civil War, Barton traveled to Europe where she became involved with the International Committee of the Red Cross (ICRC) and its humanitarian work. She subsequently established the American Red Cross as an agency that would not respond only to war, but rather would assist in any great national disaster. She served as the first president of the American Red Cross (McKown, 1966; Oates, 1994).

LILLIAN WALD (1867–1940)

A nurse and social worker who blended the skills of both professions, Wald is best known for her work on New York's Lower East Side, at the time a poor immigrant community, where she founded the Henry Street Settlement to tend the neighborhood's sick and orphans. She wrote two books based on her work: *The House on Henry Street* and *Windows on Henry Street*. Wald is recognized as the founder of public health and visiting nursing in the United States and Canada. She was also a strong advocate for another marginalized group, African Americans, and was one of the founders of the National Association for the Advancement of Colored People (NAACP), which opened with its first major public conference at the Henry Street Settlement (Yost, 1965).

ISABEL HAMPTON ROBB (1860–1910)

Isabel Hampton Robb was one of the founders of modern American nursing and is well known in nursing education for introducing a competency-based evaluation system. In 1889, she was appointed head of the new Johns Hopkins School of Nursing, and later became a professor of nursing at the forerunner of what is now Case Western Reserve

University School of Nursing. She served as president of two important organizations, the American Society of Superintendents of Training Schools for Nurses (now known as the National League for Nursing, NLN) and the American Nurses Association (ANA). She also was one of the founders of the *American Journal of Nursing*, the first nursing journal to be published in the United States and which continues today (Bullough & Sentz, 2000).

M. ADELAIDE NUTTING (1858–1948)

M. Adelaide Nutting was a contemporary of Isabel Hampton Robb, and both women were greatly involved in leading the profession. Nutting was the first American nurse to become a university professor; she also was the director of the first Department of Nursing Education (created in 1910) in a college or university, located at Teachers College, Columbia University, New York City. Although Nutting was Canadian by birth, she can be credited with substantially elevating the profession of nursing in the United States from a profession focused on training to one focused on education. Nutting believed that the education of nurses needed to be more than that necessary to satisfy a hospital's requirement for skilled labor, and established a tuition-driven, university-based model so that nurses would be educated as other university students. Many leaders in U.S. nursing education studied at some time in their educational career at the Teachers College Department of Nursing Education (Yost, 1965).

MARY BRECKINRIDGE (1877–1965)

Mary Breckinridge was initially a volunteer nurse at the end of World War I in France. While in Europe she was introduced to nurse midwives, and developed her plan to introduce nurse midwifery education and practice in the United States. She chose to devote herself to providing health care to the Kentucky mountaineer families, and founded what is known as the Frontier Nursing Service, still in existence today. Breckinridge felt that if she could demonstrate a public health model combining family-centered nursing and midwifery in the mountain communities, then it would flourish elsewhere in the country. The Frontier School of Midwifery, launched through Breckinridge's efforts and as a result of her dreams and tireless work, opened in 1939 and remains open today (McKown, 1966).

ISABEL MAITLAND STEWART (1878–1963)

Like Nutting, Isabel Maitland Stewart was also a Canadian nurse who came to the United States to study at Teachers College. She eventually succeeded Nutting as director of the Teachers College program. Throughout her professional career, Stewart supported the preparation of leaders that were needed to teach nursing at all levels, advanced the National League of Nursing Education (now NLN), and was a consistent, strong advocate for nursing education (Yost, 1965).

MARTHA ROGERS (1914–1994)

Viewed by many as a radical nurse educator, Rogers placed the science of nursing at the center of nursing education. Rogers described the science of unitary persons, a model that served as a basis for the academic programs in nursing at New York University for several decades. She considered it important to the development of the discipline to encourage and support large numbers of doctorate- level nurses, and thus expanded the New York University program to be the largest in the country during her tenure as head of the Division of Nursing.

VIRGINIA HENDERSON (1897–1996)

Virginia Henderson has been called the first truly international nurse and continues to be acclaimed by the global nursing community. Her writings and global speaking engagements affected many nurses. Most significant was her project to catalogue nursing knowledge, the Nursing Studies Index, a 12-year-long undertaking. This document—the first annotated index of nursing research—served as a key nursing reference for many years. In recognition of her global influence and of her work on behalf of the classification of nursing knowledge, the Sigma Theta Tau International Library has been named in her honor (Virginia Nursing Hall of Fame, 2009).

ELEANOR LAMBERTSON (1916–1998)

Eleanor Lambertson is known as a leading nurse educator, as well as for her writings on education for nursing leadership. Her career and influence in nursing education spanned more than five decades. She was one of the primary architects of the team nursing model, and implemented the model in several New York hospitals while holding key leadership positions in their nursing service departments. She served as director of the nursing program at Teachers College, Columbia University, and as dean of the Cornell School of Nursing; in this latter role, she advocated for the nurse practitioner movement, particularly for the preparation of primary care providers (Schorr & Zimmerman, 1988).

LUCILLE PETRY LEONE (1903–1999)

Lucille Petry Leone was the first nurse to direct the U.S. Cadet Nurse Corps, which was authorized by Congress in 1943. She remained with the U.S. Public Health Service as the Chief Nursing Officer and Assistant Surgeon General, the first nurse appointed to this position. While with the Cadet Nurse Corps, she was responsible for recruiting more than 124,000 nurses to serve in World War II. In 1949, Leone became the first nurse to direct a division of the U.S. Public Health Service, the Division of Nurse Education, with a responsibility for setting the government funding for nurse education, a program that continues to this day. Leone established support within the federal government for the role of nursing (Yost, 1965).

HILDEGARD E. PEPLAU (1910–1999)

Best known as the "Mother of Psychiatric Nursing," Hildegard E. Peplau is recognized throughout the world for her contributions to the education of nurses caring for mentally ill persons. In 1952, her book, *Interpersonal Relations in Nursing: A Conceptual Frame of Reference,* one of the first books in psychiatric nursing, was published. She served the profession as both an executive director of the American Nurses Association and as its president, and was a board member of the International Council of Nurses (ICN). Peplau dedicated her life and her work to advocate for those who were in need of much support, the mentally ill. Much of the progress in nursing care of psychiatric patients can be traced to her writings, her workshops held throughout the country, and the work of her students.

HARRIET WERLEY (1914–2002)

Harriet Werley was one of the first and strongest advocates of nursing research and its role in nursing education. She was a founder of several research initiatives, including the nursing focus of the Walter Reed Army Institute of Research, Center for Nursing Research at Wayne State University; she was founder and editor of the journal *Research in Nursing and Health* and of the Annual Review of Nursing Research series published by Springer Publishing Company. She served on many committees, including several for NLN and ANA, always advancing the research agenda. Werley also is known as the first nurse informatics specialist as she developed the first Nursing Minimum Data Set (NMDS) and advocated for its use in all practice settings (Shorr & Zimmerman, 1988).

MILDRED MONTAG (1908–2004)

Widely recognized as the founder of associate degree nursing education, Montag was also the first director of the Adelphi University

School of Nursing. She sought to alleviate a critical shortage of nurses by decreasing the length of the education process to two years and by providing a sound educational base for nursing instruction by placing the program in community/junior colleges. In 1958, the W. K. Kellogg Foundation funded the implementation of the project at seven pilot sites in four states (NLN, 1990). The success of this radically new approach to educating registered nurses is evidenced by the large number of associate degree programs and program graduates today.

FLORENCE DOWNS (1925–2005)

Florence Downs is known for her commitment to advancing nursing research. She was editor of the journal *Nursing Research*, and also held key leadership positions in academic nursing at New York University and the University of Pennsylvania. One of her greatest skills was in developing a professional community of nurse faculty at the institutions where she worked, clearly demonstrating the value of the scholarly "collective" (Fairman & Mahon, 2001). Downs never took the glory for herself; she was known for being the leader, but also for involving others, building on the strengths of the individuals for the good of the group.

MARGRETTA STYLES (1930–2005)

Margretta Styles is best known for her contributions to the credentialing of nurses, including licensure, registration, certification, and accreditation. She chaired the first ANA-funded study on credentialing, which ultimately led to the ANA American Nurses Credentialing Center (ANCC). During her career, she held a number of positions in academic leadership and in professional organizations. She was president of the American Nurses Association and the International Council of Nurses. In her many spheres of influence, she supported a global perspective of nursing and worldwide standardization of nursing credentials (Schorr & Zimmerman, 1988).

MARY ELIZABETH CARNEGIE (1916–2008)

In her landmark book, *The Path We Tread: Black Women in the Nursing Profession,* Mary Elizabeth Carnegie profiled the history and contributions of African American women to U.S. nursing. Although she is best remembered for advocating racial equality in nursing education and practice, she contributed in many ways to the profession. Over a period of more than 25 years, Carnegie served as editor of a number of major nursing journals, including editor of the *American Journal of Nursing,* associate editor of *Nursing Outlook,* and senior editor of the prestigious journal *Nursing Research,* and served as president of the American Academy of Nursing. Numerous organizations honored Carnegie for her contributions to the advancement of minorities in nursing (American Nurses Association, 2009).

REFERENCES

American Nurses Association (2009). *Nursing world.* Retrieved July 1, 2009, from http://www.nursingworld.org.

Bullough, V. L, & Sentz, L. (Eds.). (2000). American nursing: A biographical dictionary. NY: Springer Publishing.

Carnegie, M. E. (1985). *The path we tread: Black women in the nursing profession.* NY: Garland Publishing.

Fairman, J., & Mahon, M. M. (2001). Oral history of Florence Downs: The early years. *Nursing Research, 50*(5): 322–328.

Houser, B. P., & Player, K. N. (2004). Pivotal moments in nursing, Vol. 1. Indianapolis, IN: Sigma Theta Tau International.

Houser, B. P., & Player, K. N. (2007). Pivotal moments in nursing, Vol. 1I. Indianapolis, IN: Sigma Theta Tau International.

McKown, R. (1966). *Heroic nurses.* NY: Putnam's Sons.

National League for Nursing. (1990). *Vision for Nursing Education.* NY: NLN Press.

Oates, S. B. (1994). *A woman of valor.* NY: Macmillan.

Peplau, H. E. (1991). *Interpersonal relations in nursing: A conceptual frame of reference.* NY: Springer Publishing.

Schorr, T. M., & Zimmerman, A. (Eds.). (1988). *Making choices, taking chances: Nurse leaders tell their stories.* St. Louis: Mosby.

Virginia Nursing Hall of Fame. (2009). Virginia Avenel Henderson. Retrieved July 30, 2009, from http://www.library.vcu.edu/tml/speccoll/vnfame/hendersonbio.html

Yost, E. (1965). *American women of nursing.* Philadelphia: Lippincott.

2

Linda Richards (1841–1930)
A Legacy of Firsts

Debbie Ciesielka

In 1873, the first nurses' training school in America graduated its first class, and Linda Richards was the first graduate (Richards, 1911). And, twenty years later, uniform standards of training for nurses were adopted via the forerunner to the National League for Nursing's American Society of Superintendents of Training Schools for Nurses (Superintendents' Society) (Birnbach & Lewenson, 1993). At the forefront of both of these historic events was Linda Richards, a woman of "firsts" for the fledgling profession of nursing: first trained nurse in the United States, first psychiatric nurse in the United States (Domrose, 2003), first U.S. nurse to engage in international nursing (Massachusetts General Hospital, n.d.), first president of the American Society of Superintendents of Training Schools for Nurses, and first stockholder in the *American Journal of Nursing* Company (Doona, 1984). Linda Richards's story is the story of nursing in America.

At age 29, inspired by the work of Florence Nightingale, Richards resolved to travel to England for formal nurses training. This, however, became unnecessary when she learned that the New England Hospital for Women and Children was about to open a training school for nurses in Boston (Richards, 1923). Over the next four years, she focused on hospital work, spending her first year after graduation as night superintendent at Bellevue Hospital in New York City, and the following three years as superintendent of the Training School of Massachusetts General Hospital. Richards was the first graduate nurse to take charge of the school (Richards, 1903).

After two and one-half years and considerable success, Richards left Massachusetts General Hospital to gain additional training at St. Thomas's

Hospital in London. While at St. Thomas's Hospital, Richards took advantage of every opportunity to immerse herself in the Nightingale method of instruction. On the advice of Florence Nightingale herself, Richards supplemented her stay at St. Thomas's with visits to King's College Hospital and to the Royal Infirmary of Edinburgh.

In 1878, Richards returned to America to organize the Boston City Hospital Training School where, fortunately, she and the hospital superintendent shared a common vision. Shortly after Richards arrived, she was joined by three nurses, all graduates of the Bellevue Hospital Training School. The house officers did not know what to expect or how to treat these nurses. It was only after they demonstrated their value in a practical way—for example, by relieving house officers of taking the temperatures every two hours of nearly 100 patients with typhoid—did their presence gain acceptance.

Despite her success at Boston City Hospital, the experience left Linda Richards emotionally and physically exhausted. She requested a three-month leave of absence that turned into three years of recovery. She returned to Boston City Hospital in 1881 and stayed an additional four years before taking on her greatest challenge, and another "first": organizing the first training school for nurses in Kyoto, Japan, as a missionary for the American Board of Commissioners for Foreign Missions, a Congregational mission organization (Richards, 1911).

In this program, students followed a two-year course of study with lectures given by Richards, other Americans on the medical staff, and one Japanese physician. Only one textbook, *Cutter's Anatomy, Physiology, and Hygiene*, was translated into Japanese for use by the students (Berry, 1887). In many ways, the course content, with some adaptations for Japanese culture, was similar to nurses' training in the United States (Richards, 1911). In the years following Richards's departure from Japan, the nurse training school in Kyoto graduated seventy-five nurses (Doona, 1996). Eventually, the school broke away from the American Board of Foreign Missions and passed into Japanese hands (Achiwa, 1968).

In April 1891, Richards assumed the position of head of the Philadelphia Visiting Nurses' Society. With great reluctance, she resigned after eight months (Richards, 1911), joining the ranks of many who, "while attracted to visiting nursing, found the work too mentally and physically exhausting" (Buhler-Wilkerson, 2001, p. 25). Richards then returned to the task of organizing training schools of nursing. In 1894, members of the newly formed American Society of Superintendents of Training Schools for Nurses of the United States and Canada elected Richards as its first president (Munson, 1948). By age 58, she was at the pinnacle of her career.

Over the next decade, Linda Richards would re-vision nursing education by advocating for nurses' training in the setting of an insane asylum as a means to cultivate compassion. Her hope was to someday develop the care of the mentally ill as a special branch of nursing for the general nurse. She continued in this work until her retirement from Taunton Hospital for the Insane at age 69 (Richards, 1911).

More than a century has passed since Linda Richards earned the distinction as America's first trained nurse. Nursing programs in the United States have grown considerably. Innovations Richards introduced, such as patient record keeping and training in psychiatric nursing, are now standard procedures. Conditions that left Richards and others physically ill and mentally exhausted from caring for affected patients have all but disappeared. Richards gave this timeless advice: "Let the nurse of today consider it her solemn duty to raise the standard ever higher.... Let each year's work exceed in excellence that of the preceding year. Let her show to the world that her profession is one of the grandest, and that she is an honor to it" (Richards, 1901, p. 80).

REFERENCES

Achiwa, G. (1968). Linda Richards in Japan. *American Journal of Nursing, 68*(8), 1716–1719.

Berry, J. C. (1887, March 12). *Correspondence from John C. Berry to N. G. Clark* (Microfilm, Reel 337). Harvard University, Lamont Library Papers of the American Board of Commissioners for Foreign Missions, Cambridge, MA.

Birnbach, N., & Lewenson, S. (Eds.). (1993). *Legacy of leadership.* New York: National League for Nursing Press.

Buhler-Wilkerson, K. (2001). *No place like home.* Baltimore: Johns Hopkins University Press.

Doona, M. E. (1984). At least as well cared for...Linda Richards and the mentally ill. *Image: The Journal of Nursing Scholarship, 16*(2), 51–56.

Doona, M. E. (1996). Linda Richards and nursing in Japan, 1885–1890. *Nursing History Review, 4,* 99–128.

Massachusetts General Hospital. (n.d.). *The International Nurse Consultant Program.* Retrieved August 25, 2008, from http://www.massgeneral.org/pcs/CCPD/cpd_consult.asp

Munson, H. W. (1948). Linda Richards. *American Journal of Nursing, 48*(9), 551–556.

Richards, L. (1901). How trained nursing began in America at the New England Hospital. *American Journal of Nursing, 2,* 88–89.

Richards, L. (1903). Recollections of a pioneer nurse. *American Journal of Nursing, 3*(4), 245–252.

Richards, L. (1911). *Reminiscences of Linda Richards.* Boston: Whitcomb & Barrows.

Richards, L. (1923). Address at the fiftieth anniversary of the New England Hospital. *American Journal of Nursing, 23,* 282–285.

3

Sharing Their Skills: Influential Contemporary Nurse Educators

Joyce J. Fitzpatrick

There are virtually hundreds of nurse educators who could be profiled in this chapter, all of whom are known for far-reaching contributions to the discipline through their expertise in education. The educators presented are but a few of those deserving of recognition. We have not purposely excluded anyone; rather, the goal has been to take a broad view, identifying leaders from the various aspects of nursing education and influence, and highlighting some of their strengths and contributions. Each of these individuals has influenced thousands of nursing students and other nurse educators during their careers. This fact and excellence are common to all of them.

FAYE ABDELLAH

Faye Abdellah has been a pioneer in nursing education and research and is best known for her work at the federal government level. She had more than fifty years of service in the United States Public Health Service (USPHS) and served as a deputy surgeon general from 1981 to 1989. In 1993, she founded the Graduate School of Nursing (GSN) at the USPHS and served as the first dean. The GSN prepares advanced practice nurses and nurse researchers for U.S. military service (Houser & Player, 2004).

HATTIE BESSENT

Hattie Bessent has worked tirelessly to eliminate barriers for minority nurses. As an educator, her work has had a substantial influence on generations of nurses. Bessent has directed the American Nurses Association Minority Fellowship Program for many decades, preparing hundreds of nurses for leadership positions in nursing education and professional practice. Bessent's style has been to remain behind the scenes, but her colleagues in the nursing community are well aware of her work and influence (Schorr & Zimmerman, 1988).

LUTHER CHRISTMAN

A strong supporter of the unification of nursing education and practice, Luther Christman made this a reality while he was dean at Vanderbilt University and Rush University Schools of Nursing. He also fought tirelessly to advance the role of men in nursing, founding the American Assembly of Men in Nursing, which continues today. The Rush model of nursing was recognized globally—inside and outside the nursing discipline—for its integration of nursing service and education. One of the hallmarks of Christman's legacy is that he recognized the value of interdisciplinary practice and education (Schorr & Zimmerman, 1988).

RHEBA DE TORNYAY

Rheba de Tornyay devoted her career to nursing education, and provided leadership in many dimensions of the nurse educator community. She was dean of two major schools of nursing, the University of California Los Angeles and the University of Washington. She also influenced many nurse faculty members through her role as head of the graduate program in nursing education at the University of California San Francisco. De Tornyay also served as editor of the

Journal of Nursing Education and was a member of the American Nurses Association Commission on Nursing Education, roles that provided opportunities for her to have a broad national influence (Schorr & Zimmerman, 1988).

SISTER ROSEMARY DONLEY

Sister Rosemary Donley has made several contributions to the teaching and learning communities in nursing. She served as dean of the Catholic University School of Nursing, as editor of *Image* and the *Journal of Nursing Scholarship*, and as president of Sigma Theta Tau International. She has described teaching as "changing behavior." Throughout her career she has contributed much to the nursing education community (Smith & Fitzpatrick, 2006).

VERNICE FERGUSON

Vernice Ferguson had a long and influential career as a nurse administrator with the Veterans Administration, serving in the highest nursing position at the national level. However, her influence through her work with professional associations and nursing schools has been equally impressive. She mentored thousands of nurses throughout her career, following her own best advice to new teachers—find a mentor (Smith & Fitzpatrick, 2006).

LORETTA FORD

Well recognized as the founder of the nurse practitioner movement, Loretta Ford established the first pediatric nurse practitioner program at the University of Colorado in the early 1960 with a physician colleague. Her vision was that nurse practitioners could be extensions of the patient, not of the physician. As with many other leaders in nursing education,

Ford credits her teachers with significant influence on her development and achievements (Houser & Player, 2004).

CARRIE LENBURG

Carrie Lenburg is best known for her leadership in establishing and expanding the external degree programs in nursing in New York State. She is recognized for her innovative and creative approaches that incorporate self-directed learning and competency-based evaluation. Throughout her career she has assisted many schools and organizations in using her outcome-based assessment model for nursing education (Schorr & Zimmerman, 1988).

RUTH LUBIC

Ruth Lubic has had a marked influence on nurse midwifery education. Through her successful projects demonstrating the effectiveness of birthing center care for mothers and babies and their families and communities, she has provided a stellar example for midwifery students around the world. Lubic implemented birthing centers in both underserved and affluent communities, demonstrating the value of midwifery services across boundaries.

JOYCE MURRAY

Joyce Murray has made major contributions to nursing education both in the United States and abroad. She served as president of the National League for Nursing (NLN) from 2003–05, and it was during her tenure that the NLN embarked on the certification examination for nurse educators, an historic development. She also has a rich history of nursing education and practice in Ethiopia, heading a major public health initiative to prepare nurses and other health care workers in Ethiopia through the Emory University Carter Center.

GRAYCE SILLS

As a senior mentor in psychiatric mental health nursing education and professional practice, Grayce Sills has carried on the legacy of Hildegard Peplau. She has always been a strong advocate for students, and advises faculty that they are half of the learning formula for the student. She also believes that the most important outcome measures of student learning are those that are long term, and that faculty and students should be as concerned with these as with the short-term outcomes (Smith & Fitzpatrick, 2006).

GLORIA SMITH

Gloria Smith has served in many roles and has led many initiatives that served as beacons to nurse educators and nurses throughout the world. As dean of a school of nursing, she was one of the first to develop a practice model of nurse faculty. She served as director of the Department of Public Health for the state of Michigan, and as a senior program officer for the W. K. Kellogg Foundation. Her influence has been felt worldwide, and she continues to advocate for those who are from vulnerable, underserved, and minority populations.

REFERENCES

Houser, B. P., & Player, K. N. (2004). *Pivotal moments in nursing, Vol. 1*. Indianapolis, IN: Sigma Theta Tau International.

Houser, B. P., & Player, K. N. (2007). *Pivotal moments in nursing, Vol. 11*. Indianapolis, IN: Sigma Theta Tau International.

Schorr, T. M., & Zimmerman, A. (Eds.). (1988). *Making choices, taking chances: Nurse leaders tell their stories*. St. Louis: Mosby.

Smith, M. J., & Fitzpatrick, J. J. (2006). *Best practices in nursing education*. NY: Springer Publishing.

4

An International Inheritance
A Selection of Nurse Education Leaders From Around the Globe

Joyce J. Fitzpatrick

Nurses are everywhere, in all parts of the world, and most of these nurses are giving of their time, talents, skills, and services to those less fortunate. I have met nurses in Uganda who, although their own incomes are minimal, give much of themselves to raise resources for neighbors and community members who are less fortunate. Over the years I have crossed paths with hundreds of nurse educators who could be profiled as exemplary "givers." Humanitarian work is about saving lives and alleviating suffering in the short term, but it is also about planting seeds for the future development of the recipients of the services. Thus, humanitarianism contains a parallel to teaching, and nurse educators make great humanitarians. The individuals profiled here are some of the nurses whose work has been recognized as exemplary, as contributing to global health and welfare. These nurses are not alone in their giving; there are scores of other nurse educators who also could be identified as giving through their educational and volunteer work.

SUSIE KIM (SOUTH KOREA)

Susie Kim, recent president of Seoul Cyber University in Seoul, South Korea, is known as the nurse of many "firsts" in South Korea. She was the first nurse in the country with a doctorate in nursing, the first editor of an international journal, the first psychiatric nurse in Korea, and the first nurse to be president of a university. Susie Kim points out, however, that the value of this recognition is not for herself, but for the profession of nursing, and more importantly, for those served by nurses. Early in her nursing career she learned the value of interdisciplinary relationships and the importance of networking—skills that have served her well in her many roles. Prior to her current role in academic administration, Susie served as a faculty member at Ehwa Woman's University for several years, and also as dean of the School of Nursing; she is clearly a seasoned nurse educator.

One of the most prestigious awards presented to Dr. Kim is the International Council of Nurses (ICN) International Achievement Award. This award recognized Susie's contributions at the community level, specifically her United Nations Development Program (UNDP), which funded a project to deinstitutionalize the chronic mentally ill in South Korea. Through this project, she recruited many professionals and lay volunteers to help provide therapeutic services in community-based centers and made it possible for those with mental illnesses to return to live with their families. She demonstrated that psychiatric patients could lead normal lives and make valuable contributions to society. Kim's community efforts have extended far beyond this UNDP-funded project. She has developed hospice programs in Korea and China, helping many live their final days and die in peace. Susie Kim is a nurse educator who has served as a role model for many young nurses in Korea. She believes that this is one of her most important contributions—to model the giving and caring spirit of nurses who will follow in her footsteps and make their own great contributions in the future.

NAEEMA AL GASSEER (IRAQ)

Naeema Al Gasseer serves as the World Health Organization's (WHO) chief representative in Iraq, where she has worked since 2003. Prior to assuming this position, she was the senior nursing and midwifery scientist at WHO, where she championed the development of a global strategy for nursing and midwifery. As a top official in Iraq, her responsibilities include the overall health of the citizens of that war-torn nation. War, political unrest, and conflict are not new to her; she has worked previously in Lebanon, Yemen, Syria, and the occupied Palestinian territories. A tireless supporter of the United Nations' system to restore and rebuild health care services and education, she is admired by colleagues (from nursing and other health professions) as much for her creativity as for her courage. Constant stress and concern for her own safety are day-to-day issues for her. One hallmark of Dr. Al Gasseer's career is her commitment to education, not just for health professionals but also for children in crisis situations and war-ravaged countries, such as Iraq. While a senior nursing and midwifery scientist at WHO headquarters in Geneva, Switzerland, she fought tirelessly to strengthen nursing and midwifery education, particularly for service delivery in primary health care. She fights on today, focusing on needs in Iraq.

GERALDINE McCARTHY (IRELAND)

Geraldine McCarthy, the first nurse in Ireland to receive her Ph.D. in nursing, is now professor and dean of the Catherine McAuley School of Nursing and Midwifery at University College Cork (UCC) in Cork, Ireland, one of that country's largest schools of nursing. Throughout her career, Dr. McCarthy has worked to advance nursing in Ireland through participation in the redesign of the educational system at all levels. From her early qualification as a nurse, she understood the need for more education for all nurses, and has never ceased to work to expand educational opportunities in Ireland. Her experience of nursing in a variety of countries has also helped her to envision the true potential for nurse education in Ireland. In 2002, she was appointed as one of seven nurses to serve on the fourteen-member Commission for Nursing. This commission established entry to nursing at the Bachelors in Nursing (university degree) level, and regulated required clinical pathway positions for nurses and midwives, along with their necessary education. Although Dr. McCarthy considers her contributions to this commission as one of her greatest professional accomplishments, she has served on several prestigious national committees, including the Health Information and Quality Authority.

While Dr. McCarthy's professional accomplishments have been extraordinary, it is her personal commitment that deserves mention here. Since the 1980s, when she first qualified as a nurse, she has organized an annual visit to Lourdes, France, for up to 150 sick individuals and 1,000 pilgrims. She leads a team of twenty-five nurses, who are accompanied by two medical doctors, numerous volunteers, and eighty school-aged children, who also serve as helpers for the invalids and sick persons. For Geraldine, this annual trip allows her to experience the small miracles— the giving of others—and to see the importance of religious ceremony in helping people cope with difficult situations. She recounts some of these wonderful happenings: the blind man who described his young helper as an "angel" because she became his eyes for the week and described the buildings, grottos, fields, and crowds to make his visit a better experience; a woman who recounted her miracle—her husband, a paraplegic, now considers himself lucky because he saw so many people more disabled than himself; a medical doctor who, having prayed for a miracle, returned home to die in peace. Dr. McCarthy says she feels "blessed" each year as she experiences the triumph of the human spirit and realizes anew that amid suffering there is joy and peace.

SHARON VASUTHEVAN (SOUTH AFRICA)

Sharon Vasuthevan is national training and development manager for Life Healthcare Limited and president of the Nursing Education Association in South Africa. Throughout her career as a nurse educator, Dr. Vasuthevan has worked to advance nursing education and to model excellence for others. From her early career when she was awarded a Fulbright Scholarship to obtain a master's degree in nursing in the United States, to her involvement at all levels of her current organization, Sharon Vasuthevan has excelled. She considers her success in bridging the gap between the public and private sectors in South Africa a major contribution, and one that can serve as a model for other organizations worldwide.

Her appointment to the 44th South African Nursing Council by the Minister of Health was followed by an appointment as chair of the Education Committee of the Nursing Council. She has dedicated her work to providing health care for young children and the elderly. She is passionate about the development of others and believes that education is the key to success, working to provide HIV/AIDS counseling to those in her communities and to promote HIV/AIDS prevention programs. Other volunteer projects involve presentations on life skills and empowerment courses for disadvantaged women and study skills for school children, and promotion of primary health care services for children and the elderly.

JUDITH SHAMIAN (CANADA)

Judith Shamian is currently the president and CEO of the Victorian Order of Nurses (VON), the largest home care service, policy, and research organization in Canada. She is the president elect of the Canadian Nurses Association, professor at the Lawrence S. Bloomberg Faculty of Nursing, University of Toronto, and co-investigator with the Nursing Health Services Research Unit. Although Dr. Shamian has held full-time employment in service or government, she also always has maintained a very strong affiliation with academia, where she has taught graduate courses, served on student committees, and participated in many research initiatives. During Shamian's tenure with Mount Sinai Hospital in Toronto (1989–99), she established the first WHO Collaborating Centre for Leadership in a hospital environment. This group made it possible for many nurse executives from the Caribbean, Eastern Europe, Israel, and Africa to learn more about the role of nurse executives, and nursing services, through the use of strong collaborative and professional skills. From 1999 to 2004, Shamian held the inaugural position of Executive Director of Nursing Policy for the government of Canada, where she provided leadership for developing an entire generation of nurses who understand and contribute to evidenced-based policy. Shamian also was able to enhance the understanding of nursing's contribution to policy development for provincial politicians and other decision makers.

Dr. Shamian continues to promote, educate, and speak out in Canada, as well as internationally, on the extreme importance of a healthy public policy, especially in regard to advancing the health of people worldwide and the role of nurses in that effort. In addition, her ongoing work with WHO (where she previously led projects in Israel, Hungary, and Botswana) allows her to delineate the roles of nurses and midwives for the WHO Primary Health Care agenda. She is often called upon to address many issues surrounding nursing, health human resources, leadership, and health care policy by provincial and federal government departments and agencies, and internationally by other governments, academic bodies, and the WHO itself. As president and CEO of VON Canada, Judith Shamian has guided this 112-year-old organization through great transition and transformation to bring it under one organizational umbrella. In this role, Shamian champions the home- and community-care agenda in Canada, as well as works to strengthen the partnerships between professional health care providers and others who provide care, such as families, friends, volunteers, and community organizations, in order to recognize and support the entire spectrum of care.

DRAGICA SIMUNEC (CROATIA)

Dragica Simunec has served as president of the Croatian Nursing Council since 2004. She served as the chief nursing officer for the Ministry of Health Republic of Croatia from 1993 to 2004, and as president of the Croatian Nursing Association from 1992 to 2003. She was editor of the *Croatian Nursing Journal* from 1995 to 2004. However, along with thousands of other Croatian people, she left the country during its internal conflicts.

Her subsequent experience of working in a well-organized Australian hospital changed her perception of nursing, and helped with her future work in Croatia. By the time Croatia became an independent country in 1991, Dragica Simunec had completed advanced education in nursing and was in a position to assume a leadership role in the new government.

With her international nursing experience, advanced preparation, and English-language skills, Simunec was well equipped for leadership. Through her appointment as the chief nursing officer for the new Ministry of Health, she was able to delineate a nursing scope of practice as the first legal document and develop a competency based curriculum, a code of ethics, a nursing act, and, in 2003, establish the Croatian Nursing Council.

Today in Croatia, nursing is a self-regulated profession, protecting patients' rights through maintaining professional knowledge and responsibility among nurses. Dragica Simunec's current role as president of the Nursing Council is to pursue the trust of the public and to participate in decision making on the political level.

5

Two Cultures, Two Educations
One Nurse Educator

Jane Sumner

Like most educators, the way I think about my role as nurse and as nurse educator reveals the profound influence of my teachers. I am the product of two different countries and cultures, and two very different nursing education systems. I was born and grew up in New Zealand and started my diploma training at the age of seventeen; however, my university education for three degrees occurred in the United States. My story is how the values and beliefs of both education systems have shaped my thinking.

My diploma training took place within a large public hospital system; the hierarchy was based on the British system. Our teachers were demanding and exact. The focus was always patient comfort and care, and I have carried this legacy throughout my years of teaching. We learned that our communication was a totality of us giving ourselves to our patients. We were proud of being nurses, and we felt respected in our communities. The feeling of pride in the profession has stayed with me and is something I have tried to instill in all of my students.

Before I left New Zealand I spent just over two years teaching in the New Zealand system. I discovered that I loved teaching, and that it was fun and challenging to think up practical explanations to concepts students had difficulty grasping. This has never changed.

I came to the United States with family, became a visiting nurse in Pennsylvania, and again I found something I loved. I spent twelve years first as a visiting nurse and then as a home hospice nurse. My involvement with hospice work gave my life a depth that it had not had previously: total involvement. This knowledge and experience has kept me in good stead as an educator.

After moving to New Orleans in 1988, I realized that I wanted to return to teaching. I completed my master's degree in public health nursing and joined the faculty at Louisiana State University Health Science Center School of Nursing. I then pursued doctoral studies in educational leadership and administration. My mind was expanded in ways that I could never have anticipated.

I brought my own ideas to how I would teach. I wanted my students to succeed, of course, but foremost were the high standards regarding patient care that I had learned when a student. I believed that students should be encouraged to perform above what they thought they could do. I was also cognizant that students watched every interaction I had with everyone on the floor—physicians, staff nurses, janitorial staff, patients, and families. In essence, they observed my professional communication.

Although my classes spent long days on the units, I strongly believed in the importance of the post conference to consider the ramifications of patient care and how patients would manage upon discharge. I included as well discussions about ethics, moral practice, registered nurse behaviors, self-reflection, and how the students wanted to practice as a registered nurse. It also seemed important to share my own feelings after we together had endured an emotionally stressful day.

For example, one day it was clear that a patient would die while we were on the floor. I told the assigned student nurse what would likely happen and asked if he wanted reassignment. He said no, which impressed me, explaining that he had the time to give the patient quality care and be there for the patient, which he did not think the floor nurses would have time to do. I then ensured that he would always have another student with him, so he would not be alone with the dying man. All the students took turns being with their colleague, reorganizing their own work to do so. The patient's family arrived late morning, and one of the students took several of the younger children off to a quiet spot to keep them occupied. When the patient died, only the assigned student and I remained in the room with the family, although we asked them to leave briefly while we prepared the patient for removal.

It was clear that the students were shocked by the experience, so I knew that post conference was going to be focused on death, how to cope as a nurse, and the emotional toll it inevitably takes. I was as emotionally drained as they were when I finally went home that day. Still, I was proud of them. Although they were young in years and experience, they taught me that I could trust them to rise to the occasion, and that they would do their very best and they would support each other. It was a validation of me as a person, a nurse, and a teacher. My New Zealand lessons were manifested in my students.

Over the years I have found humor to be a powerful tool. Also, the ready admission that I sometimes did not have the answer demonstrated honesty to my students. My students know they can come talk to me privately in my office. They also know that, even after graduating, if they need something they could still get in touch with me, and many do. Again, this was something I learned from Sister Simpson in my preliminary school days; she was always there for us. I have mopped away many a tear just as my own teacher had, and have held to the standards that I hold most dear, which she taught me.

My experiences all over the world have shaped how I think. I am very proud of my New Zealand heritage, of growing up in a country with two different cultures, one British (Pakeha-Maori for White) and one Maori. During my training, nurses were expected to care for everyone with exactly the same amount of care and compassion. I also have been deeply influenced by my U.S. university education, particularly the intellectual challenges of my doctoral degree. But my teaching and the way I think about educating nurses is not really a synthesis of both cultures but rather something new that has emerged, something that is both and neither. In a real sense I have developed my own styles and ways of thinking, but always paramount is the patient and loyalty to the profession. I want my students to succeed and feel as proud of themselves as nurses as I do.

II

Influential Nurse Educators in the United States

Collectively and individually, nurse educators impact their worlds and work with disenfranchised, vulnerable, and suffering individuals and communities without adequate services. They offer compelling stories of their care, compassion, and engagement, often with students, to change those worlds. They create, collaborate, volunteer, and sustain humanitarian efforts. Without them, the quality of life of Americans would diminish.

Their stories describe populations, innovative curricula, issues of the heart, and simple and complex teaching-learning or service initiatives. Included are frameworks to implement change, lessons learned, and advice. A variety of experience levels in planning and development of service is represented. Stories are expressed using nurses' phrases of caring. All have made a difference.

The chapter, organized into three parts, provides an overview of nurse educators' diligent efforts to change the world around them. The first section contains changes made by individual nurse educators. The second section describes the outcomes created by a group of nurse educators. Lastly, change efforts by a program's faculty are presented. All programs and projects are based in the United States; some have outreach efforts to other countries.

—*Cathleen M. Shultz*

6

Nurse Educators and Their Individual Stories

Bozena Padykula

My fluency in Polish inspired me to contribute to the community of my cultural background. The Polish Scouting Organization (ZHP pgk), a non-profit organization in New Britain, Connecticut, was recruiting a camp nurse for a two-week assignment. The mission and work of ZHP pgk is supported by Polish communities in several different countries. The Polish community in New Britain has the highest number of Polish immigrants or those of Polish descent in the state of Connecticut and is known as "Little Poland"; 19.9% of the residents of this town have Polish ancestors.

Every year since 1974, the ZHP pgk in New Britain organizes scouting camps at a site called Stanica in Palmer, Massachusetts. The camp accommodates eighty young boys and girls between the ages of seven and eleven years old, twenty teenagers who work as junior counselors or full counselors, and ten adults serving as directors, instructors, and auxiliary staff. As well, the original camp founders continue to participate and supervise, and to provide program guidance and direction.

Initially, I was concerned that without special training in pediatric nursing I might not be qualified for the position. However, I believed that my experience as a holistic nurse and clinical instructor would help me handle this opportunity. As I observed the parents helping their healthy, happy children settle into the assigned barracks, my initial impression was that my nursing role would be minimal because all of the children appeared healthy and without medical problems. But before I could make a full assessment, several mothers captured my attention, anxious to share detailed information about their children. I listened patiently, and reassured them that if I had any questions regarding their children I would call them.

After the parents left, the children's safety and health were in my and the other volunteers' hands. I decided to organize the health activities similar to the steps of a hospital admission procedure. My first action related to medication safety. I informed the children to bring all medications to me so I could safely lock them in the nursing station area. I explained to the children that this would avoid some safety risks and prevent medications from leakage, damage, or breakage. I was also concerned that some children might not take their medications seriously, treating them as candy and offering them to other children. Another reason for my action involved the lack of air conditioning in the children's barracks, which could cause medications to lose quality or potency. Also, as their nurse, I needed to know what health problems the children had.

Next, I focused on health promotion, disease prevention, and specific health problems. Because these young campers usually performed most of their activities of daily living at home guided and supervised by their parents, I reinforced activities to maintain proper hygiene, to keep rooms organized, and to keep towels and clothing dry. Other activities that required considerable reinforcement included wearing socks during daily activities to protect the children's feet from scraping and blisters, use of sunblock and hats to protect their skin, and drinking plenty of fluids to stay well hydrated during the hot days.

Another focus was to help the children adjust to being away from home and to feel comfortable and safe. For most of the young scouts, this was their first time away from their parents—a two-week journey of independence. The time between 8 and 10 P.M. was unique—I was exposed to a massive invasion of scouts with complaints ranging from belly aches, indigestion, constipation, scratched toes, sore elbows, dehydration, to just plain hunger. They were tired but unable to sleep, feeling lost and fearful about how to survive the first few nights away from home. I often heard soft crying with statements such as "I miss my mommy and daddy," or cat or dog, or "I need to hear their voices." I felt privileged that these young scouts were brave enough to trust me with their biggest secret fears. To provide comfort, I offered two unique interventions, which I found to be effective in putting their hearts and minds at peace—mint tea and acupressure. These two interventions worked miraculously in distracting and comforting the children so they could have a night of sound sleep.

My most rewarding nursing experience was when a twelve-year-old camper, in remission after two years of treatment for leukemia, joined the camp. The plan was that he would stay for one week. I was quite surprised that a child with a compromised immune system was brought to the camp environment. His mother explained that her son was almost finished with the treatment, that his physician approved participation in the camp, and that he attended school with other children without major restrictions. Regarding the chemotherapy, the mother arranged with the physician to delay the scheduled treatment for two days to accommodate his week at the camp. Both the mother and I reviewed carefully with the child those symptoms to report immediately, and she and I stayed in frequent contact throughout his stay. The boy was surprisingly willing to report changes in his physical status. The scout stayed the week without any complications.

This opportunity to give back and to educate a community of my cultural background broadened my vision about nursing. I believe that nurses from every practice environment transform people's lives on many levels.

Marie Napolitano

Every May, I look forward to that first drive from Portland, Oregon, through strawberry and clover fields to the day's chosen migrant camp. The camp selected to start the summer program is always the one with the largest number of families waiting to begin their work in the fields, as the picking season is heralded by sweet, ripe strawberries without a predicted maturity date. When I arrive at the camp, I go to the mobile van where the Virginia Garcia Memorial Health Center (VGMHC) camp staff is registering farm workers who desire screening or need health care. The staff can register as many as 100 individuals who will be screened (blood pressure and glucose), triaged, and cared for by the nurse, and invited to attend organized classes on topics such as HIV and nutrition. I provided primary care to as many as twenty-eight adults and children during our four- or five-hour visit.

My service to this population began in 1988 when Rosalia, a registered nurse originally from Paraguay; Yvonne, an outreach worker from Jamaica; and I rode through the back roads of the county in search of camps of farm workers needing health care or social services. Through the years, the program expanded and larger vehicles were rented until a local grant enabled VGMHC to purchase its own small recreational van. The van is outfitted as a health care clinic as well as a dental clinic—it also serves the dental needs of the migrant farm worker population on alternating weekdays. The van is easily recognized, because the picture of the small child Virginia Garcia appears on its sides. Virginia, the child of migrant farm workers, died because of lack of access to proper health care; her death propelled the birth of the Virginia Garcia Memorial Health Center (VGMHC) in 1975.

The mobile van camp program is an effective and necessary outreach to migrant farm worker families who otherwise lack access to primary care. Over 1,500 migrant farm workers and their families travel to this area annually to live in one of twenty-six camps and to work in the berry fields. The VGMHC is the migrant and community health program for the county and includes four primary care clinics. Each clinic is at capacity and unable to accommodate the additional 700 to 900 migrants who are seen every summer by the mobile camp program. The upfront preparation done by the camp staff, the name recognition of the VGMHC, and the mobile program's presence at the campsites provide a more welcoming and safe inducement to these people to seek health care. Although most problems can be managed at the van clinic, the camp program also coordinates any necessary visits to the main clinics and to specialists, including arranging for transportation and delivery of medications that are not available via the van.

Migrant farm workers are an essential workforce for the agricultural sector of Oregon. The demographic of migrant farm workers is a young male, married with children. Additionally, many adolescents come with fathers, uncles, or cousins to work; some adolescents come alone. The majority speaks Spanish; however, increasing numbers speak an indigenous dialect as their first language. Families are becoming more common at the camps. Migrant farm workers in Washington County live in twenty-six identified camps consisting of cabins, trailers, houses, or bunkers made of metal. The conditions vary from decent to unacceptable with safety risks.

Predominant health problems involve the skin and respiratory and musculoskeletal systems. The most common specific diagnoses were upper respiratory infection, tinea pedis, and musculoskeletal strain. Although farm workers present with many common problems, more serious problems are also found each year. Tuberculosis, pertussis, cancers, congenital heart disease, HIV, pelvic inflammatory disease, and abdominal masses are a few examples.

The meager clinical setting, the large numbers of people seen during each camp visit, and the concern for those who chose not to miss a day of work for a more thorough workup at the main clinic contributed to my professional dissonance and stress. However, it is the lack of continuity that consistently leaves me with a feeling of an incomplete practice. Occasionally I am able to call a clinic nurse to determine if a referred individual showed up or to hear what further care was delivered or planned. Usually, the individuals I see in the van are lost to me after the camp visit. Happily, some farm workers are repeat visitors from past years and one of us usually will recognize the other. We spend a few moments talking as if we were old friends.

The need to see as many farm workers as possible during a camp visit causes a great sense of pressure and uncertainty for me as a provider. These individuals need more comprehensive workups, care, and education. But many others will be turned away if I try to provide the type of care that I want to practice. I've learned to compensate by integrating knowledge of the Mexican culture and the migrant lifestyle with insights from the camp experiences into effective communication and behaviors. I speak Spanish, which enables building a relationship within the first few minutes of contact. Asking about work and the crops, commenting on the weather, listening intently, and using humor are methods that have helped increase connectedness. I cherish as small signs of connection the handshakes, smiles, and kind words as farm workers leave the van.

I found one area of practice with this population to be challenging. Many are from rural areas in Mexico, and have maintained some degree of their traditional health beliefs and practices. For example, they might indicate that a cause of a health problem is an imbalance of temperature in the body. A young male returned from the fields with hot shoulders and then took a hot shower that he believed caused his shoulder pain. A mother kept her child home from the Migrant Head Start School because the teacher gave the child a cold glass of milk when the child was suffering from a cold. I ask what would they like to do about their problem or what they would have done back home, and often, they will tell me. The man with the shoulder pain took a pair of gloves to fill with ice to lay on his shoulders at night. The mother allowed me to write a note to the teacher regarding the need for food and drink to be at room temperature.

The most touching incident was a 58-year-old man who presented with chest pain. He placed his hand over his heart and complained of intense pain. The entire camp staff went on alert and nearly called for an ambulance while readying the crash cart. Having learned in past experience how grief can cause much chest (or heart) pain, I asked about depression and his social life. I discovered that he had a wife in Mexico who had surgery one week ago. He had been unable to talk with her since he arrived three weeks ago and he felt incredible anxiety and sadness. After a history and exam that showed no evidence of an organic heart problem, the staff assisted with phone calls home and an appointment with a counselor. This person taught all of us about the expression of personal grief through pain.

The cultural backgrounds, the unique lifestyle, and the clinical setting have left me with innumerable images of the farm workers and their children. These include the farm workers with their kerchief-wrapped heads returning from the fields on a school bus with their clothes and hands stained from the berries; the women, last in the line to enter the van, who worked the fields for twelve hours only to return home to cook dinner, care for the children, clean the cabin or trailer, and then hurry to see me for a troublesome health problem; the adolescents playing soccer after work, amazingly full of energy; the 10-year-old girl caring for her two younger siblings while waiting for her parents to return from the fields; and the 57-year-old farm worker whose wrinkled face expresses every moment of the difficult lifestyle he has lived for forty years.

The migrant camp population provided me with remarkable insights into these workers' lives. They propelled me to become more of an activist than I probably would have become otherwise. I leave the camps each year a much better person and nurse practitioner for what they have given me.

Susie Oliver

Indianapolis is the home of the Ronald McDonald House (RMH), which offers a home for families of severely ill children who are hospitalized in local Indianapolis hospitals. The RMH offers a daily place of refuge for fifty-two families. "The house that love built" is the motto that serves families 365 days a year, 24 hours a day. RMH provides care, shelter, friendship, food, and a place of serenity and hope for families. Even if a family is unable to meet the minimum charge of $10 per night, services are provided. RMH is, therefore, heavily dependent upon volunteer support and donations.

In mid-September of 1996, RMH's volunteer coordinator readily accepted my offer to help. We discussed a variety of needs and collaborated on how my graduating class of nursing students could serve those needs. Approximately one week after this initial telephone conversation, I received an unexpected call from her. The local catering company, which had provided the traditional Thanksgiving meal for almost ten years, found it increasingly difficult to identify employees willing to maintain the volunteer commitment. The coordinator inquired if our nursing students could serve the food. Then, within 48 hours after this initial call, I received another call, this time requesting that the students take over the entire project because the catering company had withdrawn totally from the project.

Within several weeks we had collected $500 from our university colleagues, and the beginning of what has turned into an annual project unfolded. When I realized that this was becoming a reality, I approached the next year's graduating class and explained how the situation evolved. The class members agreed that we would all spend the Wednesday before Thanksgiving at RMH. When our transport team arrived with the food items, we worked in the kitchen to prepare and plan our Thanksgiving Day meal.

Since we were using up much of our holiday break, I encouraged the students to involve their family members, significant others, and children. This brought not only class closeness, but also shared learning of the importance of volunteer work and of giving to others. I told the students that they needed to explain to their families that if I needed a job done, I would look for a person I thought could complete the task and call out the name with the instructions. I placed many students' husbands in the kitchen washing dishes with their children drying the dishes. Much to my amazement and enjoyment, the volunteer family members got the job done.

After successfully completing our first Thanksgiving Day meal, the students and I made a decision to continue with our project. Only the next time, the students would be responsible for the fundraising. We continued to keep our commitment to RMH for the Thanksgiving meal for thirteen years and our project has grown every year. We now have added making homemade noodles and apple dumplings to our task list. Three-dozen eggs are worked into noodles, and thirty-six apple dumplings are created, in addition to the twenty pies that were on the original menu. This menu change filled two areas of need—we needed to find more jobs to keep the students and their family members busy, and we wanted to provide a special feast for our RMH families. Many of the students had never rolled out pie dough or made noodles, but every year, I am asked by the volunteers if our recipes can be copied so they can take them home and make these items for their own families.

One area important to me is that the RMH families feel welcomed. If they had other options, they would not choose to have a hospitalized child or to spend the Thanksgiving holiday away from home. To help with this, when the announcement for lunch is made, one person is stationed at the table's end and makes name tags. The students serving the food are instructed to call family members by their names as they proceed through the serving line. This is a small but important action to maintain some sense of normalcy for the families. The smallest-sized group for our Thanksgiving feast one year was 30 people, and the largest crowd was 225. That year, we scraped the pan bottoms for every morsel of food!

Annually in April I present the option to continue our project to the next graduating class. They select fundraising leaders to discuss ideas on how their class will raise their monies. There have been unique fundraising events, from bake sales, golf outings, car washes, t-shirt sales, and dining activities with restaurants allowing a certain percentage of the proceeds to go toward the fund-raising; the list remains endless. The class of 2005 holds the record for the highest amount of yearly monies collected. That class and the class of 2006 raised enough funds to qualify for the "Family Matters" program sponsored through RMH, which requires that donors provide $3,500 to support one room at the RMH for an entire year. Our students raised and donated more than $22,000 to our Indiana Ronald McDonald House.

Service learning has opened many doors for my students and me. When a person looks outside of themselves, they see that their lives can be enriched by helping others who are less fortunate or who are traveling a different journey in life. Even though this project was begun initially to enrich the nursing students' education, I am aware that it has also touched the lives of many individuals. One such life is Louise, the youngest daughter of Cheryl Conces, the program director. Louise began participating in this project in 2000 at the age of seven. Even at that young age, Louise sensed that helping others has an impact on one's life. Louise explains this today, "I have been fortunate enough to volunteer for the RMH Thanksgiving project for seven years and have enjoyed every aspect of it. I come for two main reasons: I love the feeling that I get when the families come to eat. And secondly, I love the excitement and cooperation in the kitchen as I help prepare the food with the nursing students."

Another life touched by the volunteer program is that of ASN alumna Carol Schenk, who has participated in this project since she graduated in 1998. Carol writes, "This experience helped shape my decision to dedicate my nursing life to work with children and families in a neonatal intensive care. I learned that nursing is neither a profession, nor a career, but a philosophy of special, and even intimate, care for families in times of desperate illness and need. Nursing involves an opening of one's heart, despite the risks, and becoming part of a stranger's life. I saw those families at the Ronald McDonald House, and my future became certain." Carol speaks openly about her family's continued participation in this project. "Baking the 350 homemade yeast rolls is an honored tradition of my family now, with as many as three generations participating, daughters, sons, nieces, and my husband. Also, this project has sparked interest in both nursing and the medical field for these individuals. More futures are being determined, born from simple acts of caring, not lessons learned in any classroom."

Linda M. Brice

In January of 2003 I began teaching at Texas Tech University School of Nursing (TTUSN). As a new nursing educator and also new to the community and the culture and environment of West Texas, I wanted to involve my students in projects that would make a difference in their lives and nursing careers, as well as in the community. I saw a small ad in the community section of the *Lubbock Avalanche-Journal* that asked the question, "Would someone give us a baby shower?" The ad was placed by the March of Dimes–sponsored Stork's Nest, a nonprofit organization that helps low-income pregnant women and teens receive good prenatal care. This would be the beginning of a wonderful relationship and a growing success story for the Stork's Nest, the TTUSN, and the community of Lubbock, Texas.

Texas, and especially West Texas, have been plagued by high rates of preterm births, low birth weight babies, neonatal complications, infant mortality, decreased prenatal care, teen pregnancies, and sexually communicated diseases. One of the biggest hurdles for the medically underserved pregnant population is starting prenatal care during the first trimester. The March of Dimes has developed an incentive program called the Stork's Nest to entice pregnant women and teens to start prenatal care early in their pregnancies and to receive regular care in exchange for new baby items. The Stork's Nest is a nonprofit organization established in cooperation with Zeta Phi Beta sorority. It is open to any pregnant woman or teen, regardless of income level.

There are many ways that Stork's Nest clients can earn the incentive points needed to "buy" new baby items. These soon-to-be moms can earn points by keeping their prenatal appointments, participating in the Stork's Nest prenatal and parenting classes, maintaining a healthy diet and lifestyle, and, later, ensuring that their babies attend regular well-baby check-ups and receive all required immunizations.

The new baby items are found in the Stork's Nest "Baby Store," but are based upon availability. Unfortunately, in 2002 there were not very many new baby items available for the Stork's Nest clients to "buy." The pregnant women and teens were able put their names on a waiting list to obtain the most sought after baby items as they were donated. However, since the Stork's Nest never had enough baby items to keep the clients interested in the program, they would drop out of the program and go back to little or no prenatal care, thus jeopardizing their pregnancies and especially the health of their babies. Part of the problem was that the Stork's Nest depended upon the generosity of the Lubbock community to donate the maternity and infant supplies that could be used as the incentive items. Because this nonprofit organization was still in its infancy, most of the community members did not know about the Stork's Nest or its mission to ensure a healthy term baby for every pregnant client.

With undergraduate nursing students I developed the Annual Stork's Nest Baby Shower to support this very important community program. The first goal was to initiate a charity activity that would benefit over 1,200 pregnant women and teens per year by providing enough new baby items to keep the Stork's Nest Baby Store fully stocked. The second goal was to develop a project that could be implemented each year by TTUSN undergraduate students that would assist not only the Stork's Nest and the community, but also the nursing students in learning leadership, management, and communication skills; collaboration and community interaction skills; and health education and health promotion skills—all helped along with role modeling by the senior nursing students for the junior students. Not only would students learn the importance of helping those less fortunate, but they would also educate the community on the importance of early and consistent prenatal care.

What first started as a small ad in the local newspaper six years ago turned into a major learning experience involving over 1,000 nursing students. The nursing students develop a better understanding of what uninsured, underinsured, or low-income pregnant women need in order to receive good prenatal care, and what can happen medically to the mother and her child if they do not. Students also educate the community on the high rates of preterm births, low birth weight babies, and neonatal complications due to lack of good prenatal care.

Each year in the early spring, over 700 letters are sent to local businesses, organizations, and individuals asking them to help co-sponsor the Baby Shower. The students then go into the community to the pre-notified businesses, organizations, and individuals to educate them on the need for early and consistent prenatal care and about the Stork's Nest mission. They ask if the community members would donate new baby items, make a monetary donation to buy expensive baby items that usually are not donated, or donate an item from their business for an auction. The senior students are involved in planning and managing the Baby Shower— asking community members for donations of food for the event, talking with the media, making the auction baskets, managing the logistics of moving thousands of dollars of baby items, and setting up and decorating the Baby Shower function itself for over 300 guests. This is a project that usually takes between three and four months to implement.

The first Baby Shower was planned and completed in two months. That year, the students were able to collect $6,800 in donations of new baby items and monetary donations. In the sixth year of the Baby Shower, the students collected over $45,300 in donations. These compassionate and caring nursing students have collected a total of $130,300 in new baby items and monetary donations for the Stork's Nest during these six years. Furthermore, these students had fun, assisted over 1,200 pregnant individuals annually, and have learned many valuable skills and lessons that they will use for the rest of their careers.

Part of the funding for this project comes from small community and national grants. I have received ten community grants over the last five years, averaging between $1,500 and $3,000, and a $5,000 National Avon Hello Tomorrow Community Grant in 2007. I have worked with the local K-Mart store to maximize the grant money by buying brand-new baby items during K-Mart's quarterly baby sale; K-Mart further helps this important community project by taking an additional 20% off the sale price of these items.

Over the past six years the community of Lubbock has embraced the Annual Stork's Nest Baby Shower. Each year more and more businesses, organizations, and individuals are involved. The money is used to buy baby items such as car seats, strollers, cribs, high chairs, walkers, and electric breast pumps. Another important outcome of this project is my relationship with the Lubbock media. Each year I am invited to appear on numerous TV shows and radio programs, and to give interviews for the community newspapers to let the citizens of Lubbock know that it is time for the event. The community knows that this is an important project to help decrease the high rate of preterm births, low birth weight babies, neonatal complications, and infant mortality rates, and to assist pregnant teens to obtain early and consistent prenatal care.

Thus, a small ad in the local paper has evolved into a "labor of love" that has assisted approximately 7,000 pregnant women and teens. This project also helped over 1,000 undergraduate nursing students learn valuable lessons in caring, community involvement, and collaboration, as well as leadership, management, communication, and having fun while helping others.

Guanetta Haynes

This is a description of a program that addresses Black infant health issues in the San Francisco Bay area. The state of California, recognizing the urgency of the problem, specifically infant mortality and low birth weight of children born to African American women, passed Senate Bill 165 in 1989. The bill was designed to improve the health of pregnant and parenting African American women, and their infants and families, while contributing to the health and wellness of the entire society. As a result, Black infant health programs sprang up in seventeen local health jurisdictions where Black births were predominant. The state and county contribute to the funding of the program based on current state and county budgets and program performance. Because of budget cuts and the high demand for nurses, the Black infant health program is, in general, facing difficulty in meeting their funding obligations. Black infant health program staff also is unable to adequately address the current needs of the African American community with the current budget and with limited personnel.

The proposed intervention will enlist senior nursing students currently in the public health component of their bachelor of nursing science program to increase the nursing staff capable of conducting home visits. The nursing students will rotate through the Black infant health program, conducting home visits to assess the client's environment and care needs. This increase in staff support will enhance the delivery of client education, assessment, and follow-up. Funding for the faculty to supervise the eight students will be obtained from grants. The result of such an intervention would be a win–win situation for both the Black infant health program and the school of nursing. The Black infant health program would receive much-needed nursing help, and nursing students would participate in a valuable learning experience. Ultimately, the benefits would be to the mothers and their infants and families.

7

Nurse Educator Groups

Together, groups of nurse educators have created curricula or course projects to benefit identified populations. The synergy, evident in their work, reaches the underserved and "invisible" groups that are of minimal interest to the media. Most of these groups are geographically constrained, disengaged from mainstream America and each other, and lacking the resources or the ability to access existing health care services. These communities are recipients of the brightness, collective insight, and leadership of nursing faculty and nursing students.

Pat Tooker

"Little Liberia" is the unofficial name of the Parkhill/Stapleton sections of Staten Island, New York. These communities earned this name because they are home to what some believe to be the largest Liberian immigrant population outside of Africa. Many Liberians fled to escape persecution and the atrocities of the fourteen-year civil war that took place from 1989 to 2003 in their home country. The majority of the Liberian immigrant population is composed of refugees, torture survivors, and former child soldiers, many undocumented immigrants to the United States. In addition to the Liberian immigrant population, these areas are home to an ethnically diverse population of people from Ghana, Sierra Leone, the Ivory Coast, various Caribbean countries, and Hispanics, Latinos, African Americans, and Whites. These communities are among the most disenfranchised, impoverished, and crime-ridden sections of New York City.

In 2003, a community assessment was performed by the International Trauma Studies Program of Columbia University to help address the needs of the growing population of West African immigrants in these communities. The most critical issues identified were the isolation and disenfranchisement of the refugees from the larger surrounding community. Also identified were an environment of mistrust among community members that rose from past experiences, cultural differences, and language barriers, and a lack of access to critical social services such as entitlement programs. The outcome of the assessment process was the development of the African Refuge (Drop-In Center), designed to support the needs of these neighborhoods through community outreach, development of family and youth psychosocial programs, and social service referrals. In 2007, the Drop-In Center evolved into the African Refuge Family and Youth Center. The success of the center captured the attention of the Unithree Investment Company, which donated a larger space within the public housing complex. The staff and volunteers of African Refuge identified that access to health care was the most significant issue.

In November of 2007, African Refuge sponsored a health fair, which included blood pressure screening. Of the thirty blood pressures taken, approximately half were elevated, and half of those were significantly elevated. In discussions with the participants screened, the majority had been previously diagnosed with hypertension during an emergency department visit. Most had no health insurance or primary care health provider. Some were prescribed antihypertensive medication from an emergency physician. Many believed that once the thirty-day supply was completed, they were "cured" and needed no follow-up. Some expressed concerns about becoming addicted to antihypertensive drugs. Many had the co-morbidity of diabetes, but did not express knowledge of diabetic self-care management.

An assessment of the community identified few available health services. Some services were provided occasionally such as during flu vaccine campaigns, via a mobile unit for health insurance enrollment, and periodic health fairs. There was no location that made consistent follow-up care available. Based upon the findings from the focus group, the community assessment, and the health fair, plans for a health promotion program were launched. An Academic Community Partnership was born.

During an informal lunch, Cheryl Nadeau, FNP-C, presented the overwhelming need for health promotion for the communities to Dr. Kathleen Ahern, director of the Graduate Program at The Evelyn L. Spiro School of Nursing, Wagner College. Dr. Ahern envisioned that community needs would be met by engaging the undergraduate nursing students in experiential and community-based learning. The health promotion program was officially implemented in January of 2008, with the first group of students providing services one-half day per week.

Annemarie Dowling-Castronovo, RN, PhD, Assistant Professor, is the course coordinator for the senior-level Community Health Nursing course. This is a required course that generic, second-degree, and RN to BS nursing students all must take just prior to graduation. Under the supervision of a clinical instructor, the nursing students continue community assessments and provide health education, screening, and referrals for additional services.

In response to identified concerns, African Refuge developed a health promotion program, which was a collaborative network of community service providers now called The Partnership in Community Health (PICH) Program. The African Refuge PICH Program now provides HIV and hepatitis C testing and counseling through several avenues—a partner agency, Community Health Action of Staten Island; a licensed social worker to assist with access to social service benefits, housing, and, legal services, as well as free food pantry bags through a partner agency, Project Hospitality; on-site health insurance enrollment through a partner agency, the Jewish Community Center; provision of full-service, primary care through a partner agency, the Community Health Center of Richmond, which also provides transportation for clients to and from their medical appointments; and immigration and citizenship services through a partner agency called CAMBA.

Through a Wagner College intramural grant from the Fox Fellows International Civic Engagement Fund, medical equipment has been purchased. The equipment is being used by the Wagner nursing students to perform screening and counseling for hypertension and obesity. Through informal evaluations it is clear that the nursing students are not just performing health assessments; they are learning firsthand the importance of cultural sensitivity from witnessing how socioeconomic factors influence the health status of individuals and communities. They find innovative ways to promote health literacy while simultaneously providing care within the client's historical and cultural context. The students identify how food, housing, medications, or citizenship and immigration influence the health of the individual and community. Students make appropriate referrals within the network of providers and provide follow-up services.

The essential benefit for the community is that PICH provides much-needed service. The clients express how PICH provides needed health screening and education. Specifically, over 55% of the clients have been identified with hypertension and receive health counseling at PICH. Twenty percent of the clients express problems with medications, and receive medication education. Prior to this academic–community partnership, the older adults in the community were fearful about leaving their apartments. Now, these same older adults come to the health promotion program to engage in safe socialization.

The best testament to civic engagement is the continued service to this community by one student after completing her semester. Through this academic–community partnership, students gain a better understanding of the ways in which individuals navigate personal health issues in their living environments. Subsequently, students experience how the nurse's role makes a difference in this process.

Rebecca C. Clark, Linda Rickabaugh, Annette Strickland, and Michelle Hartman

This is the story of how a group of nursing educators worked together with students and local and global communities to change the world, one person at a time. In the early 1990s, our small college decided to offer an RN-BSN program for the working RN. Our theme became a community of nurses committed to caring, service, and scholarship. We worked to develop a partnership between students and the community to identify and address health needs.

We encountered an early challenge in curriculum development and clinical placements. Traditional placements via the health department and home health agencies were difficult to attain. These agencies had experienced either a reduction in services or were heavily used by a local nursing program. We considered alternative sites that would provide significant student learning experiences, as one of our goals was for the students to learn while providing health services.

Simultaneously, we worked with local faith-based communities to develop health services for the underserved. While our geographic area provided extensive high-level health care, many of our region's citizens were either under- or unemployed and had difficulties in accessing preventive and maintenance health services. We sought clinical initiatives to complement the traditional point-of-care health services. This seemed a golden opportunity to partner.

One of our local churches had a long-operating clothes closet and food pantry that was open once a week for three hours, and was well utilized. This group was interested in expanding services for constituents who met the poverty guidelines established for federally assisted food pantries (earnings of 150% of the federal poverty level). We began negotiations with church leaders and the food pantry group to investigate the potential for offering a health clinic that would provide health screenings, health information, and referrals.

At the time, we also successfully obtained a Helene Fuld Grant for innovations in curriculum that focused on our community-based health center. Funds enabled purchasing a computer, blood pressure cuffs, glucometers, and other supplies for the health clinic. Students and church members were intimately involved as we developed publication brochures, newsletters, and flyers to showcase the services we were offering.

So, where did the change occur? It began with each of us as faculty. We found that the partnerships with students and community leaders required that we adopt a nontraditional view of education. We continually collaborated with the community and our students to frame the services that we could provide. As guests in the clientele's world, we had to sell our services and encourage them to participate.

The RN-BSN students were all experienced RNs, many working in critical care areas. They were not enthusiastic about the perceived "low level" of care that would be offered in the health clinic. This setting required that they adapt their interventions from strong, direct-care methods to strategies that would enhance the patients' knowledge and health efficacy. The students designed health fairs and health-education campaigns that engaged the community in dialogue about health behaviors.

Two of the community's most pressing health needs were foot care and mammography and Pap smear screening services. Many church members and food pantry participants were in need of foot care, including washing and cutting of toenails. The students reviewed the foot-care literature, talked with podiatrists, and developed a screening tool for foot care needs and policies for foot care. Uncontrolled diabetics were excluded, but we provided foot care for many in the community. This particular service was a challenge for both faculty and students, and seemed to be a very intimate experience.

This nursing program–faith-based community health center has now been in operation for over ten years; over 200 RN-BSN students and many faculty members have provided a range of health services. As faculty, it has been important for us to serve as mentors to the students to showcase the wide range of skills, responsibilities, and interventions that are within the scope of practice for nurses who are not nurse practitioners, but who provide important health services for a broad section of our community. Students, after their initial concerns about the value of this type of nursing, become engaged with the patients. Students continue to comment on how these experiences help them see the complexities that their patients face, and they develop a variety of skills and a broader range of compassion that enhance nursing across practice sites.

The program has continued to develop. The college added a traditional undergraduate baccalaureate nursing program, and faculty sought additional methods to add value to nursing community-health clinical rotations. Senior BSN students participate in pilot community-health promotion projects under faculty mentorship. Working in pairs, BSN nursing students present teaching sessions on health promotion such as wellness and disease prevention, high blood pressure, nutrition, diabetes, immunizations, parenting, substance abuse, and stress management. The students teach skills such as hand washing and taking temperatures and blood pressures with supervision. Students identify community resources and teach participants how to access them. This program has moved interventions to the community level, bringing broader changes to the health of our region, one person at a time, with the power and relationships of many.

The third phase of our commitment to developing a strong community of nurses has been on the international front. One of our faculty worked with a faith-based medical mission group for five years. It was our dream to take other faculty and students abroad and, in 2008, we were able to make that happen. This unique opportunity includes new teaching methods by which students appreciate the values and complexities that are inherent in community-health nursing in an international setting. We took five faculty and six students to Honduras, delivering health screenings, referrals, and health information to rural villages.

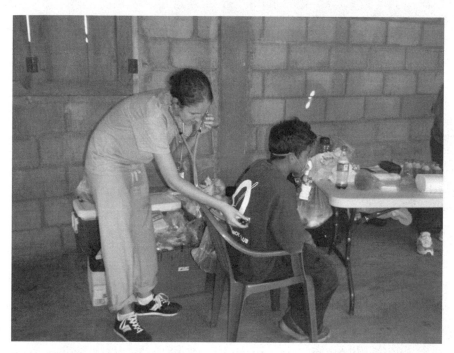

Kaylee McMahan, a third-year BSN nursing student, is assessing a Honduran patient experiencing a mild exacerbation of his asthma in the medical mission associated with Jefferson College of Health Sciences in Roanoke, VA, and Friends of Barnabas. The photo was taken by Linda Rickabaugh in October 2008.

In addition, faculty and students participated in a research project. The objective was to demonstrate increased student cultural competence through guided journaling and group reflection as a result of a cultural immersion experience in a Central American country. Nursing students examined the cultural dynamics of a global society relevant to health and the delivery of health care. Faculty assessed the effectiveness of a cultural immersion experience planned to enhance student cultural competencies.

A common thread in each teaching experience is the sense of relationships and respect we have all developed with our patients, students, colleagues, and selves, regardless of age, wealth, cleanliness, and social circumstance. This has been the gift from the local, regional, and international groups to us—changing us as much as we have changed their states of health.

Jane DeFazio

In support of the School of Nursing's community-based nursing education philosophy, a unique campus–community partnership was established. In the fall of 2004, the Staten Island Chapter of the Lay Scalabrinians developed an organization called the Scalabrinian Lay Organization. This lay persons' group is associated with the order of Roman Catholic priests who at one time used the St. Charles Mission Center on Staten Island as their seminary. The Center for Migration Studies, which is housed on the grounds of St. Charles Seminary, began in 1964 for the purpose of assisting and supporting migrants within the community. There was a collaborative effort between the seminary and the Center for Migration Studies. The Scalabrinian Lay Organization is a branch of the Center for Migration Studies, but unlike the Center for Migration Studies, the Scalabrinian focus is on working directly with migrants to support them in their efforts to assimilate into American society while maintaining their individual cultures.

In 2006, the organization received a grant to develop an educational program for migrants in the community to teach English as a second language (ESL). The program began with prekindergarten-age children and has subsequently extended to adults. The local newspaper sparked my interest about this new program. I contacted the program director, and we met to discuss and identify mutual goals for the ESL and nursing students, goals that provided a basis by which I could establish the project's purpose and objectives.

Each semester, the students are provided with the program's background information. The class project's purpose, goals, and objectives are also reviewed and a class discussion connects the collaborative goals of the partnership. My role begins by guiding the nursing students with the ESL assessment of the students' learning needs. Assessment data provide the student coherent group with information needed to develop four or five primary health promotion and prevention topics for implementation. The students plan topics and projects based on the population's needs assessment. The students' task is to deliver health information to this unique population by using teaching strategies that will enhance their learning, including use of tactual materials, auditory/visual methods, kinesthetic games, role play, and multicultural printed materials. Some of the topics introduced to the children and parents include nutrition, hygiene, need for immunizations, and safety. Additional specific adult topics include primary health promotion education for breast, testicular, prostate, and colon cancers.

After three years of a successful initiative, the School of Nursing at Wagner College maintains a community partnership with the Scalabrinian Organization. The accelerated nursing student's health-promotion projects and the community-based ESL program's successes have been highlighted in the local newspaper and Scalabrini newsletters. Ultimately, students gain a broader appreciation of the professional nursing role and lifelong civic responsibilities.

Ruth Wittman-Price, Maryann Godshall, and Angela Pasco

Our Teddy Bear Clinics were established in conjunction with local groups and parishes of all religious denominations through parish health fairs or health days, which are usually held after a religious service to foster attendance. Nursing students may be involved in all aspects of the health fair and can assist the parish nurse or organizer to coordinate the day's activities. The Teddy Bear Clinic, a clinic within a health clinic, addresses school-aged children with the goal of teaching health promotion and maintenance.

The nursing students integrated community health concepts into the development of the Teddy Bear Clinics. The activity was advertised through a parish bulletin, student-made signs, or the local papers. Children came to the clinic with a stuffed animal and pretended to be a parent with a child. The children were escorted through stations by a nursing student. The stations each had a different theme, such as hand washing, teeth brushing, injury prevention, first aid, and safety. Graduate students supervised the activities of the undergraduate students.

The following are examples of Teddy Bear Clinics' health promotion activities:

- *Hand washing*: Using a shoe box of confetti, the students taught proper hand washing technique while twice singing a short song. This helps children gauge the proper, safe duration of hand washing.

- *Teeth brushing station*: Students demonstrated proper teeth brushing on the stuffed animal. Tooth brushes were donated for the children.
- *Bandaging*: The children learn how to apply a Band-Aid or take care of "boo-boos" on their teddy bears.
- *Temperature taking*: Children learn how to take a temperature on their favorite bear or stuffed animal. They also learn the importance of what having a temperature means, and what they should do about it.
- *Car seat safety*: The importance of wearing a seat belt and, for children, of remaining in their car seat or booster seat is discussed.
- *Bicycle safety*: Children learn the importance of wearing a helmet when riding a bike and basic hand signals for turning. They learn how to ride safely on a street and to follow traffic rules.
- *Ambulance visit*: A local ambulance service brings an ambulance to the location so that children could go inside it and touch items with supervision.

After the clinic, the nursing students wrote a reflective paper on what they learned from the experience in relation to their affective experience and ability to communicate information to children and diverse groups of parents. They discussed the completion of their learning outcomes and how the concepts of human development, health literacy, cultural sensitivity, and educational principles were met and evaluated. These events are a win–win for the child, the school, church, or parish, and the student.

Another excellent event is what we call Alex's Lemonade Stand. Alex was a four-year-old girl diagnosed with cancer. She came up with the idea to sell lemonade to get money to fight children's cancer. In 2000 she and her older brother set up a stand on their front lawn to raise money for cancer. Since Alex's simple idea, many schools, businesses, and students began to raise money in Alex's name. Sadly, Alex lost her battle with cancer on August 1, 2004, at the age of eight years. In her name, over $1 million has been raised for childhood cancer research. There is a website dedicated to Alex's dream at http://www.alexslemonade.org.

The development of the Community Outreach Program, as part of the curriculum of our school of nursing, was an attempt to respond to the health care needs of the local community, and to provide services where none had previously existed. The program also meets the learning needs of student nurses who must be prepared to practice in a community-based, community-focused health care system. The goal of the program was to assist residents of the community to attain and maintain an optimal level of health and well-being. The program's general plan was to implement a community service project/clinical experience in each of the nursing courses. Services provided by the program included screenings (i.e., blood pressure, blood glucose, health status, functional status), health teaching (i.e., basic hygiene, communicable disease control, health-risk reduction, immunizations, family planning, parenting skills, well-child care, pregnant family care, problems associated with aging), management of health problems (i.e., management of common health problems, stress reduction, anger control, self-esteem, medication management), and health promotion (i.e., nutrition, assertiveness skills, problem-solving skills, health care partnerships, childhood development, management of emerging and developing families).

Students learn in various service areas, including:

- Bridge House: This program is a transitional housing service located in the community. It provides comprehensive services to persons facing long-term homelessness and a safe, supportive environment for adults and their children.
- Community Area Kitchen: The Area Kitchen provides a free meal service five days a week to a diverse group of the community's poor, indigent, and homeless adults. Abundant opportunities exist for screening, assessment, and health teaching.
- Hospital and Shopping Mall: A local hospital uses this setting to provide blood pressure screening services on a regularly scheduled basis.
- SELECT Program: SELECT (Schuylkill Education Leading to Employment and Career Training) is a program for pregnant and parenting teens. The program assists these youths to stay in school, earn a high school diploma or GED, make the transition to productive employment, and raise healthy children.

Mary P. Bourke

With a focus on the underserved needs of others, students in our program demonstrated an emotional commitment to their own education and to the community they served. Examples of typical interventions by the students include blood pressure, body mass index, and glucose screenings for fifty-eight rescue mission clients; creation of a cookbook filled with simple nutritious recipes, with the purpose of teaching homeless men how to improve their nutrition before being placed in homes; Denver II Developmental Assessments on homeless children and then educate the mothers about the results; and provision of information about immunization schedules and local resource information.

The community residents who benefited from students' interventions include persons served by the Kokomo Rescue Mission Homeless Men's and Women's Shelters, Kokomo's Housing Authority Retirement and Disability Center, Kokomo Victims of Violence Shelter, and Kokomo area schools. Groups of students collected data, surveyed their aggregate, researched "best practices," and then created interventions based on the results.

Another group installed hand dryers in the bathrooms of the women's homeless shelter and provided education on proper hand-washing techniques to prevent the spread of bacteria and viruses. The women's shelter routinely houses newborn infants and young children who are at risk for communicable diseases; consequently, prevention is imperative. At the Kokomo Violence Shelter, students painted and decorated bedrooms and bathrooms to increase the morale and self-esteem of the residents. They also screened the victims for depression.

At the Housing Authority Retirement and Disability Center, students set up a Nintendo Wii® and provided instructions on its use, operation of its accessories, and board game assembly. The goal for this intervention was to improve the residents' social engagement, cognition, and physical activity. Research from interviewing many physical therapists and nursing home staff, and research from journals led them to this innovative intervention.

Mini-grants provided the financial resources necessary to support the creative work of the students. Working as teams, the students learned the power of leadership and team work, and that knowledge is constructed within a social context of learning. Giving to others provided significant benefits to the students, as expressed by one student and echoed by many: "Our team as a whole experienced a very rich learning experience . . . that had a huge impact on our hearts. We learned things we could never learn from a book or classroom, things that we will remember forever. . . . We now understand real life circumstances that can impact a person's life, which are uncontrollable and heart wrenching."

Lynda Billings and Patricia Allen

In 2001, Texas Tech University Health Sciences Center Anita Thigpen Perry School of Nursing (TTUHSC) was struggling with the strategic plan to provide an increasing supply of nurses to the surrounding region, the state, and the nation at large. The nursing shortage was beginning to be of national concern and was publicized as a looming disaster. In the midst of diminishing clinical capacity for students and a faculty that was entrenched in nursing education delivery models of the past, TTUHSC's new Dean of Nursing, Dr. Alexia Green, and the Associate Dean of Research, Dr. Christina Esperat, took a step away from the traditional nursing education approach and took a crucial step toward uniting efforts with other educational disciplines, other nursing schools, hospitals, workforce development agencies, community entities, and private businesses to establish a successful model of cooperation and partnership. This endeavor has resulted in several community partnerships, including the expansion of an existing nurse-managed clinic, which houses a diabetes education center for managed care, and a senior house-calls nurse practitioner program for the delivery of primary care to house-bound elders in the fifteen-county South Plains area. Most recently, in an effort to battle the huge numbers of teen pregnancy on the South Plains (Lubbock and the surrounding area have one of the highest teen pregnancy rates and sexually transmitted disease rates in the country), they have established a pre- and postnatal program for first-time Medicaid mothers, as well as a program for the delivery of health-preventive information through the use of community health workers. These outcomes have been achieved through realigning academic structures, adopting innovation as a framework for change, empowering others, and developing lasting partnerships and relationships. This transformative process has resulted in benefits across the spectrum of TTUHSC and its partners, but most of all has benefited the citizens of West Texas and the state.

In 2001, this mission and the innovative vision of the TTUHSC leadership team led to the acceleration of the development of the LCCHWC, a nurse-managed primary care clinic located in an underserved and economically depressed area of Lubbock. Progress was initiated by hard work, belief in the project, and sheer faith. TTUHSC's Associate Dean of Research and Clinical Practice, Dr. Esperat, has been primarily responsible for the development and survival of this worthwhile clinic that brought primary care to the underinsured and often under-represented citizens of East Lubbock. Through efforts to establish a baseline community health-delivery system that benefits and addresses a diverse population plagued by health disparities, a collaborative arrangement with the community was established early on. It is represented by LCCHWC's Advisory Board that is made up of community members, area professionals, city officials, state and federal agencies, and TTUHSC staff and educators. Continual efforts are made to incorporate the community's needs as well as the community's preferences into the delivery of health services.

Furthering community involvement, Esperat instigated community-based participatory research in East Lubbock through a United States Agriculture Department Cooperative State Research Education and Extension Service (CREES) project on childhood obesity that involves Harwell Elementary School and a second research site in El Paso.

The Coalition and the LCCHWC are only two of many educational and community partnerships that have been conceived and developed by the TTUHSC leadership team. Texas Nursing Competency Coalition (TNCC), a state-wide group of nursing education leaders that is dedicated to the investigation and instigation of lifetime nursing competency, had its initial (2006) and third (2008) meeting at TTUHSC, and continues its research into the complexity of providing, measuring, and assuring competency in the nursing profession. TTUHSC's Center for Innovation in Nursing Education (CINE) organized the West Texas Nursing Education Consortium (WTNEC), consisting of five member universities and six member community colleges representing nursing schools from the entire West Texas region. Along with the CINE, the Center for Evidenced Based Practice, the Center for Patient Safety, and the F. Marie Hall Simulation Center have been established. These accomplishments are the direct result of the hard and dedicated work of TTUHSC's leadership.

After the horrific hurricane assaults on Louisiana, Mississippi, and Houston in 2005, over 450 refugees were flown into Lubbock to escape the destruction that faced them back home. TTUHSC assumed the lead for organizing health care providers for the refugees. Faculty, students, and medical staff from all the Coalition members provided care throughout the aftermath of both hurricanes. Having the organizational structure and the partnership experience through the Coalition facilitated the process of working together within the group.

Drs. Green and Esperat have developed a culture for innovation and have implemented processes for affirmative change. With a vision and mission that is designed as an overarching statement of what TTUHSC stands for and what it intends to achieve, they have been quick to recognize and reward the original and resourceful ideas of others. These two leaders find great ways to inspire the people they work with to achieve extraordinary results and to exceed expectations by attracting and retaining great team members whose goal is a successful and outstanding team effort. Through the combined leadership forces of Drs. Green and Esperat, a model of open-minded and constructive growth has taken place at TTUHSC.

8

Total Program Faculty

These authors acknowledge a total group of nurse educators who made substantial, sustainable changes that impacted their programs and communities. Each narrative is unique and inspiring. Each is about a group of nurse leaders with a lived mission and a legacy of change.

Cathleen M. Shultz

In 1975, an undergraduate nursing program began at a faith-based college, now Harding University, in Arkansas. Janice Bingham, from Tennessee, was one of the first nursing faculty members for this BSN program in a liberal arts setting. She was one of the early modern nurse educator pioneers to model and teach nursing care of vulnerable populations. She initiated a thirty-four year personal legacy for nursing faculty and students serving health needs of people from different cultures and vulnerable groups. Today, over 90% of the faculty and annually over 80% of undergraduate nurses participate in providing health care at domestic and international health mission sites. Community outreach service is embedded in the curriculum.

Educated as a teacher and laboratory technician, Bingham's heart was deeply touched by the plights of the disadvantaged. She turned to nursing as a second career to reach others. With experience in African countries, she took members of the senior nursing class for a summer trip to Nigeria, West Africa, in 1977. This trip began the health missions program and also launched another phase of Bingham's life as she included undergraduate nursing students and later students from other disciplines such as premedicine, prepharmacy, teaching, and ministry into the program to bring much needed health promotion, health care, and end-of-life care to the vulnerable.

The hospital served the Nigerians until its personnel was driven from the country during the Biafran War. The hospital was the first in the country to be re-opened by the Nigerian government when the tribal fighting ceased. Starvation, contagious diseases, traumatic wounds, and desolated villages awaited Janice and the students. Janice was experienced in rural clinic settings and in relating to the native Ebo tribe. Her work initiated the College of Nursing's international health care ministries, which now are in their thirty-fourth year.

No written nursing guidelines about health care in third-world countries were available to teach students in the 1970s. Immunization information for travelers was unreliable due to poor reporting and civil unrest. Janice had a phenomenal network, exuberant determination, a great sense of humor, and an innate ability to problem solve against many odds. She lived her passion as a nurse educator. Janice and others collaborated with tribal and village leaders, and government officials. Her competence and compassion were evident, and with each visit new levels of trust were established and her role was expanded. Collaboration efforts, where possible, occurred with national nurses and local health care workers. Through the years she mentored countless faculty and alumni about the role and expectations of nursing with vulnerable, fragile populations.

Most of the faculty's international nursing experiences have been in African countries such as Nigeria, Tanzania, Kenya, Ghana, and most recently Zambia. Each site had or was establishing a central clinic or hospital. Between employment periods at Harding, Janice served mission sites abroad for several years in Nigeria, Tanzania, and Ghana and also worked with relocated refugees from the Vietnam War including Cambodians, Vietnamese, and Laotians. Janice also served on the Mayor's Counsel for Refugees in Davidson County, Tennessee. Her service as a nurse and nurse educator spans over three decades.

Most of these mission sites now have paid national health workers supported by a few expatriates who were educated in Europe, the United States, or Canada. Numerous nationals were taught on site by Janice and other team members, and other natives were financed abroad to become nurses and to return to their home country. One effort she implemented during the World Health Organization's (WHO) Year of the Child was an international vaccination program. With the assistance of Mrs. Betty Bumpers (Senator Dale Bumpers' wife) and WHO, Janice took 3,000 doses of measles vaccines (donated by the Merck Pharmaceutical Company) into Nigeria. Most (80%) of the children of Nigeria were not given names until they were six years old because they often died before then. The cause of death was frequently measles. Janice and twelve undergraduate students vaccinated 3,000 children; many of these Nigerians have now grown to adulthood.

The majority of Harding nursing students are drawn to serving others. Janice has thoughtfully prepared and refined a nursing orientation and preparation program for these students. Typically, the group meets every other week in Janice's home. Topics include safety, health protection, health promotion preparation customized to the country and tribe, disease symptom recognition, guidelines on what to pack, and basic language skills. Strategies incorporate DVDs with site photos and videos, meetings with those who have had similar experiences, preparing their parents or spouses, raising funds for the trip, and best purchases to be made for their stay.

Completing health-related mission activities within a highly regulated American educational setting had its challenges. Early on, the state board of nursing and accrediting agency denied inclusion in the nursing curriculum of the term "spiritual" to describe a component of a person to be assessed because "spiritual" could not be measured. After Janice's work satisfactorily addressed spiritual concerns, the accrediting and approval bodies supported these concepts and the faculty began openly addressing the Harding School's mission of "Developing Nurses as Christian Servants."

The Harding faculty believes that each person has four dimensions (physical, psychological, social, and spiritual) to assess, strengthen, and evaluate relative to health, sickness, and dying. Our ideas, teaching strategies, and learning experiences fostered holistic care to assist human flourishing. The faculty also created a guiding philosophy to develop and evaluate health mission sites; clinical experiences also include nontraditional sites. If there were needs, the faculty created and supported ways to provide holistic care in domestic American settings. For example, early on there was limited health care for the area's Hispanic migrant farm workers. Faculty developed on-site cost-free screenings for school-age children, and facilitated referrals for care and treatment through their vast network of community providers. Also, faculty planted the seeds for area health care providers to teach and screen low-income families, and to provide prevention and referrals using primary intervention services such as breast examinations, laboratory tests, free screening mammograms, and reviews of medications. This effort led to the community's Annual Day of Caring sponsored by interdisciplinary health care providers and local businesses. In 2008, over 3,000 were served. Free clothing, school supplies, and health care were available. Nursing students and faculty were the impetus for this event, which presently has a number of corporate sponsors and over 200 volunteers; the College of Nursing remains a co-sponsor and White County Medical Center, the local hospital, is the coordinator.

Simultaneous with the international missions, domestic health care nursing mission activities were initiated in Appalachian, African American, and Hispanic communities. Some were organized through rural or ethnic-specific churches, and others through migrant worker camps. The domestic nursing focus is toward those vulnerable, poverty-stricken groups who are underserved by existing health services and disenfranchised. Often supplies were obtained, donated, or purchased by the students themselves. In both domestic and international experiences, students learned how to establish free-standing clinics and to care for vulnerable populations. Other nurse faculty have extended the program further: Dr. Helen Lambert and Jeanie Burt annually traveled to the Ukraine. Lisa Engel coordinates nursing care for the Haiti mission trip. Johnnetta Kelly created the first day-long health promotion groups with African American and Hispanic populations in the Delta region of Arkansas. Faculty have worked together, and have taught and mentored each other as well as their students.

The duration of health mission experiences abroad vary from ten days to eight weeks. All experiences are voluntary. Some experiences at sites such as Guatemala, Ghana, and Mexico are completed as an optional part of a required course. Some site visits such as those as part of the Haiti program are held during spring break, and others such as those at Tanzania and Zambia are completed during the summer. Nursing faculty travel with the students. Additionally, faculty who teach the courses and programs spend considerable time planning the trips and advising the students.

As Janice and later colleagues broadened their domestic and international nursing expertise and interests, a nursing position of Health

Missions Coordinator (initially filled by Jerry Myhan) and a standing nursing Health Missions Committee were created about twenty years ago. The Coordinator keeps the health mission program visible and collaborates regarding travel and fund raising, ensures health regulations are met, actively serves as a mentor to colleagues, plans trips, and problem solves to facilitate teaching, travel, and safety.

Over eight years ago, a health missions minor was co-developed with religion faculty. Nursing faculty took the lead in developing and teaching two courses, Culture of Poverty and Skills for Health Care Missions; the latter is for non-nursing or pre-nursing majors. This eighteen-credit hour minor is open to students in all majors. The program is overseen by the College of Nursing's Health Mission Coordinator.

Janice collaborated with other faculty to prepare nursing students and programs. Initially, the programs centered on two sites, Nigeria and Panama. In those days, no published material in English existed to guide nurses with international interests or health-related, grass-roots information about various cultures. The Centers for Disease Control's materials were dependent upon health and disease information reported by the selected countries' public health officials. These officials were keenly aware of the impact of public health reports on tourism and therefore their country's economy. Thus, those reporting from third-world countries often underreported or omitted incidents of infectious disease such as the "wasting disease" (known now as HIV/AIDS), yellow fever, malaria, chloroquine-resistant malaria, and cholera. Safe travel involved extensive knowledge of sanitary precautions and practices, as well as maintaining contacts within a country for the latest on political situations that predicted war outbreak, guerilla attacks, and marauding between tribes.

Relationships with governmental officials in the nations' capitals and with district and tribal leaders were essential to conduct clinics and travel without incidents. Often the travelers worked with the tribe's healers, shamans, or medicine men. In some countries, tribal women persuaded their men to protect the health care workers. Often, they were esteemed because of their reputation for caring for sick and dying children, pregnant women, and villagers injured from fighting and accidents. Trust was imperative to outcomes.

Other experienced nurse faculty, Dr. Nancy Clark, Janice Linck, and Mr. Jerry Myhan, emerged as nurse faculty leaders who continued Janice's work at the university while she traveled to Tanzania and Nigeria to live full-time at mission sites. The program spread to Kenya, Tanzania, and Haiti following Jerry Mayhan's five-year experience of creating and operating a nurse-managed clinic and tending the children of an orphanage in Haiti. Dr. Cathleen Shultz worked with health officials of the Luo tribe in Kenya and with people who fled from Uganda; she was in Kisumu, Kenya, when the first outbreak of the Ebola virus took place. Although the challenges were many, the faculty continued providing nursing care and teaching students, and helping those who sought care at the sites have healthier lives, prevent premature death, and adjust to chronic conditions.

As mentioned previously, Jerry returned from Haiti and became the nursing program's first Health Missions Coordinator. The health mission programs emerged as two types: short term, from five to seven days of treating and teaching all ages per trip; and long term, from six weeks to three months at one site. The latter program usually involved additional travel to even more remote sites. Hundreds are treated in the longer trips; students mainly provide nursing care at clinics, orphanages, hospitals, and mobile clinics. The illnesses are very different from the typical patient experiences that students encounter in the United States. The programs are intense and the students experience personal and professional growth.

Students and faculty raise their own travel money and money to obtain medicines, equipment, and other supplies. After a decade, the university began paying the faculty's expenses and salary for long-term programs. As well, students learn basic language skills in preparation to provide nursing care abroad, although often local translators were hired to ensure safety of care. Immersed in the cultures and living 24 hours a day with experienced faculty, students spent hundreds of volunteer hours teaching topics of sanitation, rehydration, and recognizing infectious diseases, and administering vaccinations and nursing in acute care settings and maternity wards. They have cared for patients with leprosy, meningitis, and gangrene and other third-world infectious diseases.

Required nursing courses were taught depending upon the care focus at the site. Student participation was voluntary. These required courses were pediatric, community health, and maternal–child nursing; a stateside component of each course was held on campus to ensure students had all needed experiences. The Arkansas State Board of Nursing was progressive and encouraged the nursing coursework abroad. The students' education was enriched by their nursing experiences, cultural immersion, and expert nursing faculty mentoring and teaching about other health care systems. Many graduates participate in similar programs with interdisciplinary teams through churches and other organizations. At present, several graduates serve abroad at mission sites and have become faculty for the health mission programs.

The first interdisciplinary collaboration was to create a health missions course co-taught by nursing faculty and faculty from the College of Bible and Religion. Cataloged as a nursing course, the course was approved to meet either a global literacy or a Bible course requirement for the degree. The course is open to all students and is now offered two or three times per year.

A collaborative cross-cultural strategies course offered by the College of Nursing and the College of Bible and Religion was partnered with Heifer Project International's (headquartered in Little Rock, Arkansas) global village site at Perryville, Arkansas. The world-renowned global village comprises several hundred acres and consists of dwellings representing various cultures such as an African hut, a Guatemalan hutch, and an Appalachian house. There are animals, such as water buffalo and giraffes, that are native to various cultures. Heifer is known worldwide for its humanitarian efforts to enable those in poverty to earn an income with their own hands. Families learn a cash-crop such as raising goats to eat and sell. Families are required to give the first-born of the goats to a neighbor so the wealth of survival is shared. Students and faculty live for about two or three weeks in the environment. Course content and experiences covered include brick making, animal husbandry, developing sustainable agriculture (i.e., organic gardening in small land spaces), latrine making, drilling wells, filtering water, hygiene and sanitation, first aid, nutrition, and infectious diseases.

Global decision-making strategies and survival permeate the program. Teaching strategies vary. For example, students are divided into groups as tribes, develop their own language, and learn to barter their tribe's assets (animals, crops, water) to survive. Between them, they have what is needed to survive but they learn survival is impossible without cooperation. Learning encompasses knowledge, skills, attitudes, and values. The course, held annually, is open to all students and the class numbers are limited due to space. Eventually the university built its own global village about thirty-five miles from campus where the course is co-taught by nursing and religion faculty. The Health Care Missions course, offered for thirty-two years, may be taken by students in any major and meets an undergraduate degree's global literacy requirement.

As the health missions program grew, faculty explored other ways to strengthen their work. Eight years ago, they created an eighteen-credit hour Health Missions Minor in collaboration with the College of Bible and Religion. Two additional courses were developed, Culture of Poverty and Skills for Health Missions, to provide options within the minor. Students have a menu of nursing, cultural anthropology, language, and independent, custom-developed courses to choose from and match with their interests. The minor can be completed alongside degree requirements for the BSN.

Over the past twelve years, nursing faculty was instrumental in assisting a local church to create and develop a free-standing Christian Health Ministry clinic, which is open each Sunday. Another nurse faculty, Karen Kelley, coordinates the nurse staffing of the clinic. Students participate in the clinic as part of the community health nursing course. Capstone nursing students have completed senior projects involving translating health literature, organizing the clinic's infrastructure, and developing health materials. Besides health care, counseling and nutrition services are available. The work is interdisciplinary and serves hundreds from the immigrant and low-income populations.

The latest mission service began three years ago as the College of Nursing partnered with the campus International Programs to open a site in Zambia, Africa. Janice Bingham, who returned to the nursing faculty about eight years ago, was instrumental in developing health policies and preparing twenty-four interdisciplinary students for this semester abroad. The first group traveled in the fall of 2007. A hospital has been built, and national nurses, a physician assistant, and other team members are permanently onsite. The nurses who traveled in 2008 collected over $10,000 to purchase medicine and supplies for the Zambian people.

Through her life-long commitment to underserved and vulnerable populations, Janice Bingham has encouraged and taught hundreds of nursing students and faculty to work outside their comfort zones and to share their expertise with those who desperately need health care. She is a mentor and nurse extraordinaire; numerous alumni have incorporated these practices into other nursing programs as educators and into their congregations and communities as they participate in humanitarian efforts. This quiet, yet powerful circle of nursing faculty influence has touched and changed the quality of life for thousands of vulnerable people in the United States and abroad.

By persevering and by developing sustainable programs in various domestic and global sites, and by teaching nursing students the skill of collaboration, the faculty have created, modeled, and engaged others in improving the holistic health of people throughout the world. At each site, an infrastructure was built and sustained, and every effort was made to empower native populations; most of these sites are now operated by citizens of the country. This was accomplished while providing an excellent education for nursing students. In the capstone course, students are asked to identify their most meaningful nursing experiences. Those who participated in the domestic and international nursing mission programs always mention how these experiences have positively affected and changed their views of the world. Faculty has created a culture of service within a supportive campus environment. They and the lives they have improved or saved are our legacy, a legacy that began with seeds planted by Janice Bingham. The program continues with the passion, cooperation, and support of hundreds of students, faculty, alumni, and friends of nursing.

Paula Reams

Within a small Midwestern college that offers health professions–related degrees, there was a possibility to develop a unique Honors Program. When Kettering College of Medical Arts (KCMA) administration decided to establish an Honors Program based on student assessment, the mission and outcomes of the college were reviewed. Service has been a long-standing part of the Seventh Day Adventist culture, and since KCMA is steeped in this culture, service and learning were a natural fit. Participating in a grant from Learn and Serve, which was to promote service learning in health professions curricula, the college administration and a small group of faculty at KCMA decided to incorporate the mission of service and learning within the Honors Program.

Service learning as pedagogy has been used extensively in health professions education, especially in nursing. The lure of service learning as pedagogy is present throughout the curricula because students' attitudes about it are positive. Educational leaders see service learning as a way to combine high-quality teaching strategies while supporting the community's needs. Combining an Honors Program and service learning enabled the college to begin institutionalizing service learning within the organization.

Although the college administration supported the idea of a service-learning Honors Program, it was unknown if faculty and staff did. The college participated in a service-learning conference, and two faculty received mini-grants to include service learning into their courses; still, the faculty and staff needed to fully accept a new program for service learning.

Through an open invitation to all faculty and staff, a task force came together comprising instructors from most offered programs. Representatives from nursing, physician assistant, respiratory therapy, ultrasound, and the library and research areas met weekly to create a program combining service learning and honors curricula. Initially, the task force conceived a name, developed purpose and outcomes, created a conceptual model, designed a curriculum, and wrote a bulletin description. The naming of the program ended with a tie between two college instructors who gave extensive service to their local and global communities: Anna May Vaughan, the first nursing director who had been a missionary in Africa, and Dr. Beaven, a past provost of the college with international standing and recognition in alcohol/drug addiction education.

The next step was to develop a program mission statement. The task force believed that the Honors Program should be for students who wish to demonstrate their excellence and character beyond the high standards of the college's professional programs, who have a heart for service, and who can develop leadership in service. The mission statement is: "The service-learning honors program is committed to improving communities through leadership in service learning." All courses in the Honor's Program curriculum use the same model to develop the service-learning component of the course.

The curriculum was developed for all college degrees. Local and global health care service was important to the program's and college's mission. Two courses were developed to incorporate service. International Health, an introduction to the global health care system emphasizing developing countries, includes as a requirement forty service-learning hours, with students expected to travel outside the United States for this experience. The course faculty, in collaboration with the Service Learning Honor Coordinator, plan and implement these trips.

The second course emphasizes local and national service, and is designed to introduce students to the health care needs of diverse, underserved populations in the United States. Topics consist of health promotion and illness prevention, from homeless groups and migrant workers, to the urban poor, and those living in rural settings. This course also requires forty hours of service-learning experiences in a local community.

All program students are required to take a course entitled Cultural Diversity in Health Care, which many majors at the college require as well. Numerous service-learning projects are done with peoples of differing cultures, especially in other countries. Depending on the degree program, students would be required to take a certain amount of honors courses to graduate as a Service Learning Honors Scholar. Most programs require about one course per year. All students are required to complete an amount of service learning hours, not all of which are required honors courses. Other nonhonors courses taken at the college that have service learning requirements assist with these hours.

After approvals were obtained, the Anna May Vaughan–Winton Beaven Service Learning Honors Program began. Students in the Vaughan–Beaven program participate in a course of study that critically analyzes the service needs of the local, regional, national, and/or global communities, and participate in meeting identified needs. Students who complete all program requirements are recognized at commencement as Vaughan–Beaven Honors Scholars.

The program started in the fall semester of 2002 with ten students. Today, the majority of students who start the program graduate as Scholars. Students, faculty, and staff have volunteered thousands of hours of service while earning academic credit. The department of nursing has been a leader in the Honors Program at the College. A nursing faculty member was instrumental in the development and implementation of the program, and was the first coordinator of the program. This faculty member was awarded a Community Campus Partnerships for Health fellowship. Many of the nursing courses at the college also use service-learning teaching methodologies, helping with the service-learning hour requirements and advertising the program at the same time.

In the Health Care Needs of Underserved Populations course, students develop their service-learning projects individually while the didactic portion of the course is done on the Web. Many varying projects have evolved, including food inventorying, follow-up care for underserved populations with chronic diseases, establishment of a formulary for a free clinic with free medications, disaster preparation efforts, health education programs, health fairs, and more. Although mostly on a local level, some of the projects have been done throughout the country, including California and Alaska.

The International Health course materials are also presented online; however, the group does meet at the beginning and end of the course to assist students with preparation for international travel. Most international projects consist of health fairs on topics that the hosting country has requested. Another service-learning project has been the establishment of rural health clinics in underserved areas of the world. Trips are planned during school breaks so that all students are available to attend. Currently, Guyana, Belize, and Trinidad and Tobago are the countries that are visited. Because the college is part of the Adventist health care system, there is an automatic affiliation with many Adventist hospitals located throughout the world.

The program now has requests from all over the world for students to participate in health care service-learning projects. Although there has not been a concerted effort to calculate the number of people this program has served, most health fairs in international settings see an average of 200 to 400 people. Both the nursing and health professions program have service learning in at least three courses in their curricula. Students in the Honors Program or with service learning in their courses experience continuous reflection, which encourages them to formulate new ways to view the world.

Fran Muldoon[†]

Second-semester nursing students at Delaware Technical and Community College in Newark, Delaware, embraced a collaborative experience that provided the community with a health promotion project to address Delaware's high incidence of cancer. The college's nursing program has promoted a service-learning teaching project about breast self-examinations within a service-learning model.

In the program, nursing students travel to locales where they participate in teaching, demonstrating, and mentoring the community about breast cancer awareness and breast self-examination. The experience

[†]Deceased.

provides each nursing student with exposure to the practice, and not just the theory, of public health nursing. But more importantly, this is their first experience with teaching, one of the most essential roles they will perform throughout their nursing careers. The nursing curriculum development staff at Delaware Technical and Community College thought it of major importance to educate students about the incidence of cancer and the mortality rate within the state of Delaware, while incorporating the campaign to develop the students' competencies in public health. Public health nursing consists of assessment, planning, intervention, and evaluation of community neighborhoods, and providing the knowledge and materials to educate those who otherwise would not have the resources to visit a primary care physician or gynecologist and no insurance to pay for cancer screening. Student learning includes understanding of the community's populations, cultures, epidemiology, educational competency, health literacy, and prevention focus. These specific components are a strategic part of the core curriculum.

Our course focus is the community population where we fully integrate the community nursing experience as part of our community curriculum. The program is introduced to students during orientation at the second year of the nursing program, at which point they already have had contact with patients within a hospital setting. During orientation they are introduced to the project by descriptions of the Breast Cancer Prevention Collaboration Project and then the showing of two films based on breast cancer survivors, mammography, and demonstration of breast self-exam. The most exciting program component is the introduction of Delaware Breast Cancer Coalition speakers. The Delaware Breast Cancer Coalition, Inc., started in 1991, provides resources for newly diagnosed cancer patients and establishes a mentoring program through volunteers who are also breast cancer survivors. Their mission is to educate those newly diagnosed with breast cancer by providing education, support, and individual counseling. They initiate workshops for corporate and community groups, and add a focal point to the multicultural population by offering educational classes within the community regarding breast cancer detection and treatment. They foresee creating a community where every person diagnosed with breast cancer becomes a survivor. Within this program, the Delaware Breast Cancer Coalition has incorporated a mammogram screening van to go into the communities and screen those who are unable to obtain routine mammograms. Through this program, students experience sharing the importance of breast self-exam and cancer screening. The breast cancer survivor's personal experience and journey enables students to hear about the effects of cancer, from the initial diagnosis, surgery, chemotherapy, and radiation therapy to their current lives. This is a moving and emotional experience for our students to witness, and there is not a dry eye during the presentation as students exchange open discussions with the speaker. The presentation adds to the reality of Delaware's statewide screening initiative to reduce the incidence of breast cancer.

Working in groups, students are provided with breast models to familiarize themselves with detecting nodules and irregularities. At this day-long seminar, they learn how to work together so that they can educate individuals regarding breast cancer prevention. We expect students to take a leadership role in servicing communities where there are disparities related to Delaware's breast cancer mortality rate. The proactive approach initiates maintenance and improvement of health and lessens inequities among the population groups.

Students may identify where in the community they will present their community project seminar and develop a presentation with education strategies. Working in groups, they analyze epidemiological data for the highest rates of breast cancer in Delaware. With evidence of eight or more cancer clusters within the state of Delaware, it was determined that students' projects would be useful at locations such as woman's shelters and prisons, local clinics, physicians' offices, pharmacies, exercise facilities, senior centers, corporate businesses, and real estate offices in urban and suburban locations. This allows students to experience the complexities of community health aggregates and areas of nonhospitalized nursing.

Students collect teaching information from the American Cancer Society, the Susan G. Komen Foundation, the Delaware Breast Cancer Coalition, and the Screening for Life Program. All printed material is made available to participants. Students encourage their viewers to participate in breast self-exam after watching a video, followed by practicing of breast self-exam on the models provided by the college. The presentation includes posters, handouts, diagrams, and pictures, geared to accommodate varying literacy issues relating to that particular population and individual student teaching of the audience.

The students are encouraged to practice prior to the screening and to make this a positive and fulfilling experience. They are accountable for teaching and discussing breast cancer and for acting resourcefully when approached by those seeking information. Students dress in school uniform with a visible identification. The project is a minimum of two hours with at least eight participants. Following the presentation, students provide an evaluation form for participants to evaluate the students' performance. Also included is a student self-evaluation of the collaborative community project, as well as peer evaluations. Personnel from the facility where the presentation occurs provide a letter verifying attendance and also rate the students' performance, often with commendable ratings and encouraging comments to inform faculty how well the students presented.

Following the team assignment, all students present their project by describing their teaching experience at the Breast Self-Exam Seminar Project. Faculty ask the students what worked, what did not work, and what could be done to make the presentation more interesting. They also request any ideas that students have for improvement. During the group presentation, we see team amity and camaraderie develop. Also, this is where we observe the competence of the nursing therapeutic relationships as students describe their personal teaching skills and methods of communication with individual clients. Students convey their experiences regarding the community and teaching Delawareans. The seminar offers a place for the students to relax, talk, and have an enjoyable and exciting conversation with the class and faculty about their own community experiences. We clearly see students develop an understanding of community screening and teaching while realizing what community nursing involves. Student comments are positive and enlightening. We evaluate their application of nursing theory, teaching, and integration of public health knowledge.

Many of the students take pictures of their demonstrations while interacting with the community's clientele. These pictures are placed in the official Breast Cancer Awareness Photo Album, which we provide to new students for review before developing their own plans. A faculty member also does community site visits of the student projects to ensure performance and professionalism. This is a positive experience. By participating, students apply classroom information to community health promotion, construct client education strategies, and practice community service learning. This seminar is held during the month of October, which is the national breast cancer awareness month. Students also initiate involvement in the annual Making Strides Against Breast Cancer Walk, sponsored by the American Cancer Society and supported by our

Student Nurses Association. This is a five-mile walk, and many students and nursing faculty participate, with all donations and contributions going to the American Cancer Society. The purposes of the walk are to join together as advocates for breast screening; to help people through every step of the cancer journey by initial breast screening, diagnosis, and treatment; to encourage one-on-one support programs; to provide transportation; to help self-image restoration; and, finally, to become a breast cancer survivor.

As a nurse educator I recognize that students need preparation in order to function within the community. Educational experiences should center on the community's needs and the importance of a state's health needs. As a nurse educator, I am proud to have taught and mentored our next generation of nurses and hope that they continue to advocate and teach the community about the importance of breast cancer screening. Engaging nursing students into this program has provided them insight into nursing outside the institutional domain. By assessing community innovation, students were able to identify the community needs within the program's mission and make an impact on the health of Delaware citizens.

Shirleen B. Lewis-Trabeaux

In 1999, faculty in the baccalaureate nursing program at Nicholls State University (NSU) and representatives from community agencies began collaborating to address the issue of out-of-home child care quality in southeast Louisiana. Representatives from the Louisiana Department of Health and Hospitals Office of Public Health and the Agenda for Children, a statewide family advocacy agency, participated in the discussions. The outcome of this collaboration was the Tool to Evaluate Child Health, Immunizations, and Safety (TECHIS) used to assess the quality of out-of-home child care in the region and to identify center-specific needs. Each semester, small groups of NSU baccalaureate nursing students are taught to use TECHIS for assessing child care centers in the region.

TECHIS is a comprehensive, 500-item assessment tool to systematically evaluate parameters central to child health, immunizations, and safety in out-of-home child care centers. Whereas each regulatory agency has a separate instrument and assessment procedure, TECHIS is a combination of state licensing standards, the state sanitary code, and the national performance standards for out-of-home child care programs. The tool is divided into six major focus areas (i.c., health practices and policies, physical environment, safety, feeding and eating, food preparation area, and physical plant).

Early in the planning process, the research team decided to focus on the original goal of improving the quality of out-of home-child care in the region, and not on conducting extensive tool validity and reliability studies. An expert review panel was assembled to evaluate the tool for content validity, clarity, format, variations, contaminants, and biases. As a result, TECHIS is a straightforward, user-friendly checklist requiring a minimum of expertise to execute.

While developing the TECHIS tool, the nursing faculty realized that there was a dearth of items that addressed the psychosocial component in the state licensing standards, sanitary code, and national performance standards. Subsequently, the pediatric and psychiatric nursing faculty and an early intervention specialist, developed the Psychosocial Assessment of Needs Scale for Child Care Centers (PANSCCC). PANSCCC is a 43-item instrument based on principles of quality child care that include evaluation of close and caring relationships, health and safety needs met, connection to family, and knowledgeable and responsive caregivers.

The project was piloted in 1999 and 2000, using teams of two or three nursing students and faculty with CHSC certification who visited child care centers. Prior to visiting the centers, the students were oriented to the project and TECHIS. To strengthen the data collection process of the program, today each student works independently to complete most of the assessment. Participating nursing faculty and community representatives have developed a standardized student orientation.

At the beginning of each semester, nursing faculty provides a representative from Agenda for Children with a list of available dates to schedule child care centers for TECHIS assessment. All students involved in the project attend a two- or three-hour orientation prior to visiting the child care centers. Students learn to look for consistency by observing staff and children interacting, interviewing the center director and staff, reviewing policy and procedure manuals, and perusing child health and immunization records. For example, center directors, staff, and policy and procedures manuals often identify hand washing as a priority; however, students often observe insufficient and inappropriate hand washing. When interviewing staff, students are instructed to ask open-ended questions. For example, regarding child abuse and neglect, students may ask the center director, "Is the staff trained to recognize signs of abuse and neglect?," but then would ask a staff member, "Tell me some of the signs of abuse and neglect in children."

To avoid repetition, students are instructed to interview the center director to collect specific demographic data and peruse charts as a team. Each student team is furnished with copies of the evaluation tools, business cards from participating faculty and the director of Agenda for Children, educational handouts, and a tape measure and thermometer to aid in their assessment. Students use the tape measure to assess a variety of things, such as the distance between the slats on baby beds, the distance of playground equipment from the ground, etc. The thermometer is used to test water, refrigeration, and food temperatures.

Depending upon the size of the center, teams of three to five junior and senior nursing students are assigned to assess a child care center using TECHIS and PANSCCC. Junior-level students are enrolled in a clinical nursing course entitled Nursing and the Childrearing Family, while senior-level students are enrolled in two clinical nursing courses entitled Community Health Nursing and Mental Health Nursing. It takes approximately three to five hours, depending on the size of the facility, to thoroughly evaluate a center. Students and the center's staff work together to complete the TECHIS evaluation. Historically, baccalaureate nursing students have provided a number of valuable community services such as community health education, screenings, and mass immunizations. Hence, the NSU's baccalaureate nursing program is highly regarded and community members respect and trust "their" nursing students.

Upon completion of TECHIS, students schedule a debriefing with one of the CCHC-certified project faculty. The faculty and the director of Agenda for Children discuss the results of each debriefing, and follow-up may include telephone consultation, meeting with center directors, attending a center's staff meeting, or providing in-service training for center personnel. Students are also encouraged to discuss their findings with the center director and staff if a teachable moment occurs.

All participants gain a thorough understanding of the guidelines for quality out-of-home child care centers, as well as center-specific needs. Nursing students engage in service learning, learn about early childhood care, and apply theory learned in pediatrics, community, and mental health nursing courses. As center staff and students collaborate to complete TECHIS, there is an interchange of knowledge and expertise; everyone is a teacher as well as a learner. The project evaluations identify risks concerning child health, immunizations, and safety in the region. Suitable recommendations are made and feasible strategies presented and implemented to minimize and possibly eliminate risks. Staff members in child care facilities who participate earn three hours of continuing education credits issued by nursing faculty with CCHC certification.

Participation is limited to those centers licensed by the state of Louisiana within a seven-parish region. In this area, there are approximately 187 licensed out-of home child care centers with a total capacity to provide care for approximately 12,000 infants and young children. Participation in the project is voluntary. As the project gained recognition and popularity over the years, center directors began requesting a TECHIS assessment. It is estimated that most centers in the region have been evaluated at least twice. Child care staff development programs and workshops that address health and safety practices are ongoing.

To date, only center-specific needs have been evaluated; however, project members are poised to analyze the data at an aggregate level. Additionally, changing regulations require that we readdress each TECHIS item for accuracy. Also, Louisiana is in the process of mandating that licensed child care centers be assessed using environmental ratings scales, namely Infant/Toddler Environmental Ratings Scales (ITERS) and Early Childhood Environment Ratings Scales (ECERS) designed to assess group programs for children from birth to age two-and-a-half years and two-and-a-half through five years, respectively. TECHIS project members want to examine how, and if, TECHIS will fit in this new plan to improve the quality of child care in Louisiana.

Mary M. Lebold, Darlene O'Callaghan, and Michele Poradzisz

Sometimes life surprises you and leads you down a path that you never anticipate—a path that contains challenges and opportunities to make a difference. This is a story of such a journey, one of discovery and personal change. This journey has made differences not only in our own lives, but also in the lives of other nurses and our communities—differences we had not imagined in the beginning.

Twenty years ago, in an effort to find and recruit bilingual, bicultural Hispanic nurses, we started a comprehensive re-entry program for Hispanic nurses who were educated outside of the United States. This effort was in partnership with Alivio Medical Center, Mercy Hospital and Medical Center, the Illinois Hispanic Nursing Association, Daley Community College, and Saint Xavier University. The program was a response to a need identified by the Chicago Hispanic community with courses in reading, language development, speaking, and preparation for the Commission on Graduates of Foreign Nursing Schools (CGFNS) exam and the NCLEX-RN® licensure examination. Of the twenty Hispanic nurses who completed the program, 25% to 30% passed the NCLEX-RN®. Most did not take or pass the CGFNS exam that was required by the Illinois Department of Financial and Professional Regulation (IDFPR) at that time. Needless to say, we were disappointed with the results and felt the program was not successful. This program ended for various reasons in 1989.

Fifteen years later, this feeling of not being successful was voiced at a national strategic planning meeting of individuals and organizations who had come together to develop programs for internationally educated nurses living in the United States. Again the mission was to assist resident internationally educated nurses to obtain registered nurse licensure. Following a declaration about the lack of success of the earlier program, a member of the audience stood up and said, "Don't ever call that program unsuccessful. Look at me, I was one of those students who went through the program. Without that program, I would have never passed the NCLEX® and I never would be doing what I am doing now." This was Graciela Reyes Salinas who had been a member of the original group, and later left Chicago and moved to Dallas, Texas. Since she became a U.S. registered nurse, Graciela has been a strong advocate and leader in the effort to find resources for Hispanic nurses and other internationally educated nurses in similar situations. She worked with organizations, various states, and agencies in Mexico to design educational programs; she volunteers her energy and services to assist nurses achieve their goal of becoming a U.S. RN. She is the founder and first president of the International Bilingual Nurse Alliance (IBNA), an organization committed to improving the success of internationally educated nurses with the licensure process and nursing performance in United States' health care settings, enhancing their careers, and indirectly affecting the health care needs of minority populations in the United States.

In 2002, the nursing shortage was becoming more critical and there were calls for creative strategies to recruit more nurses. Due to our earlier experience with Hispanic nurses we were asked to develop a new, similar program, as there was a serious need for bilingual Hispanic nurses. Naïvely we began to develop a new program, which was based in the Hispanic community. The program again was educationally focused on language development and preparation for the CGFNS and the NCLEX® exams. With only four days' notice presented on television and in newspapers, we had more than five hundred people attending an information session at the community college. Were we surprised! We had hoped for fifty attendees.

As we were developing the program, we were informed that funding would be available from the state to support the program and the enrolled students. The day of the information session, we were informed that the state funding was cut and we were without money to operate the program. We implemented the program anyway! Once the program was underway, we were able to obtain work force funds, funding from private foundations, and Mercy Hospital and Medical Center. To this day, funding remains a major challenge for the program.

The audience at our first information session included nurses with their families, as well as individuals who wanted to become nurses. Approximately 250 were licensed as nurses outside of the United States, but more than 50% of those were nondocumented immigrants. From the group, we chose twenty candidates after reviewing their documents, interviewing them about their work experiences, and determining their English proficiency, as well as their desire and availability to participate in a heavy four-evenings-per-week program. Since that time, the program has evolved and has been reconceptualized based on candidates' needs, as well as our experiences and available resources. We developed a not-for-profit organization to provide educational programs and serve as an advocate for internationally educated nurses and provide supportive and advising services. We are the only such organization in this region.

Over the last seven years of working with internationally educated nurses, we made many discoveries. Originally, we focused only on developing a program for Hispanic nurses living in the greater Chicago area who were educated in Mexico or other Latin American countries. This program was known as the Chicago Mexican Nurse Initiative. As we became better known, other internationally educated nurses sought our programs and services. Today, the nurses enrolled in our classes are more diverse in language and culture, contributing a broader understanding of culture and nursing practice to the other class members. English must be spoken in the program, as it is the common language. This practice contributes to the development of skills in English linguistics, medical terminology, and pronunciation. With a more diverse participant group, our organization is now known as The Chicago Bilingual Nurse Consortium (CBNC) and we have worked or are working with nurses from more than forty-eight countries. CBNC is the only centralized resource for internationally educated nurses in Illinois—and one of the few in the United States that offers programs and services to enable internationally educated nurses to adapt to the culture, structure, and function of the U.S. health care system.

We have learned that advising and social support are critical for this population. Students are frequently reluctant to share their personal issues and need encouragement to continue working toward licensure. Frequently this encouragement is not forthcoming from their spouses, families, or friends. Peers are often their primary source of support and information. This information is sometimes erroneous, which we clarify by informing them of correct processes.

The time it takes to become registered as a nurse in the United States is much longer than we anticipated when we started the program. This time lengthens with each error or incorrect application. "I did not know what to do. No one could answer my questions." "I have called and called and waited for 18 months or 2 years to obtain my credential review." "It took months for my family to obtain my papers and now I am told they are lost." "What do I do? My school sent the wrong documents." "My school did not translate my courses correctly—their translation is wrong."

With each error or miscommunication, the candidates become more discouraged and less persistent. They need and respond to peer support, coaching, and family assistance from those who are here or, more frequently, family in their home country. In one class, a candidate from Iran provided her classmates who were voicing frustration with the process, the following advice: "After several months and numerous phone calls, I just started crying on the phone — and it worked. I received the necessary documents in 2 weeks." When this story was retold in another class, a Polish candidate said, "The same thing happened to me! I just started to cry and could not stop—so if you are having a hard time—just try crying. It works."

As we became aware of the issues facing internationally educated nurses, we sought clarification of policies, procedures, and practices from local, state, and national professional organizations, as well as from Mexico and Poland. This advocacy has resulted in a positive working relationship with the Illinois Board of Nursing and the Illinois Department of Financial and Professional Regulation (IDFPR), which in turn resulted in better coordination of processes and subsequent changes in Illinois legislation regarding internationally educated nurses and nurses educated in Puerto Rico. In addition, repeated conversations with the Commission on Graduates of Foreign Nursing Schools (CGFNS) have resulted in a collegial relationship that has been exceedingly helpful in clarifying their processes and policies, as well as facilitating the process of the applicants' paper work.

As advocates, we frequently serve as a voice for candidates and assist them by clarifying their issues and interpreting the state standards and policies. Resident internationally educated nurse candidates frequently find the licensure process confusing, which leads to misunderstanding or misinterpretation on their Credentials Evaluation Services (CES) and NCLEX® applications, or prevents them from filing a licensure application. Advising is constant, requiring persistent one-on-one communication and follow-up.

A major challenge for most of our nurses is communication and fluency in English. In Illinois, each nurse who qualifies as a first-level nurse must pass the Test of English as a Foreign Language (TOEFL) examination prior to taking the NCLEX®. Many of the candidates take slow-paced English as a Second Language (ESL) courses offered by community colleges or community organizations. These courses are economical but lengthy. Most community colleges do not provide a TOEFL preparation course; therefore, students may need to be referred to courses offered by for-profit educational organizations or universities.

Students frequently become frustrated and drop out of classes, believing that they can pass the NCLEX® exam without taking any more ESL classes, as they feel these classes do not help them with nursing language and terminology. Frequently they will state that they have dropped the ESL classes because "The English class was all grammar—I need to learn conversational English." Several of our candidates have been taking ESL classes for four to six years. Tragically, for some students, by the time they are competent in English, their professional skills are no longer current. Those who have dropped out need coaching and encouragement to resume this process. The time from successful completion of ESL courses in a community college to passing the required TOEFL examination can take the internationally educated nurses eighteen to twenty-four months. Furthermore, these courses are not "English courses for a specific purpose."

Language is also a challenge for CBNC staff members, as we are not bilingual. We recognize this as a barrier to assisting our candidates. Fortunately we have been able to hire staff members who are proficient in Spanish and other languages, and we have enlisted the assistance of the International Polish Nurses Association to help our Polish candidates. We also have a list of others who are proficient in another language that we can call on when necessary. For example, we had an LPN candidate from Palestine inquire about U.S. licensure. His first question was simple "How do I become licensed in the United States?" Over the next hour, the requirements were explained to him and he stated and nodded understanding. However, at the end of the session, he again voiced the question, "How do I become licensed in the United States?" With that response, an internationally educated nurse who spoke Arabic was called and she explained the processes again to him. He left our office not only satisfied with having obtained the information he needed, but with a phone number of another nurse he could speak with if he had further questions.

The nurses we work with have an intense love of nursing and a strong desire to care for others. They want to resume their practice of nursing. Over and over we hear "I want to be a nurse again." "I thought I had lost my ability to practice nursing here." The following is one such story.

Lucy came to the United States from Mexico, first as a visitor and then in 1988 to live. That same year Lucy married and began to raise a family. She now has four children. She was a nurse in Mexico but did not become licensed as a nurse in Illinois until 2006 when she passed the NCLEX®. Lucy took several courses through the Chicago Bilingual Nurse Consortium and now works at a hospital as a home health nurse. "I thought it was impossible to become a registered nurse in the United States because of all the requirements and the paper work. The Consortium made it possible to become a nurse again. Through the consortium I met others in similar situations and made new friends. The consortium provided the support and courses that met each individual need at their level, whether it was English, nursing, or both."

We have worked with over 350 internationally educated nurses from more than forty-eight countries, the majority (65%) of whom are Hispanic, from Mexico, Central and South America, as well as a fair number (9%) who are from Poland and Eastern Europe. Other represented countries include India, Italy, Colombia, Lithuania, Nicaragua, Nigeria, Palestine, Peru, Germany, South Africa, Sweden, Togo, Taiwan, Thailand, and Venezuela. The majority of candidates reside in the Chicago metropolitan area. However, with the introduction of our Web site, we have been receiving many e-mails and phone calls from internationally educated nurses in other states asking about licensure and courses in their state or region.

Our candidates are frequently unemployed or underemployed, and have multiple family responsibilities. Similar to other new Americans arriving in Illinois, they frequently assume employment that does not match their educational backgrounds or professional experiences, for example, they become taxi drivers, nursing assistants, carpenters, housekeepers, or factory workers. Most candidates do not qualify for state or federal workforce funding, due to their previous education and the time needed to become licensed as a registered nurse in Illinois. Our programs help them achieve their desire and dream to practice their chosen profession of nursing. Once licensed, they earn a professional salary and serve as role models to their family and community. Since reopening, forty-one internationally educated nurses have taken the NCLEX® and thirty-seven have passed.

Program development was another challenge. We established a curriculum committee on which we all serve. We have invited others to join us as we develop and implement courses and services. As the program evolved, serving over 350 internationally educated nurses candidates, we identified the following stages of candidate progression:

Stage 1: Assessment of the candidate's status, orientation to the U.S. licensure process and the state of Illinois requirements for RN licensure.

Stage 2: Preparation for the requirements for licensure in the state of Illinois.

Stage 3: Preparation for the NCLEX-RN® and nursing practice in the United States.

Our achievements over the past six years are gratifying and have yielded many accomplishments. We have worked with more than 350 internationally educated nurses from forty-eight different countries, offering counseling and educational programs to prepare them for the NCLEX-RN® licensure exam and nursing practice in the United States.

We also have prepared forty-two candidates to take the NCLEX-RN®
with a pass rate of 88%. The thirty-seven RNs who passed the exam
are now practicing as nurses in hospitals, community centers, home
health, and rehabilitation settings. We have launched a Web site (www.
chicagobilingualnurse.org) and have developed a data management system to track, report, and follow up on each candidate's progress. Other
accomplishments include (a) cultivation of a positive working relationship with CGFNS, the Illinois State Board of Nursing and Department
of Professional Regulation; (b) successful advocacy for legislation within
the state of Illinois to ease the process of becoming licensed by eliminat-
ing the requirement of the CGFNS exam; (c) creation of the International
Bilingual Nurse Alliance (IBNA), a network of programs with similar
goals in other regions of the United States; (d) establishment of working relationships with governmental and private agencies that work with
internationally educated nurses; (e) development of tutoring and peer
advising seminars and other courses for internationally educated nurses;
and (f) establishment of working relationships with several community
colleges and other agencies to secure needed resources for IENs.

During the last six and one-half years, we have taken paths that were
unfamiliar and at times chaotic, filled with uncertainty and ambiguity.
Throughout this time, we have met wonderful internationally educated
nurses who love nursing with a strong desire to resume their chosen profession. For most, their journey is filled with challenges and hardship,
yet they continue to persist in the dream to resume their nursing practice. Like our candidates, we found the process challenging, and at times
confusing and frustrating. Yet we have benefited from the support from
many sources and have formed alliances that facilitate and clarify issues
and questions. Each successful step by a candidate, especially his or her
achievement of licensure, becomes a celebration of accomplishment,
patience, and perseverance. Their efforts are truly courageous and will
serve nursing and health care in ways we have yet to imagine.

Nurse Educators Who Change and Shape Health Care Globally

This section includes five chapters. In the first chapter, two separate authors raise issues about global collaboration. The first author presents a model for global collaboration for use in any country; the second identifies issues that anyone involved in international work should consider. Chapter 10 focuses on models of collaboration that nurse educators have undertaken in several countries in Africa. Chapter 11 includes descriptions of collaborative work in Central and South America. Chapter 12 describes work in other countries, while the final chapter addresses the work that individual nurse educators have initiated in multiple countries.

Many of the countries presented here have multiple health issues, including high morbidity and mortality rates, and limited resources to improve health. The needs are great. Sustainability of initiatives is fragile without partnerships, resources, consistent efforts, and the people's desires and abilities to embrace change. Nurses, through public and community health teaching and learning experiences, have known the value of working to sustain change. The nurse educators who have participated in global projects of change narrate their lived experience; almost all narratives involve students and partnerships, and all narratives convey a strong participant desire to be of service. These stories tell of these experiences, rich with encounters and challenges in many countries.

—*Cathleen M. Shultz*

9

Issues Related to Global Collaboration

G. Elaine Patterson

One approach to global collaboration is described that may prove beneficial for nurse educators assisting developing countries in their educational pursuits. Also provided are strategies for global collaboration that may be beneficial especially to American nursing educators attempting to share their expertise in foreign countries.

The concerns of nursing programs in developing countries are, primarily, lack of resources and may extend to the inability of faculty to reach professional self-actualization. The following are suggestions for intervention using sub-Saharan countries as examples.

Some of the lowest health and economic indices in the world are found in sub-Saharan African countries. Nursing educators and students are trying to eke out an existence, leading to high stress in the teaching/learning environment. It is possible to find nursing programs lacking in the most basic essentials necessary to provide quality education to nursing students. These range from no to ill-equipped laboratories, unsatisfactory learning environments, and inadequate supplies of books, to faculty who are not educationally prepared to teach at the program's level.

Providing resources is often the most easily achievable intervention to assist foreign educators. Resources can be provided in the form of books and teaching aids, but care must be taken not to raise expectations to unreachable levels. Foreign educators can arrange to give of their time and talent, either by teaching in-country periodically or via the Internet. However, the recipients must be encouraged to find ways of obtaining their own resources over time for sustainability purposes. This includes incorporating the appropriate governmental ministry in the needs assessment and assisting colleagues to convey the long-term impact of appropriate resources in providing education and building nursing capacity to produce a healthier nation.

In terms of safety, several African countries are recuperating from civil wars and are governed by leadership that may be tenuous at best. Nurses are sometimes fearful for their own safety and future employment—this is a real fear. This level of fear leads to highly stressful conditions, which ultimately affect learning and dampen creativity. Fear of a political coup is not unusual, and the uncertainty of day-to-day existence is quite stark. Ultimately, all decisions that affect changes in nursing education structures are made at the political ministerial level. Faculty become disempowered in the decision-making arenas and need support in their efforts at creating change in the educational structure. Influencing and educating politicians about the importance of educating nurses who deliver most of the health care in-country is crucial.

Some developing countries are well aware of the global advances in the delivery of nursing care and nursing education. It is difficult for them to envision when and if they will ever be able to experience nursing education at an advanced level. They reach out for help, not only for resources but also for a feeling of belonging with other colleagues in the global community. By so doing, they may seek to overcome feelings of loneliness and isolation. Some countries are attempting to transition their diploma programs to baccalaureate programs. One main obstacle to transitioning is the lack of faculty with the educational credentials to teach in degree programs.

The ideal approach would be to assist in restructuring programs to the baccalaureate level and assist the nurse educators in their efforts at improving their own educational credentials. By advancing their education, they will be able to design and implement nursing programs that will result in building their own capacities. This approach will call for partnerships with the United States and other foreign colleges and universities.

Although anxious to receive foreign help, the educator's self-esteem is at stake. Some cultures resist seeking help unless they must, and asking can lead to feelings of low self-esteem. It is important for faculty in the developed world to consistently communicate with their foreign counterparts to avoid negative feelings such as frustration and helplessness. Exchange students and faculty arrangements can also be used to bolster the trust.

Self-actualization is reached when nursing faculty have satisfied all other needs and are at a point where they can begin initiating their own evidenced-based research to address their specific country's educational and health needs. Faculty can consult nurse educators and guide them in conducting research studies and developing seminal literature. The ultimate goal is to assist nurse educators in building a level of scholarship that involves research and publication.

Nurse educators who are approached to assist in global program development must have a plan of action before beginning. Initially, it is imperative that the nurse educator forges relationships that will influence successful outcomes. In many cases this will involve meeting school chancellors, ministers of health and other leading political figures and educators who will support and influence the efforts. Once in-country, nurse educators must carefully follow established protocols. Embassy representatives, nursing matrons, and nursing sisters should be contacted and kept informed of all efforts. In many cases, nursing education is under the ministry of health and governed by the country's or region's chief nursing officer (CNO) who is responsible for all nursing activities and related nursing education. The educator must contact the CNO to garner support and advice on how best to proceed. Many foreign nurse educators are experienced nurses and midwives who hold a nursing diploma or advanced nursing certificate; these education preparations may be the country's limit of educational opportunities.

Nurse educators must bring together the stakeholders in order to define the needs and to determine the direction of change. If the focus is to improve or change the educational programs, the educator must be certain to explore the feasibility of the change from a resource perspective. Implementation must be slow using a gradual process. Key persons who will be responsible for introducing the changes and who understand that it may take a long time to see sustainable changes must be identified and used as resources.

In summary, one approach for nurse educators who are attempting to assist developing countries in advancing their nursing programs has been described. Success will be more likely if partnerships are developed with other groups who are working toward the same goal. By building their own nurse educator capacity, countries will feel a sense of fulfillment and self-actualization when the tasks have been met.

Rory Rochelle

A question that faces us today is this: Are we a just society if we are recruiting nurses from developing countries? In some countries this conundrum has been exacerbated by a slowdown in the number of people enrolling in nursing programs, creating shortages in the home country today and in the future. This is most likely due to workforce issues such as compensation and work environment.

The United Kingdom and the United States are the two developed countries that are reporting the highest shortage rates. In recent years the National Health Service of the United Kingdom has employed international nurse recruitment as a component of its strategy to alleviate the nursing shortage. In the span of three years the strategy has doubled the number of practicing foreign nurses in the United Kingdom. The United States has not pursued and organized a strategy of international nurse recruitment. This may be because nursing regulation in the United States is not at the federal level, but rather based at the state level. Yet, in the United States private recruiting firms have acted as agents for employers seeking nurses internationally to fill growing domestic vacancies.

It is clear that migration occurs. What are unclear are its long-term effects. Additional studies must be conducted in the area of short- and long-term migration. There is a delicate balance between the human and labor rights of the individual and a collective concern for the health of a nation's population. The possible adverse effects on areas in the world that are experiencing critical nursing shortages can be devastating. Placing new recruits in a dysfunctional health system is not ethical or cost effective. Some governments and private agencies have initiated massive recruitment campaigns for foreign nurses. These campaigns often delay effective local measures that would improve recruitment, retention, and long-term human resource planning.

Recent initiatives that address the nursing shortage and nurse migration include:

- Governments of heavily recruited countries have lobbied the governments of recruiting countries to stop depleting their nursing resources. (South Africa and Jamaica are lobbying the United States and the United Kingdom.)
- Governments have negotiated contracts for the recruitment of nurses for a given period of time in exchange for providing professional development of the nurses concerned. (This is occurring between the United Kingdom and Ghana.)
- Guidelines on international recruitment have been developed, specifying countries that should be approached and those to be avoided.

- Governments have introduced special immigration legislation to facilitate work permits.
- Bonuses have been offered, targeting professionals to return to their native country.
- Bond programs for education and a return of service have been developed.

There are many opportunities for future collaboration on migration issues. Sensitivity to the health service needs of all participating countries is critical in any migration collaboration.

10

Nurse Educators Who Work in Africa

BURUNDI
Carolyn Mosley

Ms. Pam Blesch is a shining light who epitomizes caring that goes beyond the walls of a classroom or a hospital. Because she volunteers her time and provides health care in the global environment, she is often characterized—as much by her students as her colleagues—as a missionary. She also is often compared to Mother Teresa because of tireless giving of herself, a path that began in 1975.

Burundi, Africa, was the site of Ms. Blesch's first missionary experience. Accompanying the World Gospel Mission of Marion, Indiana, as a part of their 1975 Summer Career Corps Program, Ms. Blesch worked with a nurse practitioner/midwife in remote areas of northern Burundi. In her three months there, she was exposed to many medical conditions, such as leprosy, advanced breast cancer (fistulas and maggots), elephantitis, and tuberculosis. One of her major duties was the reorganization of all medications in the clinic pharmacy that had been donated from other countries. Many of the drug names were in French and could only be identified using a *PDR*.

Volunteer mission trips to Senegal and Gambia, West Africa, with the International Mission Board of the Southern Baptists also occurred in November of each year from 2000 through 2002, with each trip lasting approximately ten days. Ms. Blesch traveled to remote villages and assisted with the set up of medical clinics that treated many villagers who had walked for days for access to care. Ms. Blesch effectively solicited donations of large quantities of medications from pharmacies and drug representatives in the United States. She also convinced her church congregation to donate vitamins, analgesics, and money toward the purchase of antiparasite and antimalaria medication. Other donated supplies included local anesthetics, disposable scapulae, and sterile dressings. The trips to Africa involved an interdisciplinary team of dentists, physicians, nurses, and pharmacy technicians. Ms. Blesch served in varied roles as needed, from dental assistant (disinfecting instruments between patients and assisting with extractions) to triage nurse (working with translators, sometimes from three languages, in order to determine a chief complaint). According to Ms. Blesch, the language barrier was a major challenge in caring for those needing care. Parasites, malnutrition from these parasites, and chronic pain due to arthritis in the older population comprised the majority of medical problems that Ms. Blesch treated. There also was a large group suffering from untreated diabetes, as well as many senior adults with cataracts and poor vision due to aging. Despite the tremendous contribution Ms. Blesch made during each trip to West Africa, she continued to feel helpless to meet all the needs of the community.

Ms. Blesch's next historic missionary trip was for two weeks to Dnipropetrovs'k, Ukraine, in 2003—an evangelistic opportunity for her to teach English and to present the Gospel of Jesus Christ. She taught four classes of basic English each day to enable students to reach greater fluency and to broaden possibilities for their personal and professional lives. Her classes included university students, physicians, former Communist military soldiers, and housewives.

Through Eastside Baptist Church of Fort Smith, Arkansas, and the International Mission Board of the Southern Baptist Convention, Ms. Blesch participated in medical mission trips to Ecuador in 2005, 2006, and 2007. The interdisciplinary teams during these trips were composed of nurses, physicians, pharmacists, pharmacy technicians, and social workers. Many opportunities existed to assist in feeding the hungry, as well as to identify those people who needed immediate medical treatment. Once again working with translators, Ms. Blesch was responsible for triaging all the clients and determining their chief complaint and distributed donated glucometers to the many undiagnosed diabetics.

In July of 2005, Ms. Blesch traveled to Colombia, South America, with a Christian nonprofit organization, to teach Evangelistic English. She was one of eighteen instructors who taught three to four English classes per day in a local elementary school. Bible study followed each English class. Participants in the classes included chefs, pilots, teachers, students, and lawyers.

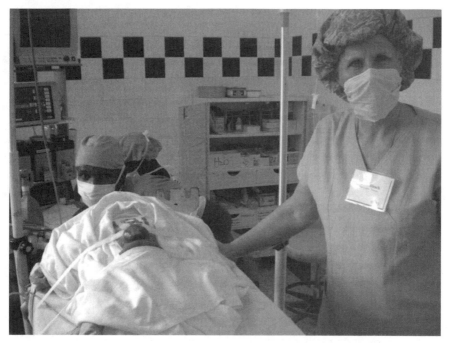

Pamela Blesch with a child having a myelomenigocele repair in an operating room in Uganda in May 2009.

Although Ms. Blesch has demonstrated an international humanitarian spirit, she mirrors this same behavior nationally and in her own community. Serving on the Froderman Foundation Board since 1976, Ms. Blesch actively solicits monetary contributions from organizations in Arkansas, Indiana, and around the world. The purpose of the Foundation is to promote religious, educational, medical, and/ or charitable causes. The Foundation has provided scholarships, built libraries on university campuses, added onto hospital wings, built rehabilitation buildings, purchased Bibles for distribution abroad, as well as funded many service organizations with a variety of needs across the country.

Ms. Blesch has also served on the Board of Hannah House from 1996 through 2005, a faith-based residence for pregnant and troubled young women. She was directly involved in all fundraising efforts for this organization that is located in Fort Smith, Arkansas. Since 2000, Ms. Blesch has served as president of the Board of One Place, Inc., a faith-based, nonprofit organization providing free services to single working parents in the Fort Smith, Arkansas, community. This organization has served over 7,000 single parents and their children with free haircuts, oil vouchers for their cars, underwear, eye exams, fingerprinting for the children, items such as diapers, laundry detergent, toilet tissue and various other basic household necessities, as well as monthly distribution of food.

Ms. Blesch's caring was extended to victims of natural disasters as well. She was one of the nurses that participated in the Hurricane Katrina disaster relief effort in August 2005, at Fort Chaffee and Fort Smith, Arkansas. Through the International Mission Board of the Southern Baptists and Global Action, Ms. Blesch personally provided buckets filled with personal hygiene products sent to Louisiana for Katrina victims and also sent overseas when the tsunami occurred in Asia.

In the Carolyn McKelvey Moore School of Nursing, Ms. Blesch is characterized by students and faculty as the prayer warrior. She was instrumental in initiating a prayer group that meets every morning at 7:00 A.M. prior to the start of the work/school day. The daily prayers are for the students and their families, faculty, and administrators.

I am sure that the comparison of Ms. Blesch to Mother Teresa in the introductory paragraph caused immediate skepticism. However, a thirty-three year history of missionary and health service to the local, national, and international communities is about as close as anyone will get to mirroring the work of this historical person.

CAMEROON
Patricia E. Zander

In 1999, I was asked by the dean of Viterbo University School of Nursing, my employer, to go to Shisong, Cameroon, West Africa, to ascertain what educational opportunities the Shisong School of Midwifery and Nursing could provide for senior synthesis students from Viterbo. While fulfilling that request, I was made acutely aware of a far more critical need, namely upgrading the education of Cameroonian nurses responsible for managing and staffing primary health care centers in the rural areas of the country. The major issues associated with health care in Cameroon included governance of the country and the health care system; questionable water, waste disposal, and food handling practices; increasing prevalence of infectious disease; and inadequate reproductive health care for women.

The Tertiary Sisters of St. Francis, a Catholic religious community in Shisong, have an effective primary health care system extending throughout the northwest province and into the other nine provinces. The system comprises eight primary health care centers, consisting of two large hospitals and six smaller hospitals. Each primary health care center has a varying number of primary health care outreach clinics, each with a number of villages under its umbrella. The primary health care centers and clinics are managed by sisters who are nurses, and are staffed by either sisters or lay nurses. Villages have health care workers, taught by the clinic nurses to provide basic health care education and to care for minor health problems. The nurses visit villages frequently to administer immunizations, care for persons with more severe illnesses; address issues of clean water, proper waste disposal, and food handling; and provide further training for the health care workers. The local population trek great distances to receive quality care from the Tertiary Sisters' centers.

The Cameroon Ministry of Health publicly recognized that community health care was needed but considered the Tertiary Sisters' program too expensive to maintain. During my visit in 1999, the key leaders of the Tertiary Sisters explained that the Ministry of Health was planning to take over their health care system and close the village-based clinics while maintaining the large centers that were great distances from the people they needed to serve. The leverage used by the Ministry of Health to close the Sisters' centers was the fact that the nurses managing and staffing the centers and clinics did not have a State Registered Nurse's (SRN) education.

The main differences between the Brevete, two-year education completed by the centers' nurses, and the three-year, SRN education was that the SRNs had more primary health care and management curriculum content. With this information, I conceived of a program modeled after the United States' continuing education programs. The Sisters acknowledged the credibility of such a program, and other reliable sources also confirmed that the Cameroon Ministry of Health would accept a certification program as fulfilling the educational requirement for the nurses.

The next questions were "What United States educational institution would offer the certificate?," "How would it be financed?," and "Who could and would teach the program?" Viterbo University accepted full responsibility as the certifying agency. The program was completely financed by the Franciscan Sisters of Perpetual Adoration through a special collaboration with two other Franciscan communities in the United States and the Tertiary Sisters of St. Francis in Cameroon. My roles were program coordinator and instructor.

As program coordinator, my responsibilities were to determine course content, establish a budget, and implement the program. The content focused on community health nursing, professional nursing behaviors, and health assessment. The community nursing content involved those areas lacking in the Brevete program and an update on new community nursing concepts. The professional nursing behaviors content was based upon differences between the two nursing programs. Because most of the work of the primary health care nurse involved preventive care and care for ill persons, a health assessment component was added to the educational program. This component enabled nurses to provide a more thorough and accurate report when they contacted a distant physician for consultation. A survey completed by the participants during the program's first day also verified the need for such content.

The nurse participants were asked to provide a written description of their primary health center's demographics and the major problems that they needed to address in their location. The nurses' information, the Cameroon Ministry of Health's initiative for 1999–2008, and community health nursing concepts were utilized to structure the community health content, as well as the results from an assignment given to the nurses to design a project that addressed the primary need of their health center. The health assessment component was a huge success. The nurses had their own assessment equipment for use during class, which they then took to their center for use in their practice. After learning and practicing assessment, each nurse completed an adult health history and then a supervised return demonstration. They also completed a Denver Developmental Screen on a child in a local clinic or orphanage. One nurse was excited when he assessed a bowel obstruction in a postoperative patient, something he was unable to do prior to the course.

The content of the professional nursing behaviors portion of the program addressed management principles as contrasted with leadership principles, with an emphasis on nursing leadership. The nurses were introduced to change theory, discussed collegiality and collaboration as a function of nursing, and individually wrote a letter to their district health officer about the needs in their area. They received a copy of the Cameroon Nurse Practice Act, which they did not even know existed. The need for nursing ethical codes and standards of practice was discussed. They were also encouraged to form a core group concerned with the betterment of the nursing profession in Cameroon. The only negative from the nurses' program evaluation was that it was too short.

A total of fifty-seven nurses received certification over the span of three summers. Two of the groups received a one-week additional session in the third summer. While I was unable to be an instructor for the second and third years of the program, my role as coordinator continued for the duration of the program.

During the initial evaluation of the Shisong School of Nursing and Midwifery, I found that the library was desperately in need of books. Viterbo University nursing faculty, with donations from another nursing library, contributed over two hundred current nursing books to help fill the empty shelves. "The library has never seen so much use in all the years of its existence. The books are being used all the time." Since that time, I was instrumental in their receiving several more shipments of textbooks—so many that the library was moved to a new, much larger, more inviting space with a part-time librarian.

A successful grant proposal based on the nurses' evaluation of the first certification course resulted in the award of $300,000 for use by the Franciscan common venture communities to further the Tertiary Sister's efforts. Three fund raisers by the La Crosse, Wisconsin, high schools resulted in over $1,000 and many educational supplies being shipped to the grade school operated by the Tertiary Sisters in Shisong. In the summers of 2007 and 2008, I fulfilled part of the original intent of my 1999 visit by taking twelve BSN completion students to Cameroon for their public health nursing clinical experience. It is the efforts of communities such as the Tertiary Sisters and the nurses working for them, along with private communities such as the FSPAs and their colleagues, who are truly the ones who make the biggest impact.

ERITREA

Sylvia Fox, Angela V. Albright, and Ghidey Ghebreyohanes

As guests of the Minister of Health of Eritrea, Africa, and funded by the One Tribe Foundation of Malibu, three nursing faculty from California were privileged to work for over two years with the faculty of the College of Health Science and the Ministry of Health Diploma School of Nursing in Eritrea. We recount here some of our experiences and observations from the collaboration with the director of the university's BSN program.

It is impossible to visit Eritrea without quickly becoming aware of its rich historical and political story—a story vital to our understanding of Eritrean nursing. Ghidey Ghebreyohannes, the director of the School of Nursing, graciously and patiently oriented us to the area's history, while escorting us to its beautiful locations. This small, young country established its independence in 1992 after a thirty-year arms struggle with Ethiopia. Border tension remains even today with Ethiopia continuing to challenge the arbitrated demarcation.

Many active nurses and nurse faculty, all veterans of the struggle, have remarkable stories. An impressive story involves delivering care via a huge hospital set up inside a cave. With few resources, they manufactured IV fluids, bandages, and essential drugs to cover 60 of the combatants' and civilians' needs. Surgical care was available within thirty minutes from the front line using innovative techniques that are revered in surgical texts even today. Nurses, after intensive training in medical and surgical skills, provided various necessary care including performing simple surgeries and cesarean sections, as well as providing primary and acute care. The significant leadership by nurses imparted a high value to the profession that still exists in Eritrea today, as evidenced by the many nurses at the Ministry of Health in leadership positions such as division heads, department heads, regional medical directors, and hospital administrators.

Currently, nurses and doctors are in short supply in Eritrea. Thus, BSN nurses are assigned by the Ministry of Health to cover the physicians' shortage and function in expanded roles, which include diagnosing and treating medical conditions, prescribing medications, and administering electroconvulsive therapy in the psychiatric hospital. The BSN curriculum includes advanced health assessment, advanced pathology, and more units than a U.S.-based BSN program requires.

There are great differences in the education and nursing practice roles between BSN nurses and diploma and associate nurses. While it is taboo for non-BSN nurses to use stethoscopes, BSN nurses do and are identified by others and by even themselves as "doctors." These gray areas are pervasive and difficult to untangle; even today there are no written regulations defining the scope of practice for any nursing level.

Reflective of the "can-do" spirit that won the war with Ethiopia, the maternal and infant mortality rate, once one of the highest on the African continent, dropped more than any country in Africa within the last five years. Eritrean methods of malaria control and increasing vaccination rates are models for other developing countries. Since independence, the number of health facilities increased from about 100 to over 300, making health services more accessible to all citizens within one hour's walking distance to a health facility. In other East African countries, this distance to adequate health care is measured as over three day's walking distance. The Ministry of Health also involves the National Union of Eritrean Youth and the National Union of Eritrean Women in health promotion and disease prevention activities such as HIV prevention, malaria control, and tuberculosis treatment. These grass-roots organizations reach the general population within short periods of time and in very cost-effective ways.

Armed with these facts, we engaged with the faculty. Before arriving in Asmara, the capital city, we spoke with Dean Azieb Ogbaghebriel of the University of Asmara College of Health Sciences, and the Director of the School of Nursing, Ghidey Ghebreyohannes. They requested assistance in faculty development in the area of pedagogical methods aligned with the philosophy of active learning and development of critical thinking. In addition, they requested that we assist them to further refine collaborative research proposals, to consult with the university faculty regarding curriculum, and to conduct an assessment of their skills laboratory.

In the second year of the project, we assessed usual teaching practices, course syllabi, and teaching resources, and visited classes and clinical sites before we actually began classes with faculty. This period of discovery laid the groundwork for our goals. We found in Eritrea a teaching paradigm based on a very traditional "sage on the stage" model. Instructors were, without exception, the most active class participants.

They lectured while students listened respectfully and took notes. Some faculty used PowerPoint slides and others wrote the entire lecture on the blackboard while students copied the words. Textbooks were housed in the library, although there were no textbooks on nursing education, management, ethics, and mental health. The textbooks were shared, often with only one for every four students, or the students would read different textbooks from those that were required or were given handouts. We had a difficult time imagining students without their own books.

Our assessment of other teaching and learning resources revealed a computer laboratory for students with limited speed access. These computers were provided by an earlier grant that facilitated twelve BSN nurses to earn master's degrees from SUNY via distance learning; however, it was clear that depending on the Internet for literature research was troublesome because of the slow Internet speed.

We decided that the best way to teach strategies that invoke active learning was to role model the principles of active learning. Our class consisted of twenty-eight to thirty-eight faculty from the departments of nursing, pharmacy, clinical laboratory science, and public health. The nursing faculty consisted of instructors from both the diploma program and the university BSN program. The heterogeneity of the group created interesting dynamics. This was the first time that faculty from the different nursing programs met to collaborate on issues important to all programs. This initiated a process of working together and sharing ideas, which continues. Daily, we were impressed with the high level of participation, the thoughtful and receptive attitude, and an obvious commitment to teaching and learning.

Over a two-week period, we held nine three-hour classes, with a break for morning tea, a practice we enjoyed as it gave us an opportunity to get to know our students. Initially, we were reluctant to leave the classroom and go to another building or room, worrying about time and the vast amount of material to be covered. However, we learned an important lesson as we adapted to the cadence and rhythm of the Eritrean way of life. Morning tea was one way that people demonstrated their appreciation for being with one another, giving to others, and spending time to communicate.

We organized the classes so that everyone sat in a circle and began each class by presenting the day's objectives and agenda as a way of modeling and engaging the students in an active learning process. We wanted students to understand what would be accomplished in each class, and where they could be by the session's end, and that they would accomplish these objectives by participating in learning exercises, activities, and discussion. Initially, it was difficult for them to shift from the respectful student position to a questioning and participatory position.

On day one, introductions served as an icebreaker as we repeated their names, and inevitably mispronounced many of them. We laughed at ourselves and were relieved when they laughed with us. After this warm-up, we presented the principles of active learning and its impact on both the learner and learning, and in particular critical thinking. We utilized PowerPoint slides to present the didactic material, modeling best practice guidelines for slide development. Each day we ended the class with a mini-evaluation such as a "one-minute paper" on the "muddiest point," or the most important thing they learned plus the one thing they did not understand. We directed them to take exactly one minute to write these responses and then submit them anonymously. Each evening, we read these one-minute papers and discussed among ourselves the raised issues and collaborated in preparing responses. At the start of the next class, we addressed their concerns and revisited areas needing clarification. We demonstrated consideration of their comments, showing the importance of on-going teaching evaluation to student learning, and emphasizing that continuous evaluation of teaching improves teaching as well as student learning.

Throughout the nine days, we presented major concepts and then had the faculty practice using them. Sometimes they worked alone but most often in pairs or small groups. For example, we gave them an assignment to find and read the mission and philosophy of their institution as well as the educational philosophy. We asked them to determine if and how these were part of their course objectives and to present specific examples. This was a stimulating exercise—many faculty did not know that the institution had mission and philosophy statements and how these might relate to specific courses.

One of the course objectives was to train the faculty to develop objectives and to demonstrate a corresponding teaching activity using principles of active learning. Each day we helped them see how each element could be integrated into their teaching. We encouraged them to choose simple topics and to concentrate on using active learning principles. As we neared the final days of class, we gave them opportunities to work in teaching groups, while we circulated among them to provide assistance. The final class session, when they each demonstrated their learning, was incredible. They were very excited, and their enthusiasm was contagious. In evaluating one another's demonstration, they applied active learning principles. They were respectful during their written and oral critiques, which helped everyone see what they might have done differently to be more effective as teachers. We cannot adequately express our enjoyment in working with this consistently warm, open, and eager faculty.

In addition to teaching methods, the director of the BSN Program requested that we work with faculty on refining their curriculum, over-all program goals, and individual course syllabi. Before we arrived, faculty mainly relied on a disease-based medical model and, in fact, we observed them using medical textbooks as their primary resources. The BSN curriculum supported this orientation with its inclusion of a strong science core, including chemistry, biochemistry, and physics, as well as advanced physiology and assessment courses. The impetus seemed to flow from a desire to prepare students for the advanced roles required of BSN graduates. We challenged them to articulate their thoughts about what makes nursing unique from medicine and from advanced nursing practice.

Friendly debate helped the faculty determine what they believed was essential and what they could relinquish. Listening to this discussion encouraged us to ensure in our own students the importance for seeing the world from the other's viewpoint. Informed by reading and listening to many struggle era stories, we respectfully understood the history that gave rise to their medical model point of view. We also wondered if the focus on disease management might coincide with a silo approach to health problems, which has been typical in Africa. We remained adamant in our consultation that a nursing framework is necessary for a nursing curriculum. This remains a consultation theme that will be ongoing.

While it was clear that a paradigm shift will not be swift, there are new forces that will facilitate a revised orientation. For example, the Eritrean Nurses Association was admitted to the International Council of Nursing in 2007. This membership will ensure the Eritrean voice in conversations about nursing in nations with histories and circumstances both similar and different to their own. Also, more faculty are gaining opportunities for advanced nursing education from schools throughout the world through distance learning. Over time, we are confident that a self-delineated Eritrean nursing paradigm will emerge.

Both the consultants and the Eritrean faculty became invested in one another and continue to work together today. Since our initial visit, the consultant team, along with another nurse, a psychologist, and a specialist, have gone to Asmara for staggered visits over a five-month period. Building on the initial teaching/learning seminar and curriculum work, we continued to advance the objectives of enhancing teaching and learning, building curriculum, and bringing the faculty of all nursing programs together for more collaborative work. Dr. Angela V. Albright, who stayed for five months, joined a task force composed of all the nursing education program leaders. The goal was to mainstream nursing education programs in Eritrea and make recommendations for future directions. The document produced by the task force is now used as a reference for the nursing programs and the Ministry of Health. There were several other outcomes of this phase of consultation that are too numerous to describe here.

Another way we stay connected is through Sigma Theta Tau International. The School of Nursing at California State University, Dominguez Hills (CSUDH) inducted the Eritrean BSN faculty into their Xi Theta chapter. The California-based members have enjoyed learning about Eritrea and the challenges shared in teaching and providing nursing care to our respective populations. The Sigma Theta Tau publications are welcomed as a current source of information about nursing trends in education, research, and practice. Currently, one of the Eritrean Diploma Program directors is completing the MSN program at CSUDH via online classes in the Parent-Child Clinical Nurse Specialist option, funded by the One Tribe Foundation. We are exploring other sources of funding to provide similar opportunities for additional Eritrean nursing faculty.

We look forward to future endeavors together, such as, perhaps, establishing visiting professorships and student visits to Eritrea. Whatever develops in the future, we as consultants and the Asmara faculty continue to connect via e-mail and telephone about curricular issues and research proposals. We all enjoy the chance to hear one another's voices and to feel close again.

GHANA
Jennifer L. Morton

For two weeks every August, the international mission in Sekondi is home to a primary clinic. The clinic represents the only health care available to many in this community. For Blessing, a young woman who arrived in the clinic with pernicious anemia, the treatment is simple—B complex vitamins; however, the vitamins we can give her will run out in two months.

Over the course of subsequent missions, my desire to know my African patients, their culture, and their health issues has transformed my thinking. My patient encounters through the use of interpreters are centered on cultural assessment, community health education, available resources, and how these resources can be best integrated into their lives. Blessing needed long-term strategies different from prescribing vitamin supplements: Malta, 1 bottle Q.O.D. Malta, an inexpensive and accessible carbonated beverage (many describe its flavor as molasses-like) is rich with B-complex vitamins and has long been revered for its healing qualities with Ghanaians. Other ways to treat anemia in developing countries include cooking in iron pots and adding iron nails to the soup pot for the cooking process. Community health education serves a secondary role by teaching iron fortification strategies that are culturally responsive and sustainable. Such strategies will also benefit Blessing's children. Although this mother of four left the clinic with multivitamins for herself and her family, she also left with the knowledge and skills for sharing valuable health education information with family and friends.

Kwame, a young boy, presented in the clinic alone; not knowing his own birthday or even his age, he appeared to be about seven or eight years old. He reported that his mother had died some time ago and he was living with his grandmother and several other children. He appeared malnourished with a protuberant abdomen. Upon further inspection, he was noted to have a very large umbilical hernia, atypical of U.S. children as this type of hernia is surgically repaired prior to reaching such a size. His facial expression seemed shameful and embarrassed while I reduced the hernia that draped up and over the waistband of his soiled shorts. Kwame's quiet melancholy and his maturity beyond his years captured everyone's heart. Some were sad; some commented in judgment wondering why he was alone. Kwame represents yet another case that has adjusted my worldview about what is accessible to a global, vulnerable population. Knowing that this type of uncomplicated hernia, although large, would be a fairly urgent surgical procedure in our culture, in a developing country, it just is not a priority. Changing our thinking to provide Kwame with strategies for and understanding how his medical situation can be managed until he is contacted for the surgical referral was the culturally responsive approach. Our strategies included creation of a device and strap to keep his hernia reduced at all times, as well as some age-appropriate counseling on high fiber diet choices. As we advocate for Kwame to receive the necessary surgery, we also understand that many more patients need surgery, and that priority is given to acute problems with the best probable outcomes. Despite having provided Kwame with palliative options for the short term, he continued to visit the clinic daily. This young boy that touched so many hearts provided a valuable lesson for the faculty and students of this mission, lessons of hope and resilience.

Participating in a global health experience such as transcultural health missions has transformed my practice twenty-one years into my nursing career. After becoming a nurse, I settled in a tertiary care hospital that served patients from many cultural groups, although today my definition of culture has changed greatly from those early days of practice. I soon became aware that something did not feel complete. I was finishing my master's degrees in nursing and public health and, although I had spent many hours giving back through service with vulnerable populations, some of which included diverse and immigrant populations here in the United States, there remained a void. My desire to gain knowledge outside of what was comfortable was my impetus for further exploration.

I began to explore options. Through graduate study, I became aware of opportunities for cultural immersion and soon realized that West Africa could be my instrument to grow into the most culturally attuned nurse that I could be. Five trips later, this two-week immersion experience is now something I long for personally and professionally. Moreover, it has become something I value as an important component to health profession education, and I have modified and reconstructed aspects of this very immersion experience to share with my own students. Such an experience represents "a gift" predicated on the belief that being immersed in and caring for a culture so far away can heighten our skills as health professionals and, in turn, provide our patients with optimal health outcomes. Moreover, being acculturated to this other culture helps us to truly understand and subsequently embrace the others' cultural beliefs that at one time may have rested outside of our comfort zone.

Transcultural mission programs tend to fundraise extensively in an effort to transport medications, medical technology, and health care services to populations that would not normally have access to such services.

Although meritorious, they represent strategies that cannot always be sustained over the long term and beg the question, is it culturally sensitive to deliver "Western" health care services to a population in urban West Africa that does not have consistent access to such health care? Moreover, what happens when the mission is over, the medications have run out, and the symptoms have returned?

Blessing and Kwame's stories are important examples that we, as educators, can use to help transform our thinking. This occurs by desiring to know our patients, becoming knowledgeable about them, their health care beliefs, their religion, what their supports are, and most of all, to understand this while putting all judgment and bias aside. Although it seems natural that being seven years old and alone is somehow "not okay," it is only "not okay" according to a Western paradigm. Furthermore, it is imperative that we become educated about the social and family norms of the cultural groups we are treating. This knowledge will assist us in transcending bias and judgment. It is an innate quality of the nurse to nurture and to be concerned, yet this cultural transformation will serve to help us to "be okay" with what we formally thought was "not okay."

When we stop and think of the barriers that prevent the underserved in the United States from acquiring health care, we quickly recognize that most of our underserved still have access to over-the-counter analgesics, vitamin supplements, and basic health education. Moreover, they have been socialized in some format to health information and have developed some sense of health literacy. Media dissemination through newspapers, television, and the Internet are ways by which those of us living in Western cultures embrace some forms of community health education. Schools are yet another mechanism. In many parts of western Africa, media dissemination is often limited and unreliable, and school attendance and literacy are low, resulting in low health literacy overall.

Transcultural health missions are a way to transcend health literacy through community health education. Although meritorious, it is clear that disease management strategies often associated with health missions do not provide long-term, positive outcomes. HIV/AIDS is on the rise, and there are persons living with chronic malaria and endemic infectious diseases—these are but a few examples of health disparities that are far from being eradicated.

Community health workers represent one of the most important contributors to positive patient outcomes for mission work. They are interpreters, providing an important link to effective communication.

They are also educators for the area's health professionals, as well as for the patient and community. The community health workers and participants (health professionals and students) of the mission represent their media channels. This serves to reinforce the importance of just how a health promotion model, complete with education and opportunities for dissemination, can be empowering, while at the same time providing strength and resiliency.

Coordinating such an experience for students and faculty is enlightening and challenging. It is important that we experience our own gaps in knowledge as important parts of the cultural competence process that help to transform our thinking. We must never forget that all of us require mentoring and nurturing with the unfamiliar.

As I recently returned from my fifth trip, exhausted by flight cancellations and delays, and for a fleeting moment feeling like it was too much to incorporate into my already busy life, I reflected back on Blessing and Kwame and all of the other patients. A sudden calm came over me. How could I give this up? This mission empowers a community to take charge of their health with their own resources.

KENYA
Sandra L. Hould

"Wewi ni mjonjwa wapi?" "Where are you sick?" This is a phrase we would ask many patients in Kiswahilli at St. Joseph's Mission Hospital in Kilgoris, Kenya. Quite often they would respond, "Ninahoma, kuhara, kutopika." "I have fever, diarrhea, and vomiting." We would then suspect malaria, which would often be confirmed under the microscope.

Malaria outbreaks occurred at least twice a year during the rainy seasons in Kenya. During this time, census in the pediatric ward soared from the normal 10 patients to 150 patients, with an expected stay of one month. Babies and children with malaria are placed everywhere! Once all the cribs and beds were occupied, mothers with sick children would place them on top of tables, counter tops, or any flat surface they could find.

St. Joseph's Mission Hospital, located in the Rift Valley Province of Kenya, was founded by a group of Dutch Sisters in 1963. The hospital first started as a dispensary and grew to a 195-bed facility, serving as a medical center for at least 150,000 people. There was no main electricity or water supply in Kilgoris. A diesel-fueled generator, however, provided electricity to the operating theater throughout the day and a larger generator provided electricity until 10 P.M. at night, which allowed both operating room accessibility for emergency surgeries and lighting throughout the hospital's wards. Kerosene lanterns were used after 10 P.M. Normal activities such as gaining intravenous access were challenging in such poor lighting. The duties of the day nurses included ensuring that lantern wicks were trimmed and filled for the night nurses and the collection of rainwater warmed by solar panels for patients' baths.

Moreover, nursing staff made do with practically nothing. They created their own bandages and surgical drains. They would cut into layers of gauze and make 4 x 4 drain sponges. In addition, they would save used rubber gloves and, after careful washing, would cut off fingers and fingertips and use them for Penrose-type drains. Dressings and drain sponges would then be wrapped in gauze, placed in metal containers, and autoclaved for sterilization.

The nursery accommodated premature babies with hand-made incubators known as isolettes. A Bunsen burner placed underneath kept the isolette warm. Temperature control was crucial, but had to be monitored manually by observing a built-in thermometer within the isolette. Humidity "control" was provided via water held in a metal dish built into the upper left-hand corner of the isolette and from underneath the isolette where there was a drawer to hold a tray of water.

Inventory of antibiotics—but not narcotics—were counted at the change of every shift. Antibiotics, regarded as a valuable commodity, were legally controlled, whereas counting narcotics was not necessary as they were too few available. One reason for the many drug-resistant organisms was thought to be the wrong prophylactic use of antibiotics, which attributed to the government regulating control.

Diet consists of *ugali*, a cornmeal, and *sukuma-wiki*, a spinach-type green. In the pediatric ward, porridge was served for breakfast and a hard-boiled egg added if the child was on a high protein diet. Usually, a high protein diet was implemented if the child was diagnosed with kwashiorkor, often seen after a severe bout with measles.

One remarkable attribute evident in the nurses at the Mission Hospital was their acceptance of the amount of work left to do from the previous shift. When consulting the work-list generated by physicians' rounds, they would inquire what the previous shift had completed and start right in with any pending duties.

St. Joseph's Hospital in Kilgoris was well staffed because of the Oloosagararam School of Nursing, which was located next door to the hospital. Every year, twenty-six students began a two-and-one-half-year preparatory course, finishing with a Kenya Enrolled Nurse (KEN) certificate. Of ten different categories of nursing practiced in Kenya, KEN ranked sixth. Students were trained in clinical nursing skills beginning with an eight-week Introduction to Nursing course. Following this course, students were assigned to wards and by the time they completed their studies, they had acquired such skills as suturing and episiotomies. In contrast, during periods when the hospital census declined, students were held responsible for washing walls, windows, and organizing supplies.

Kenya gained independence from Great Britain in 1963. In prior years, the English influence prevailed both in health care and in the language spoken for professional purposes. For example, Kiswahilli was considered the national language, but English was spoken in hospitals and schools. Students were usually trilingual, as many of them also spoke their own tribal tongue.

Government requirements concerning patriarchs and foreigners working in Kenya obligated them to work in a government facility for a period of time before "going out into the bush." During the process of fulfilling this requirement, and while working as a nurse at Kenyetta National Hospital (KNH) in Nairobi, Kenya, it was apparent that some English customs were still practiced. Tea was served to nurses and staff at three o'clock in the afternoon every day.

As a staff nurse and nurse educator for one year in Kenya under the auspices of a Catholic missionary society, Mill Hill Missionaries, the Nursing Council of Kenya, Ministry of Health initially assigned me to two months at Kenyetta National Hospital before going to the mission hospital in Kilgoris. For the first month I was assigned as staff nurse in a pediatric ward, and for the second month in a pediatric emergency ward. While working in the pediatric ward I saw just about every disease I had studied in college—from Burkitt's lymphoma to tetralogy of Fallot where children were seen in the typical squat position.

For the most part, the type of nursing conducted was task-oriented in the hospital setting. The census in pediatric emergencies normally would be at least 250 patients. These children would come through the main hospital's emergency department to await placement in the wards. Remarkably, every child was seen daily by a physician. Four times a day, mothers with their sick child or children awaiting treatment would "queue up" on benches in the hallway. In groups of two, they would then enter a treatment room where four nurses would administer medications. Each parent had a card given her from the physician. Panadol elixir or IM antibiotic would often be the treatment of choice. My idea of bringing "primary nursing" to this setting quickly vanished as the task-oriented approach was the most successful in dealing with so great a number.

In summary, nursing in Kenya continues the charm and dignity of the English nursing profession, but is now establishing its own sense of nursing, which portrays the culture in a gentile and unique way.

KENYA
Amy Toone

Three pastors traveled on foot two full days to ask me, for the third time, to come to their Burundi refugee camp. My mobile clinic staff was reluctant, as this area was known for roadside hijackings, lion attacks, and biting tsetse flies that carry African sleeping sickness. I realized that this area needed medical help desperately, as most of the population were refugees from the violence and genocide in neighboring Burundi. I worked in Kigoma, Tanzania, for my four years and had the reputation for providing a full health clinic during the day and showing a religious film in the evening. The regional government authorities assured me that they would monitor my transport, as they knew this was one of the worst roads in Tanzania. It was a desolate and rough area that acted as a natural barrier to keep refugees in the camp. Driving around this camp, there was nothing except forest, tsetse flies, and prowling lions. I talked my staff into taking the trip and we left for a week of clinics and church services and living roughly in tents.

I loaded the clinic and camping items in the trailer. For this trip I took a mechanic along, as I knew this trip would be rough on the vehicle. Things were going well until about five miles from the camp, the car's electrical system died. During numerous attempts to roll start the car, we landed in one of East Africa's notorious soft-sand spots on the roadways and quickly sank to the axles. We were bitten numerous times by tsetse flies as we worked on the car, hoping that the biting flies weren't carrying African sleeping sicknesses. The tenacious tsetse flies do not respond to repellent. After dusk we heard a lion's roar and realized that we needed to enter the vehicle for safety and to remain there for the night.

Aware of the dangers of hijacking, the staff advised that if a vehicle approached that we should scatter and leave the keys in the car so the hijackers will just take the car. We each agreed to enact that tactic, and I ended the long day with a prayer. I prayed that God would send an English-speaking diesel electrical mechanic. My staff laughed and commented that the more fatigued I became, the worse my Swahili was. They thought my request for an English speaker was quite funny, as no one in that area of Tanzania spoke English.

At three in the morning, headlights approached and we jumped from the car and scattered as planned. To our amazement, the Across Africa Open Air Safari truck stopped and someone yelled "Good day, Mates." This Australian man was a diesel mechanic and while he could not fix the problem, he diagnosed it, and told my friends what parts were

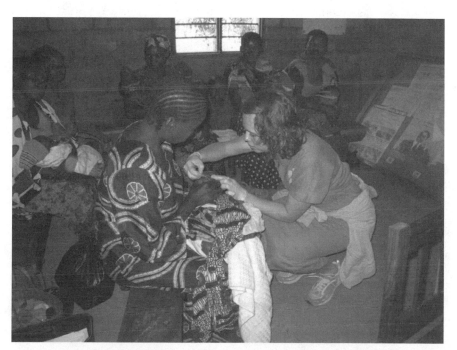

Jessica Snell, nursing student at Harding University, administering polio drops at an immunization clinic. (Note: WHO is working to eliminate polio as they did smallpox.)

needed and then he pulled us from the sand. My nurse midwife was so impressed that God answered the prayer that she immediately had us stop to pray for a good husband for her. By the time we finished attempts to work on the car, a new dawn arrived. We walked the final five miles to the camp and shared our story of how God answered our prayers.

The local pastors were correct in that the medical needs in this refugee camp were enormous. When we stepped from our tents in the morning, there was a line of waiting patients that stretched as far as I could see. The clinic was held in a school building for five days. One morning, a young boy was in line and he had what looked like a huge parotid abscess. Believing that white people might know more than local medicine men, the grandfather brought this ten-year-old for me to examine. I could find no obvious cause for this abscess and took a picture to show my colleagues who might know what it was, as I had heard about future continuing education conferences for doctors and dentists in neighboring Kenya. When I later attended this over-packed seminar and showed the parotid abscess picture there, the physicians diagnosed Burkett's lymphoma. We were able to get the child treated and he recovered fully. I asked if nurses could attend this seminar, as there is an average of five missionary nurses for every doctor. Unfortunately, the conference organizers explained their conference center was at maximum capacity.

It was at this time that I realized we needed a continuing education conference for nurses and nurse practitioners serving in transcultural areas. Little did I know that my life would change drastically in the next few years and I found myself teaching in Texas and directing an FNP program, although my heart for missionary nursing never wavered. I was delighted when the head of a mission agency asked me to arrange a continuing education conference specifically for missionary nurses and nurse practitioners.

The primary goal of these conferences was to educate missionary nurses in what they would need to practice in Africa and the Middle East, which are topics not usually covered in traditional nursing programs. We also educate about the latest drugs, technology, and developments in the management of illnesses so the missionary nurses remain current while working as nurses and nurse practitioners. I realized that in teaching others to do their jobs more effectively, I would have more influence on the nursing world than if I returned as a missionary nurse to only one specific area of Africa.

My five-year experience as a missionary nurse practitioner in Tanzania enabled me to identify relevant topics for the first conference. We wanted to make the conference affordable, as the average missionary family with two children lives on an income of $18,000 per year. We offered forty-eight continuing education hours for a registration fee of $50. The conference lasts a week and is held in a safe and family-friendly environment. Due to the continuing education requirements of the missionary nurses, we offer this conference biannually in odd-numbered years during spring break. Many of the initial faculty were U.S. nurse educators; as the conference continues, the faculty is becoming increasingly international.

Our first conference was in 1998, and we had eighty nurses from six basic geographic areas. In 2007 we had our fourth conference with 121 nurses attending, with most of the participating nurses from Africa, as the conference was held in Kenya, East Africa.

Surprisingly we also had a large number of nurses attending from the Middle East and North Africa, which is separated from the east and west of Africa by the Sahara Desert. This is significant because many tropical diseases found south of the Sahara, such as plasmodium falciparum malaria, are not found north of the Sahara. Another major difference between the regions north and south of the Sahara is the religions that weave the fabric of the various cultures. North of the Sahara is almost exclusively Islam; south of the desert is a combination of Islam, African traditional religions, and Christianity. The governments north of the Sahara are predominately based on Islamic law and the southern governments vary from dictatorships to democracy, Islam, and tribalism.

The religions, governments, and common diseases affect the conference participants and their conference needs. When we realized at the first conference that one-third of the nurses were from war-torn areas, we started a day spa and counseling service. Both were very popular by the end of the conference. When faculty were not teaching, they were giving pedicures, manicures, haircuts, and listening to fellow nurses with compassionate hearts. The nurses enjoyed the plush conference center located in the Ngong Hills of Kenya, which is the area where the film *Out of Africa* was produced.

The conference agenda provides educational offerings during the day, some afternoon free time, and a worship service each night. As a former British colony, the British influence on the Kenyan culture remains, and there are morning and afternoon teas. We also offered parallel lectures with some tracks focused on specific patient populations like pediatrics or obstetrics. Attendees liked these various areas of the conference: educational offerings, physical renewal, spiritual focus, and fellowship/networking.

One need identified by the participants was fellowship and networking opportunities. Several nurses were from remote areas and wanted to meet other nurses. This led to much of their free time being consumed by impromptu regional meetings and networking, where newer nurses were able to receive valuable cultural advice from the more "seasoned" nurses. Topics such as female circumcision and how nurses could culturally respond emerged that we had not placed in the agenda. Because 90% of attendees were from countries ravaged by AIDS, another unscheduled topic was the psychological toll of dealing with so many patient deaths from AIDS. This was addressed in both group and individual therapy provided on site for attendees. We realized at the first conference that to best benefit the participants, we needed less lecture time and more networking time. Over the years this has resulted in continuing education being limited to 40 hours and arranging more free time for networking.

These International Nursing Symposia are offered only in the odd-numbered years, so to date we have had five conferences. As with most conferences, the first was organized by the coordinators, which were primarily myself and a few other fellow missionary nurses. My faculty colleagues volunteered their expertise and spring break time to teach. I based the agenda of that first conference on topics I wish I had known before serving in Africa.

The second through fifth conferences were planned by the conference participants using the feedback from previous conferences. An evening to plan the next conference is on the schedule of all conferences. Participants present desired topics and suggest international experts in those areas as potential lecturers. This conference does not call for abstracts but rather matching faculty for the requested topics, which leads to a more international faculty better able to address the international nurses' needs. The 2007 nurses came from sixteen countries. All conference teaching is in English. The countries where most missionary nurses were educated were the United States (50%), Great Britain (25%), Germany (15%), Sweden (5%), and other countries combined (5%).

The schedule follows the cadence of Africa. Three days of study and then a day to play. On the play day, many go on a safari in a nearby game park, have a formal high tea, go shopping at a local market, or just walk through the tea plantations that surround the conference center.

The topics often requested are: suturing physical assessment; refinement of differential diagnosis by history and examination; how to set up a mobile laboratory; how to treat common diseases with reliable available products; AIDS care; zooanotic diseases; and pharmacology updates. I have been amazed at the zest for knowledge and skills updates by these nurses. One nurse, Marcie, came to one of my suturing skills lab sessions. When she explained where she works in Nairobi, I thought she would never need suturing skills and I could not determine why she picked my lab that afternoon. I gave away all the sutures and instruments after the class. Shortly after this class, the Embassy in Nairobi was bombed. Marcie headed to the site to assist rescuers. She sutured people until all the supplies I gave her were exhausted. After this event, I learned to just trust God to have us teach the right subjects to those who will need this knowledge.

We only teach requested topics and pharmacology updates at each conference. The topics from past conferences ranged from how to handle abnormal uterine bleeding with just a condom and an IV bag, to the treatment of malaria. The attending faculty often commented that they learn as much from the nurses as they teach. We realize anew how much we can all learn from each other. This fellowship of spirit and knowledge is central to the conference. Each of us leaves with gratitude for their sacrifice as well as awe at their resilience. Together, nurses can improve the communities we serve worldwide.

SOUTHERN AFRICA
Lee A. Perry

When I lay in bed during the stillness of the night, I reflect on my trip to Africa. I am still deeply affected by the massive number of shanties and people idling about with nothing to do and children scattering here and there. But go a mile farther down and the scenery changes to one of hope and prosperity. I saw that although they were poor, the people in these villages were humble and patient. They were always smiling, warm, and eager to praise God every opportunity they had, even though they had so little. Poverty was not used as a reason to be dirty; the villagers were always neatly dressed and clean. The red dirt did not cling to the feet of those who traveled along the roads.

Our group traveled to Gaborone in southern Africa, where a group of villagers had waited more than five hours for our arrival. Once there we had some uplifting spiritual interactions. Their prayers were no different from ours. They prayed for jobs, marriages, healing, salvation, faith in God, building a home, delivery of family members from prison, strength, and further studies.

The next day we went to a different village. Many of our staff did spiritual teaching, medical education about HIV and safe sex, and engaged children in active questions and answers. The medical team members did triage and medical screening. We had one doctor in our group who saw patients until he was at the point of exhaustion. We distributed all of the clothing and supplies we had. Then five of us left to visit the HIV hospital. Some of the patients were so emaciated that their rib bones were very prominent. One, a child in the hospital, did not know my language, nor I hers, but she knew the universal sign of prayer and said "amen" at the end of the prayer I recited and smiled. Other lifeless bodies lay before me wretched in pain and unconsciousness. Yet, we prayed that our Heavenly Father would touch their bodies and deliver them from pain. There was no privacy; all the patients were grouped together— men, children, and women or maternity patients.

This hospital scene was so different from our familiar hospital setting. There was no automation, no beeping IV pumps, no piped-in oxygen, no electric beds, no fancy bed clothing or bedside curtains, no modern-day chest tubes. The patients just lay there in stillness. One young man simply cried when he received our prayers—I don't know if it was the prayer itself, the fact that he was dying, or simply that someone had come to see him. Although the appearance of the hospital was cluttered, the nurses stood out in their white uniforms.

There is a saying "everything happens for a reason." That reason became crystal clear when we learned at Sunday worship service in one of the villages that the villagers' customary hospitality—feeding their guests first—resulted in approximately 115 people not eating at all because they ran out of food. Out of this came the good. Our group and our bishop pledged to feed for a full year those villagers who attended the center. We gave what we had that day and continue to carry out our pledge today. Also, Bishop Sarah, an American citizen helping the people in Africa, was given a check for $72,000, which enabled the purchase of an SUV to travel to outlying villages and reach more people.

We also visited Scottsdene, a poverty-stricken area in which there is a facility called A Healing Center for Women and Children or A Balm in Gilead Center, dedicated May 16, 2004. At this center there were classrooms but no teachers or desks—and no children. We identified the need for computers, telephones, health education classes, and sewing machines to support the goals of the center—to give the people good nutritional food, health assistance, Pap smears, HIV testing, and breast exams. Sewing machines were requested so that the women could make things useful for the community. If they sold something for five Rands, they had to give one Rand back to the center. Another hope was for villagers to come and learn, and then to recruit others.

The ladies who visit the center usually have no more than a fourth grade education. They are trained to do domestic work so that they can get jobs that will at least pay minimal wage (800 Rands per month, approximately $110 in U.S. currency). They receive training twice a week for three months. We also distribute condoms, toothpaste, toothbrushes, crayons, soap, and clothes for all sexes. We also visit the homes of villagers who are incapacitated and unable to come to the center. Our travels also took us to Cape Town, Langa Park, and Robben Island. It was quite a wonderful experience to see so many different aspects of southern Africa and to connect with the people. Everywhere there were warm embraces from those humble, hardworking, and beautiful people.

In addition to my work in southern Africa, I have volunteered in Hurricanes Katrina, Rita, Gustav, and Ike. Each encounter presented its own unique situation. With Hurricane Katrina there were massive evacuees who needed health care, but some just needed to talk and to tell their story of how they survived. Most were still in a state of shock. If you looked into their eyes, you saw emptiness and helplessness, and an insecurity of which direction to go or who to talk to for help. I found that my nursing skills were of great benefit. Besides administering health care, I spent endless hours talking to families and listening to their sad stories. Many recounted how they sat on rooftops awaiting help. One individual explained that he was a dialysis patient and did not have treatment for seven days, and how grateful he was just to be alive.

My involvement in Rita was a little different, in that people were evacuated before the hurricane made its impact. The health care need exceeded the resources available, however. As nurses we had to be creative, using our triage skills and the nursing process to meet the demands.

Gustav had yet another set of challenges. I was working at my hospital as charge nurse on night shift when I was informed that we would receive thirty patients from Port Arthur, Texas, via ambulances. Some paperwork was sent ahead, informing us of diagnoses, ages, and sex. Preparing to receive such a large number of patients made me remember my days in the military. I quickly gathered my staff together and we developed a strategy for admission. The nurses employed sound leadership skills and organization.

Hurricane Ike also brought numerous patients and we received help from our sister hospital in Port Arthur. The nurses and respiratory therapists who came to help immediately became very close to our staff. This was a great demonstration of how nurses can bond and work toward our common goal—great patient care, no matter where the location. A group of nursing students also volunteered at one of the shelters for exceptional patients. Such encounters—whether in Africa or Louisiana—demonstrate that nurses are ready, willing, and able to respond to many situations and disasters, always putting the patient first.

SWAZILAND
Evelyn L. Acheson

In 1995, I was selected as a curriculum consultant/advisor to a mission hospital in Swaziland, Africa, as part of a USAID foreign aid project in that area. This was my first international assignment and I was keen to do a good job. I worked closely with the school of nursing tutors (faculty) as a peer to accomplish the curricular revisions needed in the program. Soon after I arrived in the small southern African kingdom, it was graduation time. At a faculty meeting on that hot summer day, assignments were made for the graduation preparations. I quickly learned that in southern Africa, graduation and other such celebrations had a high level of expectations, especially because the Royal family was invited to attend. In the British tradition, the reception was referred to as "tea." As the newest member of the group and the only foreigner, the duty of preparing graduation tea fell to me. I agreed, thinking, "How hard could it be to plan a party?"

"How many do you expect to attend the tea?" I asked, and was told about five hundred people. That sounded like a very big party, but I was assured that many people would help and that the budget was adequate. In addition, they told me that a large beast had been donated. Then they informed me that I would need to slay the beast! "I'm not slaying any beast!" I exclaimed.

"Oh, no problem, the students will do it," I was told, and slay the beast they did. On the hospital grounds the week before graduation, a large bull was delivered in the back of a small pick-up. The students were rounded up and the beast was slain and field dressed on the spot. The meat was hauled to the hospital's kitchen and cut for cooking. Big chunks of meat were cut and boiling continued all week. I supervised from afar. A couple of days before graduation, the kitchen staff began slicing the beef for sandwiches. They were concerned that the beef would not be sufficient, so they also boiled fifty chickens, and one hundred eggs. I supervised, this time a little closer. Looked like quite a lot of food to me, surely enough for five hundred guests.

The day of graduation, we began making sandwiches. We made sandwiches of beef, chicken, and eggs—I've never seen so many sandwiches. I went to the bakery and picked up the huge sheet cakes, seven of them. Enough to feed five hundred, the bakery staff told me. All afternoon we made more sandwiches, enough for five hundred, the kitchen staff told me.

Graduation night came. We were to have begun the ceremony at 8:30 P.M. but were stalling for time, waiting for the Royal family to arrive. Nine o'clock came, but no appearance by members of the Royal family. As ten o'clock came, the decision was made to proceed, knowing that if any of the Royal family came, we would stop and begin again. By eleven P.M., the ceremony was over and no Royal family. The building was packed, and the crowd spilled outside of the building. Time for tea!

The crowd was tired and hungry and they made a rush to the reception building. Sandwiches and cake disappeared in record time. By midnight, all the food was gone, and the line was still very long outside. That year, one thousand people attended graduation, and we had prepared for only five hundred!

What to do? Without food, the only choice was to close the door, turn out the lights, and go home. The crowd outside became cranky and demanded food. The food was finished, however, so I quickly got in my car and drove home.

The next day, the only talk was about how embarrassing it was that people were turned away hungry from graduation tea. It was very humiliating for Africans to turn away guests without giving them meat, I was to learn. Anger turned toward me, since I was in charge of the tea. No problem; blame the foreigner. What does she know of African customs? She didn't even know how to slay a beast!

I continued my work with curriculum development, even though my reputation for organizing tea was ruined. When I asked about the existing curriculum, what I thought would be a good place to start the task, they responded with blank stares! "What curriculum?" "The plan for courses you follow to teach the students," I said. "Well, we know what they need to know," I was told. I persisted, "Let's have a look then." Nothing was in writing, so we went to the senior class and asked, "What courses do you still need?" The class recited, "Gynecology, orthopedics, and pharmacology." So that became the curriculum for the senior class. The exercise was repeated with the other classes of the three-year program, and thus I had my "curriculum."

As was the custom at that time, the freshman class was selected from a list of qualified students who themselves might not have chosen nursing as their career. These students came to the school of nursing and moved into the dormitory, even though some had chosen education or mechanics or something else. Once at the school of nursing, they began classes right away. The freshmen had classes for one month, and then were sent to the wards to work, unsupervised, on night duty. The one-month class comprised the proper way to clean a sluice room. For those not acquainted with the British vocabulary, the sluice room is also known as the dirty utility room, where bedpans and other items are cleaned. The upperclassmen were very happy to see a new class because that meant they were relieved of night duty. The juniors were then sent to class for one month, then the seniors.

One day I thought I would sit in on a class taught by another tutor. The tutor had transcribed her notes on transparencies and instructed a student sitting near the overhead machine to change pages when all the notes had been dutifully copied.

I learned that only the tutors had access to a textbook. The tutors copied material from a textbook onto a transparency, or sometimes read it to the class. Students stood when the tutor entered and broke out into a hymn singing in perfect harmony. They sat when the tutor gave permission. Study hall was from 7 to 10 P.M. each night and was mandatory.

I saw that my work would be challenging, and since the embarrassment with the tea incident, I knew I would need to proceed with caution. I first proposed that the freshmen stay in class for several additional months to learn how to give medicines since they were doing that on night duty. I was advised that pharmacology was not taught until senior year. I did not understand why they bothered, because by senior year, students had already been giving meds for two years. And I was told that freshmen could not stay in class any longer because the hospital counted on them for night staffing.

Next, in my naïve state, I approached the matron (director of nurses) at the hospital. When I proposed an extension of classes for the freshmen, she voiced the same protest, "Who would staff the hospital at night?" Who, indeed?

The principal tutor (dean) of the nursing program and I began work the same day. We inherited the "curriculum" with all of its shortcomings. The tutors had trouble seeing the problem: "This is the way it had always been done." The principal tutor and I negotiated with the matron to allow the freshmen a total of two months in the lab and classroom—a compromise, but a slight improvement to the existing plan. In order to accomplish this, however, the juniors were required to stay on nights another month. Needless to say, I was even more unpopular.

I made a decision to sacrifice my focus on the senior class and to concentrate on the freshmen class, also increasing time in the classroom for juniors when possible. I taught classes on curriculum development; I skipped over any theoretical underpinnings or conceptual framework and went straight to basic knowledge and built on that. Such a simple plan just might work, I thought.

Not as easy as I had supposed, because the tutor of "sluice room 101" was unwilling to give it up. She had seniority and in a culture where age is respected, I was treading on dangerous ground. I decided to take a different tact and "promoted" the senior tutor to teach the skills lab with a junior tutor, disguising the arrangement as a mentoring/teaching/role model assignment. She liked the idea, and graduated from "sluice room 101" to fundamentals. Together we planned the class, but ran into another snag. The hospital needed all of the sheets and supplies and couldn't lend them to us for practice. Another compromise: We practiced in the hospital. The senior tutor was not happy with this arrangement because as a tutor, she did not need to go to the hospital. Her uniform as a tutor was a navy skirt with white blouse; nurses wore all white. Then another snag... by now I was known as the troublemaker. Why teach students to give basic patient care when that was not the nurse's responsibility, but that of the patient's family?

Somehow we were able to keep the freshmen for two months, providing training for some basic skills before sending them to staff the night shift as charge nurses. I learned many things that year. I learned how important it is to consider cultural beliefs, traditions, and individual personalities when introducing change. I had to think long and hard about what the nurses in Swaziland *really* needed to know, and not just what I believed was important based on my own background. I compromised more than I thought possible, and most nights I went to bed thinking about how to introduce change in a nonthreatening way, how to help the tutors to do a better job, and, in general, how to impact the system in a positive way while preserving their traditions and cultural beliefs. Other nights I just wondered what I had gotten myself into.

Nurses in much of the developing world do not provide personal care to their patients. That is the job of the patient's family. As well, patient education is not a nurse's job, rather they see their role as an authority figure giving orders to patients. Hospitals and nursing schools must work together, and separating the two is like performing surgery on conjoined twins; one must be careful to give each the essential organs for life. We experienced the same growing pains in the United States when diploma schools were closed and nursing education moved into universities.

A few years later I accepted an assignment at the University of Botswana as a senior lecturer. Botswana is also in southern Africa and only a couple hundred miles from Swaziland. Botswana had a longstanding democracy, and nursing education was primarily taught in diploma programs under the direction of the Ministry of Health. A career ladder program was offered at the University of Botswana in the Department of Education for practicing nurses and led to a Bachelor's of Education (BEd) degree. Most nurses who were selected for this program had completed three years of the hospital-based program, plus one year of midwifery, and often, another year or two of specialty training. This totaled four to six years of education. The BEd degree required three more years of university education.

My assignment was to teach research and medical–surgical nursing, which included health assessment. Both courses lasted nine months, or two semesters. The research class required students to conduct an independent study in their home country, collecting data while at home during

Christmas holiday. Students at the University of Botswana came from the surrounding African countries of Swaziland, Malawi, Zimbabwe, Lesotho, and others. During the two years at the university, I supervised sixty-three research studies.

What I had learned in Swaziland made me better equipped for this assignment. I considered that the nurses came to the university with as much as seven years of education and a minimum of three years of experience. My goal was to present new material in medical–surgical nursing that would be a challenge to these students. I decided to organize my course by body systems, beginning with assessment of each system, followed by assigning care of hospitalized patients with conditions of that system, and finally having one or two students present case studies using their patients. For example, we began with nutrition. We studied all the assessment methods available to measure the nutritional status including BMI for adults and older children, and upper arm circumference for one- to five-year-olds. They were assigned patients such as children with growth stunting and adults with anemia. Two students chose this for their case study and presented it to the class.

I found this approach to be very effective in some ways and a total failure in others. First, the assessment part required a place to assess each other in a practice mode. No such rooms were available, so I enlisted the help of the Student Health Service using their equipment, rooms, and beds and patient gowns. That worked out well, but the nurses who had completed family nurse practitioner training before coming to the university were unwilling to participate, stating that they already knew how to do an assessment. I compromised and made the assessment lab voluntary. After a short while, all students participated willingly.

Going to the hospital for clinical application was a total failure. I did not know that the students felt that going to the hospital was degrading for their station within the government system. When I first announced the clinical assignments to the class, I was told that they didn't have transportation. I then ordered a university bus to take them to the hospital that was only two blocks away. Then I was told that they did not have uniforms for such an assignment. I found a way to have them each fitted for a white lab coat, paid for by the university. I worked feverishly to arrange with the hospital matron for these clinical assignments. She kept asking what the students would be doing. I told her my plan for case studies of patients with afflictions of the specific systems. I laid out the plan for her for nutrition conditions the first week, and then skin conditions the second week, and so on. She seemed amused, but promised me the arrangements would be made with the various ward supervisors.

After a month or more of preparations, the bus arrived to take the students to the hospital located for the first assessment. Students each had a new white lab coat, and the ward supervisors were expecting us . . . or so I thought.

Only a few of the students showed up and each was given a ward assignment. They walked to the various wards and turned around and came out almost immediately, each saying the ward supervisor wanted to know what they were doing there! I was embarrassed and angry, but persisted by going to each ward supervisor to explain. When I had this all settled, I returned to my students and found they had all gone. The next morning at class, I said, "I was at the hospital yesterday to participate with students in a clinical learning experience, but I was there alone!"

Students apparently were reluctant to explain their indignation at being asked to go to the clinical area—they were university students with as much as seven years of education. I didn't understand, but realized it was a futile battle—white lab coats, bus, coordination with the matron, and all. I compromised and suggested that the students would only go to the hospital wards when it was their turn to present the case study.

The case studies were a huge success, although students had no experience presenting to their class previously, and found it a frightening experience. I gave them a template to use to guide their preparation. I soon realized that these case studies were really stories, and the students loved stories. I also learned with them. When a student presented a case study of a man with burns received when he had a seizure and fell into an open fire, the class burst into laughter. I was appalled; I didn't see anything funny about this. (I eventually learned that students laughed when they were uncomfortable, and not just at humorous things.) I asked why they were laughing. One student explained that they believed that if a person had seizures, it was because he was possessed by the devil. If he fell into a fire during a seizure it became proof positive of being possessed. I talked to them about that and asked if they believed that to be true. Most said they did not believe it. I then asked what it must be like for a person with seizures to live in Botswana. After class a student told me that she had a cousin with seizures and that she believed it would be awful to have that condition given how people treated her cousin. The next year, in my research class, this same student chose as her research topic, "The Lived Experience of People with Seizure Disorders." She was able to interview several people with seizure disorders and wrote a poignant report of the pain they experienced being outcasts from society.

Another case study was about an infant who had a broken leg because his mother dropped him. Again the class erupted in laughter. At least this time I realized that this was not a case of sick humor, but of being ill at ease. When I asked what the laughter was about, I was told that it was only a stupid mother who would drop her baby off her back. Babies were carried on their mothers' backs until they were nearly two years old, wrapped tightly with a towel, cloth, or blanket. I had observed mothers putting their infants into this position, and it required skill to lean forward, toss the infant onto their back, keeping him there while they wrapped him securely. My students had no tolerance for error with this skill. I listened and learned about the culture.

Research class was a wonderful experience for me. I was able to guide and learn from the sixty-three students throughout the process. Most of the studies were concerned with aspects of AIDS as that was and is the most urgent and perplexing problem in southern Africa, especially Botswana. During those years the students studied caregivers, most of them mothers caring for their adult children along with their grandchildren. The old mothers cried and told my students that they did not know what their children had, but they knew it was bad. They were not told that their adult children had AIDS. The old mothers said it would be good if someone could help them carry water or firewood once in a while to lighten their workload. Nobody talked about AIDS, although there were many funerals in each village every weekend, and the number of orphans grew every year.

I taught students how to use computers to make graphs, to enter and analyze statistics, and to write reports. The first year we had only one computer that was the personal property of a senior tutor. She banned us from using her computer when she learned we were using it on Saturdays and at night, although I had asked permission before we began. I was so frustrated and angry. After stomping about for a few days, I set about finding access to computers for my students and was granted access to a computer lab from another department. It was very rewarding for me to hear students squeal with delight at composing a document and seeing it printed, and every research paper included several pie charts.

I also introduced poster presentations, inviting all the nursing leaders from town the first year and those from throughout the country the second year. The first year, the posters were made by hand, with careful printing on large pieces of cardboard. The second year, the students printed charts, graphics, and text in the computer lab and the results were astounding, even to them. I collected their abstracts and printed them in a little booklet, cajoling the university print shop to copy them. I sold them to the visiting nurse dignitaries, and used the proceeds to give cash prizes to the winning posters. Poster day was a highlight of my time in Botswana for the students, faculty, and nurses in the whole country because we helped illustrate the importance of nursing research.

From the success of the poster presentation, I realized that, after seven years and over 210 research studies conducted by BEd students at the university, a database of the studies with several search fields would allow other researchers to utilize and build on them. I found a library science student who needed a project, and presto—a database was developed for nursing studies. I continued my earlier education about influences of culture, the real worth of nurses in the world, the place of nursing research, and also the use of stories in education. I am much wiser now.

UGANDA
Karen B. Drake and Jemimah Mary Mutabaazi

This story began in January of 2002 when my Bethel University nursing colleague Dave Muhovich visited Uganda with a dozen senior nursing students during an international option for the course Cultural Diversity in Health Care. Dave previously spent nine years as a nurse in community development projects, often taking students to visit the projects and its people in a setting where he had personal experience.

While in Uganda, Dave was asked what a nursing department like Bethel's could do to help nurses in Uganda improve the standard of nursing and health care in the country. Uganda is a country of thirty million people. The majority of nursing programs prepared nurses and midwives at a minimal education level in hospital-based programs. The nurse–patient ratio, even in an acute care setting, is often one nurse to forty patients. Baccalaureate nursing education is a relatively new concept, and it was only available at two government universities, Makerere and Mbarara. Other nursing education programs were post-basic nursing courses offering diplomas in public health nursing, pediatric nursing, nursing/health administration, and nurse/midwifery tutors. There were no graduate programs in nursing at that time.

I personally was drawn to the collaboration idea in Uganda when my colleague presented this to interested nursing faculty. Contributing to professional nursing development somewhere in Africa was still my passion. I spent seventeen years teaching nursing in Zimbabwe. There I found joy in introducing rural young people to the profession. Discovering potential nurse educators in my graduates, mentoring them to teach alongside of me and eventually to take leadership roles was particularly rewarding.

My colleagues and I began formulating a plan for me to visit a rapidly growing, private Uganda university that had expressed interest in a partnership to expand nursing education in Uganda. When we contacted the U.S. embassy in Uganda, they were enthusiastic about the idea and suggested we consider the Fulbright Senior Specialist mechanism for support. I applied and was accepted by Fulbright for three consultation visits to work with Uganda Christian University (UCU), a newly chartered (accredited) university, to develop a baccalaureate nursing education program.

My first consultation visit with UCU was in January of 2005. At that time, UCU did not have academic courses in science or health care, so there were no nursing or health care colleagues available for collaboration. A newly arrived volunteer from the United States, Douglas Fountain, with a masters' degree in public health administration, was assigned by the university to work with me. He came with a wealth of background in administration and project management, plus a willingness to learn about my passion for developing a university-based nursing program. This was encouraging, because many academic settings throughout the world placed nursing under the leadership of related professions when nurse educators did not have recognized academic degrees. This often resulted in longstanding, stifling situations, especially when nursing education was placed under the field of medicine. In many countries, the historical relationships between medicine and nursing have hindered the nursing profession from flourishing, even after nursing faculty acquired doctoral degrees.

Doug and I set out to discover the state of nursing education in Uganda. Between 1991 and 1994, the first six Ugandan nurses to earn master's degrees were sent to Case Western Reserve University. Most did not have a bachelor's degree so arrangements were made to complete the dual requirements. On their return to Uganda, they were the first and only nurses in the country with graduate education. The first nursing baccalaureate program began in 1993 at Makerere University, the country's premiere university. In the following year, a similar baccalaureate program was started at Mbarara University of Science and Technology. Later, Aga Khan University (2001) started its program. Initially, these programs were designed as degree-completion programs to enable the large population of diploma nurses to obtain baccalaureate level nursing education. Even in 2005, there were still fewer than ten nurses in the entire country with master's degrees in nursing, and no nurses with completed doctorate degrees.

Doug and I were surprised to discover that the critical mass of several hundred nurses with bachelor's degrees was struggling to develop as a profession. While there was talk of a pay structure related to education in the future, graduating with a bachelor's degree did not provide a new opportunity for advancement in most work settings. Many nurses moved out of their jobs to work for nongovernmental organizations in research, but then were lost to the mainstream health care system.

One of the first official visits made was to the Commissioner of Nursing at the Ministry of Health. Mrs. Margaret Muura Chota and her deputies gave us their recommendations and encouraged us to visit the existing baccalaureate nursing programs. We visited two of the three existing nursing baccalaureate programs, as well as government and private hospitals and hospital-based nursing programs. In addition, we spent time studying the mission, vision, and educational philosophy of UCU. One of the progressive steps that UCU had taken was to include a number of core courses for all undergraduate programs. Some of these included Writing and Study Skills, Basic Computing, Ethics and Worldviews reflecting the Christian perspective of the University.

At the first visit's conclusion, I submitted a proposal to UCU for the development of a degree-completion program initially, followed by a master's program and later a direct-entry program as the numbers of master's-prepared nurses increased. This proposal reflected the evidence we had collected from visits with the Commissioner of Nursing, the two schools of nursing, and UCU officials. It contained suggestions for collaboration with Bethel University's Department of Nursing.

After my return to the United States, a Memorandum of Understanding was signed between UCU and Bethel University, confirming our partnership and the recognition of our desire to work together to forward nursing education in Uganda and at UCU. In a meeting with my colleagues at Bethel, it was also decided that if any of our nursing programs or course syllabi could be adapted for the Ugandan context, it would be available to UCU with proper acknowledgment to Bethel University.

The second consultation visit was in June of 2005. The primary focus was to further develop a curriculum overview, course descriptions, and outlines for the degree-completion program, and create a ten-year plan for nursing education at UCU. It was helpful that my colleague from Bethel, Dave Muhovich, was present during this time to work with me on the enormous task of curriculum development, and that we had permission to adapt courses from the Bethel nursing programs. The wealth of our previous experiences in Africa provided the necessary context as we adapted U.S. coursework to the realities of the nursing profession in Uganda. An advisory board was convened and included several significant and important individuals in Uganda, including Mrs. Chota, the Commissioner of Nursing, as well as key nurses, multidisciplinary health care personnel, and administrators of UCU. We were pleased with their positive feedback and some excellent suggestions for additional revision of the proposal we submitted to them. Certainly the seeds for advancing the nursing profession and the health care system in Uganda were sown in these early collegial collaborations.

My third visit was in January of 2006. Between the three visits there had been extensive consultation by email, online chats, and voice over the Internet. The UCU nursing program had received approval from the administration and preliminary approval from the Commission for National Council for Higher Education of Uganda. A wonderful nurse educator who had played a significant role in the development of two of the other bachelor's programs in nursing in Uganda, and who had been a member of the advisory board, Mrs. Mutabaazi, was now hired as the director of the program.

Jemimah Mary Mutabaazi, a nursing legend in Uganda, had struggled in her own journey as a professional nurse. Educated first as a diploma nurse in a hospital program, she went on to study midwifery and to obtain a post-RN nurse-tutors' diploma. She had obtained a baccalaureate nursing degree from the University of Zambia in Lusaka and, in 1992, a master's nursing degree at Case Western Reserve University in Cleveland, Ohio. She was one of the original six nurses to obtain graduate education. Mrs. Mutabaazi specialized in community health nursing and nursing education and had been a nurse educator for more than twenty years; however, she could not get released to undertake a doctoral program because of the acute shortage of educators in the country.

Jemimah began her official role as Director of the Nursing Program in December 2005, just before my third visit. It was delightful during January of 2006 to work together with her on many of the details for the start-up of the program scheduled for May of that year. The collegiality of our working relationship was satisfying to both of us. Jemimah had a good understanding of nursing education in the United States since she had studied at Case Western, and my years of teaching nursing in Zimbabwe gave us common ground in understanding the needs of nursing education in Africa. Jemimah had the vision for specifically applying our ideas to the Ugandan context, and we both worked to understand the academic context of UCU. We met with UCU administration and teaching staff to outline logistics and necessary resources, as well as to educate them on the differences and uniqueness of nursing. We introduced administration to "clinical" nursing skills labs, and the expensive necessity of student/teacher ratios when in the clinical setting.

We again used every technical means of communication to continue developing the baccalaureate degree-completion program. Jemimah developed an entrance exam to assess prior learning in nursing and the ability to learn in the university environment. The decision was made to start with a first class of very experienced nurses from throughout Uganda. The first class of fourteen students began in May of 2006. Many of these students already held significant roles in administration, education, and community health. Jemimah was the sole teacher in the first semester, with a few part-time lecturers.

In March of 2006, I was awarded a Fulbright Scholarship to spend a year at UCU. We were excited, as Jemimah had shouldered this alone and we could now work together for the year. The commitment of both universities to this project was important. I had taken a sabbatical only two years earlier and thus was several years away from another sabbatical. However, the administration of Bethel was committed to the success of this unique partnership and granted an unusual, extra sabbatical at this time. I arrived in late August of 2006, just as the second semester of the program was beginning.

The first semester included a number of university core courses and nursing assessment with only a minimal amount of clinical experience at the very end. The second semester now included weekly clinicals. A part-time clinical instructor also joined us, and the three of us and fourteen students went to clinical every week. I had been granted licensure as a nurse in Uganda so I could teach and practice. We spent our time working with students as they applied the nursing process to their knowledge and experience of nursing care.

While English has been the language of the classroom for many years in Uganda, numerous patients spoke their own tribal language. We taught classes and worked with our students in English, but they communicated with many of the patients in their own tongues. At times students did not know the language of their patients and then needed a classmate to interpret for them. Language and culture are a very real challenge for nursing in Uganda.

The Ugandan higher education system required a formal research project and a written thesis for the baccalaureate degree. This presented a considerable challenge for us. When teaching students that research develops from existing knowledge and prior studies, I sent them out to find previous Ugandan research. We discovered that this is almost impossible as there are no databases similar to Medline or CINAHL that we take for granted in the United States. The students went to the various libraries and browsed through past research projects on the shelves. Jemimah was helpful as she had a wealth of memory about research projects that her past students had completed. The process was tedious and yielded very little.

Searching the Internet for global research projects in their areas of interest was also a problem. The World Health Organization has a wonderful resource called HINARI, but obtaining full text articles was problematic. The computers were slow, the bandwidth was narrow, and both were shared with many other students, faculty, and staff. Electrical power was also unpredictable. In January 2007, we were able to obtain seven new computers that at least addressed the computer availability issue.

One innovation that the nursing program at UCU has undertaken was to provide the nursing students with computer competencies. In addition, students were required to type all papers using American Psychological Association (APA) format. Computer literacy and APA formatting were particularly difficult for the students; however, as nurse leaders in Uganda, they are important skills. In addition, students were taking a course in Nursing Informatics. Understanding the process of turning data into information and knowledge, and using it to inform wise decision making through technology has been transformative. Community health nurses who have been calculating immunizations on paper, and nurse administrators who keep all statistics by hand were delighted with the power of spreadsheets. Some of the nurses reported that a few computers exist in their workplace, but no nurse knew how to use them. Computer competency, so taken for granted in the United States, is one of the keys to rapid change and improvement in both nursing education and the health care system in Uganda.

Repeatedly students told me that nurses are not respected in Uganda by physicians or the community. One student wrote, "It is very difficult to get appropriate and necessary higher education in Uganda because nurses are marginalized in development of their career." Nursing does not yet fully support its own development as a profession. "It is not very easy because you may apply and get admitted but your employer may refuse to release you citing the acute shortage of staff and also with the hidden reason that just in case you obtain higher qualification and take his/her job," said another student. Nurses also struggle financially. Nurses are poorly paid and also have families of their own. "One would rather pay fees for the young ones instead of undertaking BNS with such competing demands." "Even those who have struggled to attain higher education are demoralized because of lack of recognition and promotion." Students who have been able to study in this program have written, "We are learning to reason out things and find out why things are the way they are." "There are many new things being taught and I would encourage more nurses to come for this course."

Jemimah and I constantly reminded students that they need to advocate for their profession and for their patients. Students who have come to study at UCU tell us that they have very high goals—"become articulate in defending the nurses, and patients, rights, be empowered with knowledge, become an effective administrator of nursing services when given a chance, teach other nursing students, lobby for other nurses to be supported for higher education, make a difference in the health care system, contribute to a better image of nursing in this country, manage nursing information through nursing informatics, and training at UCU to pave a way for a master's degree and probably a Ph.D."

Bethel University has discovered a number of ways to connect faculty and students with this project. Each January, for the past two years, we have taken approximately twenty-five students enrolled in Cultural

Diversity in Healthcare Course to Uganda to take the course. Bethel students have been paired with UCU students for a variety of activities and shared clinical experiences together. Ugandan students have served as cultural guides for the Bethel students. Bethel students have learned much from UCU students about building relationships with patients and giving spiritual care. In turn, Bethel students have helped UCU students with Internet searches, editing of papers, and APA formatting.

Bethel faculty colleagues, Diane Dahl and Dave Muhovich, and I have led these student trips. We have found time to consult with Jemimah and her staff as the program developed. Diane recently served as an external examiner, part of the required evaluation for recognition by the Ugandan educational system.

Bethel faculty and students have collected nursing textbooks and raised money to ship the books to UCU. Bethel students entered the books into a database that provided information about the books. Our local chapter of Sigma Theta Tau (Chi-at-Large) has also taken an interest in our partnership by collecting books and raising money. It has been fulfilling to see U.S. nursing students become interested in global nursing, and to invest in these seemingly small contributions that make a huge difference in a developing country.

In June of 2008, UCU graduated its first baccalaureate class. On this occasion our Bethel department chair, Dr. Sandra Peterson, came along to share in the celebration and to extend congratulations. It was a delightful time of celebrating their successes and our joy in partnership. On this trip, we launched the next step of our partnership, a master's program. Two of the fourteen graduates joined five other students to make a class of seven.

The first phase of the master's program is designed to prepare nurse educators. Because there are no doctoral-level nurses in Uganda, this program is dependent upon our enlisting Ph.D.-level colleagues to teach by modules or online. The first class of UCU master's students plans to travel to Bethel University for part of the 2010 spring semester. This will give the UCU students an opportunity to take one course with Bethel master's students, appropriately the Global Health course. In addition, Jemimah Mutabaazi has been invited to speak at our annual research symposium in 2010. The vision is that ultimately some nurses from Uganda can obtain doctorates and be able to continue to lead in the academic and professional arena. Nurses in Uganda struggle to be recognized as professionals and to take their place in the multidisciplinary aspect of health care. Education and the acquisition of degrees in nursing will do a great deal to empower Ugandan nurses as professionals. Empowered nurses can advocate for better care for the population, and ultimately health care is improved.

There is one more aspect of our partnership that is very exciting. Bethel University has developed a new curriculum with a very strong focus on communities around the world where individuals are underserved by health care systems. One of the provisions of this curriculum is for some of our students to choose a semester abroad at UCU. UCU is now an affiliate of Bethel's accrediting body, Consortium of Christian Colleges and Universities. Bethel faculty such as Dave Muhovich and myself who accompany students will partner with UCU faculty to teach each other's students on site in Uganda. The potential for ongoing collaboration and partnership is limitless. The benefits to both institutions and their faculty and students are immeasurable. While perhaps change is slow, it begins one nurse at a time, one program at a time, and ultimately affects individuals and the systems around them. It has been rewarding to play a role in preparing nurse leaders in Uganda to take their place as professionals in the health care team in Uganda and globally.

UGANDA
Jennifer Gray, Jackline Opollo, and Lori Spies

We began our work in Uganda with the belief that we were the ones rich in resources to share with the nurses in Uganda who have few material resources in their practice settings. What we have learned, however, is that despite health care settings with few material resources, nurses in Uganda had extensive personal resources of resilience, commitment, and altruism. They have inspired and benefitted us through our partnership well beyond what we have contributed.

We describe workshops implemented through the collaboration of the North Texas Africa Health Initiative Uganda Team, the Ugandan National Association of Nurses and Midwives (UNANM), and Makerere University School of Nursing. The Africa Program was founded in 1994 at the University of Texas at Arlington. Dr. Allusine Jalloh, history professor and founding director of the program, and Dr. Jennifer Gray,

Associate Dean of the Ph.D. in Nursing Program, University of Texas Arlington School of Nursing, convened a group of health professionals and community leaders in 2006 to discuss opportunities to work with health organizations in Africa. Dr. Jalloh is a native of Sierre Leone and Dr. Gray worked as a missionary nurse in Cameroon, West Africa, in the late 1970s. A team was comprised of persons with an interest in Uganda. In addition to Drs. Jalloh and Gray, the team included David Mureeba, an entrepreneur in telecommunications who was born and raised in Uganda; Jackline Opollo, a student pursuing a joint master's degree in nursing administration and public health; and Lori Spies, a doctoral student who was on faculty at another school of nursing that provided its nurse practitioner students with international clinical experiences. The team articulated their dream of a long-term project to improve health outcomes in Uganda, but quickly realized that first-hand knowledge of the culture, nursing profession, and health care in Uganda was prerequisite for seeking funding.

In the summer of 2007, we traveled to Kampala, Uganda, accompanied by the Perezi Kamunanwire, the Ugandan ambassador to the United States and hosted by UNANM. The purpose of the twelve-day trip was to meet with leaders in government agencies, nongovernmental organizations, schools, churches, and health care organizations. Because of UNANM's and the team's network of connections, we met the Queen of Buganda, the AIDS Commissioner, the Commissioner of Health, the Nurse Registrar, and other dignitaries.

With the help of the UNANM officers and members, we held an all-day workshop at our hotel on the last day of our trip. Prior to our visit, we asked our UNANM contacts to suggest HIV/AIDS topics to include in our workshop. We presented sessions on basic pathophysiology, antiretroviral medications, communication, and human resource management. The room secured for the workshop could comfortably seat 100 people, but approximately 180 people registered. With limited financial resources, we were able to provide the attendees only with a snack and soft drink during the six hours. We did provide small gifts to the attendees thanks to the generosity of Ms. Opollo's employer, a large urban hospital. We asked the participants to list other topics of interest for future workshops.

We returned home and began seeking funding for a larger project in Uganda. As time passed, we decided to return to Uganda in the summer of 2008 with the goal of assessing a rural health district and learning more about Uganda's health care organizations. UNANM agreed to make many of the meeting arrangements. We included in the itinerary three workshops to address research, entrepreneurship, and curriculum.

For the research workshop, UNANM secured a theater-style room at the government hospital and arranged catering for a noon meal. An in-country nurse researcher was asked to be the keynote speaker on the role of the Ugandan nurse in research. We obtained permission from the publisher to copy the article the researcher had published and distributed copies of the article along with the other handouts we prepared for the workshop. To supplement the keynote presentation, we provided content about the steps of the research process and how to critique a study. After lunch, the sixty-five nurses who attended the workshop were divided into small groups and each group was assigned a specific component of the study to critique. Following lively discussion, each group reported what they determined to be the strengths and weaknesses of the study. The nurses were very engaged in the process and urged us to provide another research workshop on our next trip.

The Makerere University School of Nursing provided the space for the half-day entrepreneurship workshop with presentations by Dr. Jalloh and professors from the Makerere College of Business. Our team facilitated the contacts and worked closely with UNANM to secure the speakers. The twenty-five nurses and nurse midwives introduced themselves and gave an outline of their experiences with owning a business, several of whom owned multiple small businesses over several years.

When we met in 2007, the faculty of the School of Nursing expressed a desire to know more about curriculum development. In the time between trips, Ms. Opollo wrote her professional paper for degree completion on factors shaping graduate nursing curricula in Uganda. Ms. Opollo presented her professional paper at the beginning of the workshop, and Ms. Spies shared how she developed and implemented a graduate-level assessment course. Dr. Gray guided a review of the master's program curriculum that another group of visitors had written for the school. The interaction and discussion over the course of the two days provided a foundation for continued collaboration.

We have made mistakes. At the first workshop, we learned the necessity of providing adequate food and other refreshments to workshop participants. This fact is especially relevant in a culture in which social amenities create the context for effective communication. We also learned of the incompatibility of computers, projectors, and electrical sources, minutes prior to the beginning of a workshop.

On our first trip, our schedule was intense with little time between multiple appointments each day. The Ugandan culture requires time for tea at the end of a visit or meeting. Add to the longer-than-expected meetings the challenges of unpredictable traffic and poor roads, we spent most of our trip rushing to the next appointment. Our schedule in 2008 was planned with these factors considered.

We also have experienced success. Collaborating with the professional nursing organization has been the critical factor in our work. UNANM ensured that, for each visit, the chief nursing officer in the Ministry of Health was informed of our visit. Their endorsement of our visit opened many doors. In addition, the UNANM officers and members distributed workshop information, assisted with registration, and recruited participants. UNANM has also benefitted through our collaboration. They made connections with government officials known to Mr. Mureeba that they had not had before. They visited organizations with us and learned more about resources within their own communities.

The inclusion of in-country speakers had multiple benefits. Few nurses knew that the well-known nurse invited to speak for the research workshop had conducted a study and published her findings because the researcher had not been asked previously to be a keynote speaker. The nurses and nurse midwives who attended the entrepreneurship workshop had the opportunity to meet business experts who were locally accessible. The relationships that were initiated through these activities have continued and will benefit the profession in Uganda.

Three principles have guided the collaboration with our partners in Uganda: building on shared values and common goals; approaching situations as cultural learners; and committing to long-term relationships. These three principles are intertwined. Shared values and common goals were shared with our nurse colleagues in Uganda by partnering with the professional organization, UNANM. We asked many questions about nursing practice in Uganda during visits to different clinical facilities and in our informal meetings with our colleagues. Demonstrating respect and a willingness to understand the context laid the foundation for mutually beneficial relationships. What we learned is not unique to this project. Returning to Uganda and following through on our assignments were just the beginning steps in demonstrating to our Ugandan colleagues that we have a long-term commitment to working with them.

UGANDA
Diane Yorke

We arrived in Uganda on Sunday, October 5. Several of us wondered if we were appropriately prepared for the shared learning we had scheduled with the nurses from Mulago. However, we knew that we could present this teaching–learning experience well and were all very keen to do so. What we did not know were the learning needs of the nurses who staff the Uganda Heart Institute.

For several of us, this was our first participation in the combined University of North Carolina Chapel Hill (UNC-CH) and the District of Columbia Children's Hospitals' Uganda Heart Mission. On the UNC-CH side, this project was conceived in 2005 when a team traveled to Kampala to set up a pediatric intensive care unit in Mulago Hospital. The unit is still operating today and sees an amazing array of children suffering from illnesses common in Uganda: extreme malnutrition, extreme dehydration, malaria exacerbations, sepsis, meningitis, and hydrocephalus.

In 2007, several of the original planners from UNC-CH, along with several interested RNs and other health care team members, joined the DC Children's Hospital team and traveled to Uganda to perform surgical corrections on children with a variety of congenital heart defects and to select children with congenital heart defects to travel to the United States for surgical correction. The joint efforts of UNC-CH and DC Children's performed surgery on more children during the two weeks of the mission than could travel to the United States for surgery. As well, more training and education was provided to a larger number of the Uganda Heart Institute's health care team than could have been provided during one overseas training session.

The first joint mission was very successful; ten children had their heart defects corrected—patent ductus arteriosus, atrial septal defect, and ventricular septal defect. Children with these defects frequently have difficulty eating, which results in poor weight gain and poor growth.

On Monday we rose at 6 A.M., had breakfast, and got to the Mulago Hospital before 10 A.M. Boxes and boxes were emptied and the contents organized and set up to resemble a fairly complete, if limited by U.S. standards, pediatric intensive care unit. The U.S. nurses had set up a core course of lectures and presentations that mimic the core cardiothoracic orientation offered at our two pediatric intensive care units—pediatric assessment, introduction to pediatric heart defects, review of monitors, care of chest tubes, review of common intensive care laboratory values, care of central and arterial lines, management and care of patients on ventilators, cardiopulmonary bypass, and fluid and drug management—delivered in what would be considered eight hours of continuing education–type presentations. However, we quickly learned that more time was needed.

Tuesday we were up bright and early once again and ready for action. When we reached the hospital we were told that the first patient's chest x-ray indicated he had pneumonia so his surgery was postponed. The second patient, a young active girl with a significant patent ductus arteriosus, had an uneventful surgery and was off the ventilator before coming out of the operating theatre. She did extremely well and was smiling at her mother and at the nurses before the next morning.

The third patient was a tiny, eleven-year-old boy. He told his mother that he was nervous and wasn't sure he wanted to have his heart fixed. As he was walking down the hallway toward the preoperative workup room, he was introduced to the first heart surgery patient from the 2007 mission trip. This patient had acted as ambassador to the nine patients last year, and assumed that role again this year and eased the anxiety and fears of this boy of similar age and stature. Beside him was his grandmother who also was a great support to patients and families last year. She offered words of encouragement to this patient and also to his family.

At dinner that night, some of the group were talking about the trip and the reasons they were here. All of them considered it a professional responsibility to share their expert clinical skills and to have this extraordinary opportunity. They are thrilled to have this experience on so many levels—to share their knowledge, to help develop a new program, to meet different people and make far-reaching, professional, and personal relationships. Many expressed that every health care worker should have the opportunity to experience the need of others, the opportunity to serve, the chance to demonstrate their caring in a completely different society and medical system, and the opportunity to bring this experience back to their own practice at home. Many of the Uganda staff had years of experience and were quite capable of caring for these pediatric patients, but they required reinforcement of the specific concepts that we were presenting: cardiac medications, calculations, coronary anatomy, and pathophysiology.

The next day, we were off to the hospital very early once again. The plan was to present the lecture on care of the ventilated patient, but the speaker, a respiratory therapist, was called away to the NICU. No formal lecture took place and the staff nurses were disappointed, particularly the nurses who switched shifts to attend. But these nurses stayed until the middle of the afternoon, asking questions, assisting in nursing procedures, and demonstrating great interest in learning everything we could show, teach, or tell.

The two surgical patients from the previous day were visibly better and progressed so well throughout the day that they were both transferred to the step-down unit by the end of the night. The patient with pneumonia had recovered and was being made ready for the OR. The nurse on his case was taught the importance of checking the physicians' drug orders doses and calculating the correct amount of medication to give. When this patient returned from surgery, a Ugandan nurse assumed his care. She was taught about the importance of pain control and sedation for children and, as the day progressed, she assumed all of his care with little prompting from us.

The second admission required much preparation and there were many nursing activities to be taught, reintroduced, or reinforced. However, the critical nature of this patient's condition preempted many of the possible teaching moments: drugs for intubation needed to be prepared too quickly for a complete discussion of the purpose and indication of these drugs, and the staff RN pair were not provided enough time to independently perform all calculations or to physically draw up the medications.

But we have achieved some visible influence. The nurses at Mulago Hospital wear the traditional white nursing dress and white cap. But on Wednesday it was fascinating to see the Ugandan medical staff provide the Ugandan staff nurses with green OR scrubs to wear so that "they could be more like us." Later in the week the nursing manager, Sister Grace, was asked if this dress code would continue after we left. She told me that there had been a meeting of the nurses and hospital management and a unanimous decision had been made to not only accept this change in dress code but that the Heart Institute was going to have new blue scrub uniforms made for the nurses.

The next morning we were in the hospital once again and the U.S. nurses were able to present another lecture, this time about cardiac defects that were being repaired. The staff was so attentive and asked so many detailed questions that at one point, the presenter decided to demonstrate how they could research the information. The UNC-CH nurses had obtained a donation of nursing and cardiac nursing textbooks for Mulago, and had emptied these boxes at the beginning of the week. By the end of the week, however, the Ugandan staff nurses wanted the books handy in the pediatric intensive care postoperative unit, and by the next heart mission, we saw these books up on a display shelf.

The following day we found time to provide another of the prepared lectures, this time on cardiac medications and maintenance fluid calculations. The content was reinforced during the night shift and the Ugandan staff was able with little assistance to summarize the most important aspects of cardiac medications and of fluid balance and monitoring.

On the night shift, patient care and nurse education continued. Patients were monitored and a few of them slept through the night. Their mothers came in at 6 A.M. to give the children baths and to assist the nurses in getting them repositioned and out of bed as appropriate. The pace of the night shift work was not any slower than that of the day shift, but the flow of traffic was much less. The only persons present were the patients, sometimes their parents, and the nurses. During these quiet times, the Ugandan nurses were introduced to and participated in the structured learning activities on a computerized pediatric cardiac care program. They loved this format, and asked for and were given a copy of the heart and lung sound modules so that they could continue to practice and refine their assessment skills.

Later that same night, discussion came around to nurse charting. During this past week all charting had been recorded on charting sheets brought from the United States. The Uganda Heart Institute has its own charting sheet but it does not permit good charting of fluid intake and output, and the Ugandan nurses preferred to use our charting records. Mulago Hospital also has a useful standardized charting sheet used in the intensive care units, but this was not available to us during this visit. Similar information is presented on all of these sheets and it makes sense to chart on the institution's forms to facilitate staff's learning to document per the Mulago Hospital protocol. The Ugandan and U.S. nurses looked over all three sheets to pick out the best aspects of each in order to design a more useful nursing charting document. This project will continue online as our time here was almost finished. It is hoped that a finalized version of the modified and improved document will be completed within the next few months, so that the Ugandan staff nurses can present it to the medical staff.

There are some cultural differences that have been interesting to observe: tea time, scrubbing in for work, changing shoes within a six-foot-square transition zone, multiple electrical extension cords, and so on, but similarities are also apparent.

As in the United States, Uganda faces a nursing retention problem. Nurses frequently leave their hospital positions. A minister of the health department came to speak with us about nurse training, especially wanting to know what programs or training could be offered to have Ugandan nurses prepared *and* willing to stay at the bedside providing patient care. I explained to him that the United States experiences much the same problems he described.

During the last shifts of the last few surgeries, the Ugandan staff nurses were able to talk about the things they felt were urgently needed to continue to make the Heart Program successful: better nurse staffing, a dedicated pediatric intensivist, specialty-trained respiratory therapists, and more intensive care training, as they have "been building [their] skills from the ground up." The U.S. nurses also spoke of what they felt was needed to continue to make this and other health missions in Uganda successful: education, enthusiasm, and equipment. Education is needed for the Ugandan health care workers, but also for foreign health care workers so that we can better understand not only the practical but also the historical and political situation of health care provision in Uganda. For this mission we prepared a core cardiac care curriculum and were able to deliver all but two of the twelve planned lectures. We provided all content on several flash drives. For the interim, plans were laid to continue course development that can be offered online and to provide certification as well as professional development. Much enthusiasm is needed to make an education mission like this one successful. The volunteers on this mission were enthused, dedicated, and persistent in sharing their knowledge and skills with the Mulago Hospital health care workers. We came to recognize both the similarities and the differences between our educational and health care systems. The enthusiasm was palpable.

UGANDA

Meg Zomorodi, Brooke Bailey, Jamie Cash, Sarah Day Dickson, Alison Helmink, Katie Horrow, James Ludemann, Kristen Poe, and Jenna Woodruff

I've always wanted to participate in a mission trip, so when I was approached about traveling to Kampala, Uganda, for two weeks for a neurosurgery mission, I did not hesitate. Without knowing any specifics, my neurosurgeon husband and I agreed to be a part of a twenty-eight–person medical team, all determined to make a difference in the lives of the Ugandan people. We had no idea of the impact that Uganda would make on our lives and how determined we would be to maintain a relationship with the people in this beautiful country.

What we found there was a flashback to the 1960s where physicians operated with ether and the operating room nurse was the true canary in the coal mine—when the nurse passed out from the ether fumes, surgeries stopped for the day. There was one ventilator in the 1,500-bed hospital, and it was only used for new admissions. If a patient came into the hospital and the ventilator was being used, the family of the patient using the ventilator had to decide to either withdraw life support or manually ventilate the patient. Our plan quickly shifted to one that included donating medical equipment and education, and ultimately we donated nine tons of equipment to Mulago Hospital. With help from the University of North Carolina at Chapel Hill School of Nursing faculty and students, more than 100 textbooks were donated as well. This was especially important to me since education was my top priority.

When we arrived in Kampala, word spread about the U.S. mission and more than 100 people drove across the country to have access to this free service. When we realized we didn't have a phone or any way to stay in touch with the operating room, I donned a mask and ran back and forth between the three operating rooms in order to maintain contact between them and the recovery room.

When I first arrived in Mulago Hospital, I met Agnes, the only recovery room nurse. She told me her role was to ensure that the patient was still breathing, and then send him or her to the floor, where the nurse-to-patient ratio was one to fifty! I provided information on assessment and postoperative recovery, and my audience grew every day. By the end of the week, we had a full-time recovery room staff of eight nurses who performed full head-to-toe assessments, monitored vital signs, and determined when, and if, the patient was stable enough to be discharged from the recovery room.

On our last day in Mulago, the chief nurse told me that these nurses had been hired for the recovery room; their plan was to transform the recovery room into an overflow intensive care unit. I spoke with her about continuing my relationship with Uganda and made a promise to her to never forget the wonderful nurses.

During our second trip to Uganda, we implemented the first continuing education program for nurses in the country. Nurses from both Uganda and the United States collaborated by e-mail to discuss the planning. We decided that this continuing education program would focus on the nurses' role in the care of neurosurgical patients—the purpose of our mission. This program provided an opportunity for the nurses to describe their role and to receive education on the current standards of practice for the treatment of traumatic brain injury and tumors, and for the assessment of these patients.

I coordinated with eight BSN students from my nursing school to travel with me to Uganda and work at Mulago Hospital as part of their summer work experience. Students between their junior and senior years are required to intern in a hospital setting where they must work closely with the nursing staff. I coordinated with Makerere University and Mulago Hospital, and they assisted me in setting up housing and work experiences for the students. Together we decided where and when the students would work, and I assisted the students in submitting grants for funding and in raising money for their travel.

Each student was given the responsibility of following a patient before, during, and after surgery. They were instructed to conduct a baseline neurological assessment and prepare the patient for their operating room procedure. The student would then scrub in for their assigned patient's surgery. This served a two-fold purpose: The students would establish a rapport with the patient, and the health care team would have an individual who could provide continuity of care. After surgery, the student followed the patient in the recovery room, the intensive care unit, and the nursing floor.

My life, the students' lives, and the lives of the nurses, patients, and physicians at Mulago hospital were all touched in ways that are difficult to describe. The following are the students' descriptions of their summer work experience in Uganda.

James' Story: The Beginning

This mission trip and its opportunities have been the highlight of my studies at the UNC School of Nursing, as well as the most exciting five weeks of my life. Our team was welcomed, and the medical care, performed by Americans, focused on the hands-on education of local professionals. I was surprised how I underestimated the time it would take to feel accustomed to the local medical environment of Mulago. I had not anticipated the cultural shocks that are encountered in a developing country, and how a student's expertise can seem limited in the face of these obstacles. While these barriers seemed discouraging at first, they set the stage for some of the greatest learning I experienced, where I was required to face my discomfort and cultural incompetence on my own and problem solve. I soon realized where I could help, and I found ways that I, as a nursing student, could contribute to the health and wellness of the patients around me. The opportunity to problem solve coupled with the chance to see an international health team achieve great educational and medical goals made this experience so rewarding. I am excited to see how this knowledge guides my career as I graduate and begin my practice.

Jenna's Story: The "Art" of Nursing

My experience helped me to grasp how little I know and how much more experience and knowledge I have to gain. The Ugandan health care workers are extremely knowledgeable. Mulago's doctors know there is a gap between their system and industrialized nations, and they are eager to absorb as much knowledge as possible. The doctors are forced to make the best of the few resources they have. I gained so much respect for the Ugandan doctors and nurses as they deal with this dilemma every day. Their pay is less than desirable and the situation seemingly hopeless; yet, they persevere, push on, and come in each day with a smile on their faces and with passion for patient care. The majority of the world faces health disparities every day and by working at Mulago, I was able to see this gap. I had to rely heavily on compassion, patience, and love to support the patient. I always knew those were important concepts, but I never grasped how far they really go. I know that I will take with me what I learned about humility, putting the patient first, and compassion, and apply it to my practice. I realized that compassion and empathy know no borders. Humor, respect, and dignity know no boundaries. Simply taking a patient's hand in yours and making eye contact lets them know that you care about them. There were many experiences that brought this message home to me. One night I was taking care of a pediatric patient who they did not expect would live. There was nothing that anyone could do so I just sat and held the baby. At one point the child quit crying and stared at me. I realized that even if this was this child's last night, at least he learned what it felt like to be loved. Another night, I had a patient who was struggling to get his cup and I walked over and handed it to him. He looked so shocked as if having someone care for him, in this way, was foreign to him. This experience made me aware that simply touching a patient gently on the back or sitting with a patient can bring great relief. Through compassion I can let patients know I care about them. That is nursing at its finest.

Alison's Story

Prior to my trip I had no idea what to expect. I planned to go in with an open heart and mind, and this experience became the greatest adventure of my life. Of all the hopes and expectations I had for the trip, I would say that my top two were that I would have the opportunity to know and love the people of Uganda, and that I would somehow make a difference. My expectations were met in ways I could never have planned. I had the opportunity to live in Kiwangala Village for one week, among local Ugandans, and living with them was unique and amazing. The experience was humbling and opened the door to several learning opportunities. I had the same feelings in the hospital setting. When the physicians and nurses saw that you were willing to work *beside* them and that you were working toward the same goal, relationships grew. I now have an appreciation for how different cultures truly are, and how important this difference is. Communication was difficult, even though the majority of Ugandans speak English. Although we used the same words, these words did not necessarily have the same meanings. This experience taught me how to look at various cues, not just words, to analyze whether or not a patient understands what I am saying, or whether or not I understand what the patient is telling me.

Brooke's Story

I had feelings of anticipation and nervousness before I went to Uganda, but I knew that the trip would undoubtedly change the way I viewed myself, the world, and nursing. I was excited about being able to use my clinical skills to help care for the Ugandan patients. At the same time, I was worried about the risks of traveling to Africa, facing cultural and language barriers, and not being clinically prepared. I was able to focus on my learning goals and recognize the opportunities for professional and personal growth. What was most amazing was to see how members of the United States health care team improvised with limited medical resources. Calculating drip rates, reading glass thermometers, and making our own warming bags out of gloves and hot water were some of the things we did to care for the patients. As part of my experience, I was paired with a Ugandan nursing student so that we could discuss the differences and similarities of our nursing education. In Uganda, the nursing role is much less defined. I took in as much as possible during the trip, but it took me a few days after returning to the United States to sort through my thoughts and feelings about everything I experienced. I returned from this trip with a huge appreciation for the United States, for our health care system, and for all the conveniences we have in America. I have also dealt with feelings of guilt and questions about why I am blessed with a comfortable life, while there are so many starving and hurting people in the world. I have not been able to come to any conclusions about these questions, but I have re-evaluated what is important in life, and I know that I want to use my career in nursing to help underserved populations.

Katie, Kristen, and Jamie's Story

Although the surgeries we performed in Uganda improved the lives of many, there is so much to do that we could spend a lifetime there and still want more time. This experience illustrated many differences between health care expectations in the United States and Uganda. We constantly compared the Ugandan methods of providing care to ours. With few resources and less education, the Ugandans have little to work with, yet still work twice as hard to help others. They are proud of what they do. Upon arriving home, we realized that we learned and experienced more than we thought we ever would. Everyone who volunteered for this trip did so knowing it was for a good cause and were all eager to teach. The graciousness that the Ugandans expressed after their surgeries had an emotional impact on us. Immediately after the surgery, the patient and family would express how grateful they were that we had come over to do this for them. We have learned to be more sensitive to why patients do some of the things they do, the decisions that they make, and their fears or pain. We think that spending time in a country with few resources opened our eyes to some of the issues that people face, not only in a country like Uganda, but also in the United States. After having this experience, we will continue nursing with a more open mind and flexible attitude. We cannot begin to describe how valuable our experience of working as a student nurse in Uganda has been on our future nursing practice. Every day that we spent in Uganda, whether it was with the newborns at Mulago, or just the time we spent with some locals, we felt we were becoming more culturally competent. Working in a medical system that is vastly different required us to constantly be creative, flexible, and adaptable. One of the most valuable skills we gained was learning the true meaning of empathy and compassion. This experience emphasized how important caring, presence, kindness, and understanding are in nursing care.

ZAMBIA
Helena Stanaitis

Early in 2003, a friend asked me, "Would you like to go with us on a vision and medical ministry trip to Zambia, Africa?" This question caught me by surprise because my only international medical ministry experience was to the Dominican Republic the previous year. That trip's goal was to provide medical care in collaboration with local health care professionals. Most trip members served together as medics-on-call at our church, and most were registered professional nurses.

On the vision trip to Zamtam, Zambia, the select group planned to travel to Kitwe, Zambia, collaborate with Christian agency personnel who serve in many third-world countries, and tour some villages and meet with the villagers. Some team members would visit village schools and meet with village council members. Those interested in health care issues and/or health care professionals would meet with village health care providers, perform home care visits, visit an established health clinic and hospital, and attend church services. Other opportunities to visit with community members, health care professionals, and government representatives would probably emerge. The portion of the trip that was personally important was to use my nursing assessment skills and determine the health care needs of a community.

My friend and her husband are not health care professionals but have serving hearts. They sponsor many health care initiatives and served in environments that support human justice and humanitarian efforts.

My teammates were the "select group" and we all brought to the table a different set of skills, experiences, education, and vision. On this team were a physician, business professionals, high school students, school principals, pastors from various congregations, and myself, a nurse. After a few moments of reflection and prayer, my only response was, "If you can use me as a friend and my skills as a health care professional, I will serve with you." She said, "Thank you, we need your skills and experience on our team." As a nurse, the word team was intriguing.

With these simple words and within ten minutes, my life took an amazing turn toward discovery, self-fulfillment, and exploration. It is in this discovery that I began my journey to Zamtan, Zambia, and a continuing relationship with a caregiver community. During an orientation program, we were introduced to our teammates and the culture of Zambia. Our agency provided vital information for our global adventure—personal safety information, immunizations, food, passport and visa requirements, money transfer and rate changes, flight plans, residence accommodations, as well as ground transport. This information was vital as we journeyed with some barriers. Learning about the country, health statistics, mortality and morbidity rates, the HIV prevalence rate, fertility rates, and the people's life expectancy assisted our transition to life in Zambia.

Upon arrival at the International Airport at Lusaka, the capital of Zambia, my eyes viewed all that was dark, in fact, brown in color. Brown trees, plants, buildings, uniforms of security personnel, planes, asphalt, dirt roads—and the people. On the road to our accommodations it was difficult to see through the brown haze emitting from the mines or the burning brush. During the hour's ride to the first village we talked about our roles. The Zambians who would be with us during the journey explained that a tentative schedule was prepared and how that schedule might be affected by the Zambians' unique attitude about time. The schedule of activities is not always followed, and, as in many cultures, Zambians do not have the propensity for being "on time" as we do in the United States. So we learned flexibility and taking opportunities to listen to our hosts and to join their prayers and songs of worship.

At the first village, we were greeted by the entire village council and the community. The scene resembled a whirlwind of color, music, and people of all ages. Hands were touched, smiles were shared, and greetings were acknowledged. The color brown had changed to chocolate, coffee, bronze, tan, auburn, russet with mixtures of red, yellow, green, blue, and purple; truly a mosaic of joy. There were smiles and tears expressed during this celebration. We had gifts for the children, as well as medical and educational supplies for the health care staff. Our first visit was to the school to work with the primary school-aged children. We read stories, played games, and listened as they recited poems and sang songs of welcome. We were prepared to give our gifts to the teacher, but she asked that we distribute some of them to students she had chosen because they were obedient and leaders in their class. Two male students who came before me and I gave the first a book and a packet of crayons. The young man turned to his classmate and gave him the book. I was in awe as I saw the sharing and love that was demonstrated. I said, "Thank you very much for sharing and I have some gifts for him also." It was hard to stop the tears from flowing.

In the villages there were health care providers called nurse aides, who visited the chronically ill, the elderly, and those with HIV, AIDS, malaria, tuberculosis, and chronic lung disease. Members with health care experience were invited to work with them while they made home visits. I was paired with a 19-year-old woman who had been trained as an aide in Lusaka and returned home to care for her people. I offered to carry her medicine box, made of wood and weighing more than the medications and supplies that were inside, as she made her home visits. She introduced me to patients, provided nursing care, taught what was needed, documented her findings, planned for future visits, and prayed following each patient. I asked her, "What did she need to support her in her duties?" She replied, "I have no needs." Yet I saw the need for food, clothing, medicines, and other basic essentials, and it was difficult for me to comprehend her response. Other members visited schools and met teachers and children; some went to the church and met the pastor and some congregation members, while others met with the clinic staff consisting of one nurse, one physician assistant, and a certified midwife. The clinic comprised a two-room cement block building with an entry/admitting room that also stored minimal medications and supplies, and an adjacent treatment room. This clinic served four villages with approximately 19,000 people. A tall, deep well edifice stood close to the clinic and supplied clean water to the clinic school and village. The clinic was a central meeting place for health care, clean water, and socializing.

Each night, team members discussed their day's experiences that included providing health care, visiting with school children and sponsored children, praying with the council members, talking with teachers about attendance requirements, meeting traditional birthing attendants (village midwifes), touring the hospital, and meeting with administrative and government officials. Each day we assessed what we thought were the community's needs. Yet our question to those we met did not elicit a list of needs; rather, the most frequent response was, "Thank you for coming to us." Were we asking the right questions? Following three days with our hosts in different environments, we rearranged the nursing process and its assessment element. We needed a response and validation as to what we could do for their community. We decided to ask, "If there was one thing that I/we could do for you and your people, what would that be?"

The following day, armed with that question, we learned that this was the right path. Each day in Zambia is filled with joyful activity. I never heard a child cry or saw a child alone; many a child was carried by another child; all gifts were shared; and only quiet socializing was heard as the people queued waiting for meetings or classes to begin. This time, when I asked the Zambian health care aide the revised question, she answered, "In an emergency we carry our people to the hospital on our backs or place them in a wheelbarrow to get there. Is there some way you can help us?" Transport, even in the best of times, is difficult in what is considered the "bush" in Zambia. I was so happy; here was something that was a need, defined by one who knew the community best. The next step was the planning stage. I almost ran back to my team to tell them this good news. Communication is a wonderful tool when one knows what and how to ask and to involve others in planning.

In all, the Zambian aides' responses were for the community: clean water, schools, transport, and health care. Most focused on vulnerable women and children. We asked one health care provider, "If you could have the clinic made larger, what would it look like, and what would it provide?" She proceeded to draw on plain white paper a new clinic as she envisioned it. She requested care for vulnerable women and children, such as those made widows and orphans by the ravages of HIV and AIDS, and means for preventing transmission of the HIV virus from the mother to the child at birth. We saw, heard, felt, and validated their needs, and now had a vision to pursue with them into a reality that required great understanding, patience, and resources.

We were captivated by the people of Zamtan, a former "squatters camp." Our short experience enabled us to further study the ways we could assist. It was a plan to offer a "hand up" and not a "hand out." We would partner with a people who creatively used their own resources to meet their needs.

Later, in the United States, we sorted requests, defined priorities, sought resources, and best of all, made new alliances with agencies and people who supported the desire to serve others. We worked in an environment where all things were possible. The year following our journey to Zamtan, our leaders obtained a small, flat-bed truck to transport villagers to the hospital and bring supplies to the community and clinic. Soft-sided carry bags for all homecare providers were obtained and filled with needed supplies, medications, and requested materials. Medications and supplies for the clinic were obtained, financial assistance to build a second well was received, and a meeting room and classroom were designed and scheduled to be built. None of us lost sight of a "new" clinic but we realized that it would take much time, energy, finances, partnership, and commitment from the Zambian government and the villagers. We returned in 2004 to implement our collaborative plans, bringing desired items, architectural plans, and support for building some of the structures, and commitments from some members of the first team as well as new, enthusiastic invitees. Partnerships and commitments were made and discussions regarding the possibilities and logistics surrounding the clinic's construction began. Intense discussions and prayer guided our decision making and communications. Strategies were planned, and long- and short-term goals were made. Always, these were completed in collaboration with the villagers.

As part of our commitment, we returned every year to serve as assessors with some of the original team and others invited to see and hear the "vision." Annual visits involved evaluation of goals and necessary changes with adjusted time lines and business alliances. Additional support materials, medications, and supplies were provided, as well as education as requested by some of the villagers.

Early in 2005, the financial support goal was finally reached; we had sponsors committed to the vision of providing care, not only for the vulnerable women and children, but also for empowering the Zamtan community to provide health care services to all who seek it. Plans were agreed upon by the involved agencies as well as the government and the villagers—the people who were to be served and who also served each other. Groundbreaking occurred in the fall of 2005; within two years of the initial planning, plus negotiating for land, supplies, and workers, and involving Zambians in the physical as well as developmental stages of building their clinic, the clinic was scheduled to open in the summer of 2006. Calling the opening merely a celebration would be an understatement. With all of the villagers, supporters, workers, professional staff, and government officials attending, it was a grand opening beyond all expectations. Where did all of the banners, music, costumes, platforms, food, and people—yes, people—come from? When we first arrived in 2003 there were approximately 19,000 people living in the four villages surrounding Zamtan; the census had now reached 21,000. The services provided within the clinic campus were a regular office clinic; an immediate and urgent care facility; an immunization clinic; total prenatal, delivery, and postnatal care facility; an HIV and AIDS clinic; a tuberculosis clinic; counseling and laboratory services; and a pharmacy.

In 2007, another "vision" trip was planned and I again had the opportunity to become involved in not only using my nursing skills, but also as nurse educator to work with the traditional birthing attendants and pastors from surrounding villages. With an educator, the certified nurse midwife from the clinic, and myself sharing the teaching responsibilities, we provided a two-day workshop for all traditional birthing attendants from the four villages, a total of sixty dedicated women. This was the first time these women had been gathered together at the same time, in the same place, for an educational meeting. Some walked five or six miles each way to attend the classes. With much celebration and songs of worship and joy, education was provided in a professional and simple manner. With the past influence of traditional birthing attendants and the present acceptance of certified nurse midwives, protocols were established and ideas discussed for future meetings.

A pastors' workshop focused on HIV and AIDS education and the ways that their congregations could make a difference. Many pastors took this opportunity to personally connect themselves with the other pastors they met and to create ways in which their churches, together, could respond to the HIV and AIDS pandemic. What a great pathway for pastors to journey on together.

What started as a "vision" trip to assess the health care needs of a distant community in sub-Saharan Africa launched the development of a medical and health care facility that now serves the children and families of Zamtan, an oasis that has contributed to families moving into the area, the building of schools and churches, and the continued commitment by many agencies internationally. The area was visited by numerous learned and inspiring individuals who chose to see true partnerships and the potential for growth and development.

As a nurse, I thought I had experienced the spectrum of patient pain and suffering, and unanticipated acts of caring and compassion. None of my professional or life experiences had prepared me for the caring of brothers for brothers, the acceptance of a simple life, sharing meager resources, love and joy easily expressed, prayers for experiences and just for being alive, government collaboration with people and the community, all levels of professional staff sharing information and visions, and all persons taking a servant's hand for the good of all.

Some of the lessons that I learned were that the true provision of total nursing care requires the integration of all aspects of the body— physical, emotional, and spiritual. Also, I identified that change can only be accomplished *with* the people and not simply for them. Success on such a journey evolved with understanding, patience, commitment, and partnerships to support the vision of improved health care for marginalized people through sustainable, community-based partnerships and interventions.

ZIMBABWE
Mackie H. Norris

As an associate professor of nursing, I was privileged to operate a nursing center located at a low income housing complex. As a part of that responsibility I directed student nurses' experiences and engaged in nursing practice during times when no students were present. The population served was primarily elderly residents. My major task was health education and health promotion, and also involved managing chronic illnesses. The center was a collaborative partnership between the university and the county health department. What prepared me for that responsibility and a future opportunity was my education and practice in the field of community health nursing. This narrative discusses my participation in a team charged with making a recommendation concerning an educational program at an international university. As a team member,

I was intricately involved in determining the most efficient and effective approach for establishing a much-needed educational venture that had the potential to change the lives of people from many nations, immediately and for many years to come. The story follows.

Throughout the region known as sub-Saharan Africa, wars for independence and other reasons influenced residents' lives. Many of the countries gained their independence but paid a great toll on their desired quality of life. In 1980, the country once known as Rhodesia became Zimbabwe following its successful fight for independence. The country was seen as a regional jewel, but political unrest, droughts, and other factors reversed any gains. The current conditions in Zimbabwe are widely publicized; the fighting placed the quality of life in great turmoil with a scarcity of jobs, food, and supportive care, along with an inflation rate that is the highest ever experienced anywhere, estimated at over 11 million percentages by some accounts. All of these factors impacted the quality of life and set it in a continuous decline. Yet, amid all the struggles stands an institution contributing to the betterment of life. Africa University is strategically placed to meet unique and evolving regional needs.

I first visited Zimbabwe in 1994 for the official opening ceremonies of Africa University, a United Methodist–related institution chartered in 1992. In 1988, The United Methodist Church's governing body approved institutional funding in response to dialogue at the World Methodist Council in Nairobi, Kenya, and a proposal presented by two United Methodist bishops serving the 1985 African conferences. The proposal requested that The United Methodist Church establish an institution of higher learning on the African continent. Thus, the journey began to create the Africa University, whose mission statement is "to provide quality education within a Pan-African context through which persons can acquire general and professional knowledge and skills, grow in spiritual maturity, develop sound moral values, ethics, and leadership qualities."

The institution opened its doors in 1992 to forty students enrolled in either the Faculty (College) of Agriculture and Natural Resources or the Faculty (College) of Theology. The master plan called for the addition of other faculties over time, including but not limited to, the Faculty of Medical Sciences. Since 1992 the following have been created: Faculty of Management and Administration, Faculty of Education, Faculty of Humanities and Social Sciences, and the Faculty of Health Sciences. Additionally the Institute of Peace, Leadership, and Governance was opened in 2003.

The introduction of major educational units is aligned with the institution's governance and regional needs. The university's student population is not limited to Zimbabweans, however; enrollment is international with students from twenty-two African nations and beyond, including several United States' students matriculated to this institution for a degree. The teaching faculty represents ten African nations with periodic visiting lecturers from European and Western nations.

I was merely a spectator in this critical, historic development. But that changed in 1998 when I was invited to join a feasibility study team whose task was to conduct a needs assessment with analysis, perform on-site visits to existing health care delivery institutions and organizations, gather information relative to the existing educational opportunities and their offerings, and craft a recommendation, including a time table for implementation, budget, and proposed curricula. The team was headed by a physician with expertise in medical education and public health, and included four other physicians, including two from China and one from Zimbabwe, as well as a college president and its nursing school dean, a dentist, and myself, an experienced nurse educator with community health and care delivery experiences. My role was to provide a nursing perspective to this mission's responsibility.

Our work as a team began in late 1998 when we met in Mutare, Zimbabwe, to develop a feasibility study plan. Although the team mainly consisted of U.S.–educated health practitioners, it was essential to understand the historical characteristics of non-Western, post-colonial health education practices. One team member, a Zimbabwean neurosurgeon, was invaluable to our understanding. Her insights came from dual experience and education—a native Zimbabwean with a Harvard education and training. At the time of the team's visit, she had been working in the United States due to nonexistent opportunities to practice neurosurgery in Zimbabwe, which lacked skilled personnel, hospital facilities, and other support resources.

The British education system is evident in post-colonial Zimbabwe. Points of cross reference were incorporated into our task. For example, the term "faculty" is called "college" or "school" in Western educational systems. Also, many programs offer diplomas and certificates rather than degrees after four years of matriculation.

The name of the faculty (school) was changed to reflect the curriculum intent, which was to prepare health practitioners who would impact the lives, health, and environment of sub-Saharan Africa populations.

The new name became the "Faculty of Health Sciences," rather than "Medical Sciences." The term "health sciences" represented a broader mission and focus than merely preparing physicians. This change had the support of the entire study team and ultimately the governing body. The name change enabled the creation of an advanced training curriculum for persons already holding nursing certificates. The vision for a medical curriculum became part of the program's second phase, with dental education completing the third phase. These development phases were based upon available resources, consideration of long term and immediate impact, and recruitment of potential students.

The study team also explored available resources supportive of health-related curricula, such as laboratories, technicians, in-patient facilities, clinics, and qualified lecturers and professors. Also, the university needed support from existing training institutions as collaborative partners. We visited nursing and medical faculty at the University of Zimbabwe Faculty of Medicine and Dentistry in Harare, Zimbabwe, and spoke with faculty members at institutions in South Africa, Mozambique, and Tanzania. These institutions were chosen because of their general proximity to Africa University and their reputation as schools of choice for health practitioners, a fact supported by data collected in our Health Practitioner Survey.

Some needed data were available through the World Health Organization and the Zimbabwe Ministry of Health. These agencies provided information about life expectancy rates from chronic and infectious diseases and causes of death in the region served by Africa University. Also, the Zimbabwe Ministry of Health had invaluable information about the number and type of personnel employed in health occupations throughout the country. These data informed the final recommendation by the study team.

In early 1999, the study team developed and disseminated a Health Practitioner Survey. Anticipating difficulties in distributing and returning the document, the decision was made to utilize existing contacts for distribution. The surveys were distributed through the offices of regional resident bishops and medical missionaries assigned to sub-Sahara Africa by The United Methodist Church. These routes were used because of the affiliation between The United Methodist Church and Africa University, and the interest of the church officials in supporting a Faculty of Medical Sciences. Attempts were also made to distribute the survey through existing training institutions with very little success. The survey collected information about medical/health training by practitioners and the desire for further training through continuing education and other means that might be provided though the Faculty of Health Sciences. Also, the survey gathered information about the practitioners' perceptions of the region's health needs. The survey shaped the final recommendations offered by the study team.

Eighty-seven surveys were returned for analysis. Because of the routes and methods of distribution, it was impossible to determine the return rate as the distributed amount was unknown. Five sub-Saharan nations were represented by the returned surveys: Angola, Burundi, Kenya, Sierra Leone, and Zimbabwe. The Pan-African response was encouraging. The team met in late 1999 to begin analysis of survey results, compare health data for the region, and draft preliminary options for the Faculty of Health Sciences. Results supported that the region's health needs could best be addressed by practitioners with public health skills and knowledge, and who would be available for an immediate impact on infectious diseases and other chronic health problems in the region served by the university.

Another task of the team was to determine the adequacy of the proposed medical facilities to serve as training sites for students needing clinical placement. Several team members, including myself, visited the Provincial Hospital in Manicaland, one of the seven provinces in Zimbabwe, and some outpatient clinics operated by The United Methodist Church at mission stations throughout the region. Other religious bodies also had hospitals and clinics in the area and at least one private corporation planned to construct a new 120-bed facility in 2001; this construction has not yet begun. Another privately operated hospital facility in Mutare was visited, and its management was receptive to developing a collaborative agreement with university officials. The team determined, at the time of the study, that available local resources were not adequate to support medical, dental, or basic nursing training.

Exploration of possible clinical facilities was not limited to Zimbabwe or sub-Saharan Africa. Because of the connected nature of The United Methodist Church, other United Methodist institutions had opportunities to engage in some manner with the Faculty of Health Sciences.

In the fall of 1999, the feasibility study team reported the following recommendations to the General Board of Higher Education and Ministry: (a) The Faculty name should be changed to The Faculty of Health Sciences to capture the anticipated broader health education and training focus; (b) initial course offerings should be developed for currently certified or licensed nurses and other health professionals seeking to increase their knowledge and skills in public health; (c) a degree program should be developed in Phase 1 for currently certified or licensed nurses to obtain a Bachelor of Science degree; and (d) medical and dental education and training should become part of Phases 2 and 3, respectively. All recommendations were approved and work was begun to secure funding and select a dean for the Faculty of Health Sciences at Africa University. Following the dean's selection, completion of the curriculum with course descriptions, credit hours, prerequisites, and other scholastic duties were addressed. In 2003, the Faculty accepted students for a Bachelor of Science degree for currently registered or certified nurses that required two years of study and an eighteen-month postgraduate diploma in public health for practitioners interested in public health practice. In 2004, the official opening of the Faculty of Health Sciences building was celebrated. The facility construction was funded from various sources. I had the honor of participating in the celebration and of meeting the dean of the Faculty. The first students (four) from the Faculty of Health Sciences graduated in 2006.

Academic year 2008–09 found a total of sixty-four students enrolled. They are fairly equally divided among the programs offered in the Faculty. Full-time faculty and part-time lecturers provide instruction. Enrollment is projected to increase as more funds are made available for student scholarships. When the university enters Phases 2 and 3 of the curricular plan, the projection is that even greater numbers of students will enroll.

From an idea conceived in 1985, to an official opening in 1992, to an exploratory study in 1999, Africa University with its subsequent Faculty of Health Sciences had already made a significant impact in its short history. Collaborations were formed to address the eradication of HIV among children, and vaccines are being tested through the university and the Faculty of Health Science in cooperation with St. Jude Children's Hospital. Public health principles are taught and then applied throughout the region by health practitioners; hopefully, the graduates will help raise the life expectancy of children, decrease the infectious disease rates of sexually communicated and other diseases, and improve the health of others.

I continue to be engaged with Africa University and the Faculty of Health Sciences. My last visit to the campus was in July of 2007 as a part of a Volunteer in Missions team. While there, I worked in the library sorting health and related literature and textbooks for use by students enrolled in the health sciences curricula. I had extended an offer to teach some courses while there, but the school was out for the summer session at that time. In the future, my plans may include spending time at the university during sessions where I will be able to assist in instruction in the health science curricula, particularly for those who have nursing backgrounds and interests. Repeating the words of the mantra describing the existence of Africa University, "The dream is alive!"

11

Nurse Educators Who Work in Central and South America

ARGENTINA

Catherine R. Coverston and Erin Maughan

The shock of entering an open hospital labor room with no form of privacy for the fourteen women was astounding. There were no sheets with which to give them privacy, no hospital gowns, and no family allowed. The stark white tile walls, the stained floors, the beds covered with torn and stained sheets, the women half dressed, and only medical residents and students to care for them made some of us feel ill. The pictures we had seen, the stories we had heard from faculty and students who had been there before us, did not prepare us. After recovering from the initial impact, we went to work. Yes, it was easiest for the students fluent in Spanish to approach a woman and begin to provide labor support, but compassion moved even those of us whose vocabulary would never get much beyond "dulce de leche" to lend to the women the caring support of nursing that crosses all barriers.

The women immediately trusted us. The medical personnel, however, who had never worked with nurses in the labor room, were skeptical. They appreciated the supplies and equipment we brought, but, having never worked with nurses and believing that nurses were only good for giving shots and changing dressings, they had no idea what a difference an educated nurse could make. They soon learned otherwise and were amazed at the knowledge and insight we had. We demonstrated simple techniques to help the women cope with the pain of labor, to read the progress of labor by watching the woman rather than by painful and embarrassing physical exams. Our willingness to listen, learn, and teach led to many changes in attitude and behavior by the medical staff toward the laboring women.

Since 2000, we have been working in a large maternity hospital in the northwestern province of Tucumán in Argentina. Tucumán is one of the poorest provinces of Argentina with a population of almost 1.5 million people in only 22,524 square kilometers, an area smaller than the state of Vermont. The hospital is a public maternity hospital and serves as a referral hospital for surrounding provinces. In 2000, the birth rate at the facility was about 14,000 per year. The Neonatal Intensive Care Unit (NICU) had 60 to 70 occupied beds, and postpartum, 120 beds. Our college was invited to the hospital in Tucumán through a humanitarian organization, Deseret International Foundation (DIF). Our college had been involved in international work since 1995 with sites in Guatemala and Jordan.

The economic situation was already dire in Argentina in 2000. Provinces were printing their own money in order to pay their bills, but the money was only good in the province of origin, so destitution grew as the people were unable to meet their obligations. Public hospitals showed clear signs of inadequate funding. Sterile gloves were hoarded for surgery; water taps, except in the surgical suite, ran only cold water; linens were scarce; and infants were covered with plastic, not blankets. There was no end to the shortages.

In addition, not all the "nurses" had a nursing education. Despite an excellent university with both a medical and nursing school, funding was inadequate. Most nurses who had graduated from the university were in administrative positions. Others who were actually doing nursing work had varying amounts of education and some had only on-the-job training. Most of the staff nurses were in the NICU. Mothers of infants who were stable but not ready to go home were expected to stay in the unit and care for their infants, supervised by a nurse who gave medications and treatments. Midwives provided triage in the labor area, but there were no nurses providing care for patients in labor. Postpartum also had few nurses. There were three floors dedicated to postpartum where mothers stayed twelve to twenty-four hours after a vaginal birth and forty-eight hours after a cesarean birth. Each floor had at least forty patients staffed with two nurses who each worked a twenty-four–hour shift. In postpartum, although the nurses passed medications, their work was mostly record keeping. They did not do regular rounds or assess mothers or infants.

The hospital administration had two requests: provide education for the nurses and investigate why so many women did not come for prenatal care. When we arrived a few months later with twelve undergraduate and three graduate students, we were still unsure of exactly what we would do. Bolstered by the optimism of DIF's leader, we had brought donated supplies we knew would be helpful, including gloves, sheets, baby blankets, patient gowns, and a variety of other supplies donated by our local hospitals. Although the hospital had agreed that our students could rotate through the labor rooms, postpartum, and the NICU, we were unsure about what we would be able to do. Because we had seen the lack of support on our initial assessment visit, we had spent time preparing the students not only to provide support, but how to look for maternal behaviors that signaled advancing labor. It was not long before the residents were asking us how we knew a woman was ready to deliver and they began to trust us and appreciate our presence. Soon we were incorporated into performing maternal and fetal assessments.

One day we came upon a woman who had just delivered and was hemorrhaging. We learned this was not an uncommon problem. After birth, women were left unattended in the delivery room until someone brought her clothes to her to prepare for transfer to postpartum. Once they were in postpartum, there were no assessments or teaching done until medical rounds in the morning or evening. We began our first teaching intervention: We taught the mothers to massage their uterus and why they should. We taught all of our students how to teach this in Spanish. With every delivery, we taught while the residents and medical students were still present. Before long, they were teaching the mothers as well. When we returned the next year, we found the residents and medical students were still continuing the teaching. Because they did not chart postpartum hemorrhage consistently, there was no way to collect data to determine whether it made a difference, but the residents reported to us that it had.

Over the years we have been able to collaborate with our Argentine colleagues to solve many problems. The hospital administration wanted us to help provide education not just to their own hospital, but also to the larger community of health care providers. Working with DIF, LDS charities in Utah, Educar, an educational foundation in Argentina, and the school of nursing from the University of Tucumán, we were able to put together a three-day nursing conference during our second year. The conference included various lectures and interactive training on cardiopulmonary resuscitation, advanced life support, neonatal resuscitation, STABLE, pediatric medications, loss and grief, wound care, and many other topics. This event solidified our acceptance in the community.

As the trust within the relationship grew, we were able to help the hospital staff articulate problems as they saw them and help them work toward interventions. Many of the interventions were student driven as they identified areas that could be improved and discussed them with the staff. For example, the students investigated parents' satisfaction with infant care in the NICU. Over the years we taught developmental and Kangaroo care. We also trained community women to work as doulas and provide breastfeeding support. In 2005, an Argentine graduate nursing student working at the hospital decided to make implementation of developmental care her thesis. Her involvement greatly increased compliance with this important care.

One of our greatest concerns for several years running was poor growth of preterm infants in the NICU. The hospital has "baby friendly" status and all babies receive breast milk if at all possible. We have supported this program with supplies, buying a larger refrigerator and sterilization equipment. However, many preterm infants were not growing adequately. When we raised this issue, we were told there was nothing that could be done. However, we had noticed an inconsistency in feeding practices. We discovered that there were discrepancies among what was ordered, what was given, and what was charted. Because several hospitals in our hometown area in the United States had been researching feeding protocols for preterm infants, we asked our local team of researchers to help us with a protocol to take to Argentina. The implementation of a feeding protocol was a wonderful learning experience. Although the physicians in Tucumán were well educated, they had no access to current research even though they could read English. Our university's online library resources allowed us to do searches for the literature about feeding practices. The Argentine physicians were then able to read the literature themselves and decide what they believed was possible considering their financial restraints. Once the physicians agreed, our graduate student was able to work with the physicians and nurses to implement the protocol, turning it over to them so they would have ownership. Data have shown that implementation of the protocol saved lives, reduced the incidence of complications, and increased infant weight gain.

Most recently, at the request of a patient and staff committee, students created posters about intimate partner violence and posted them in all the hospital bathrooms. Calls to the help line increased significantly after the postings. In addition, the group wanted some written literature concerning family planning, again a student project. We provided enough brochures for one year and identified local funding sources so that the creation of brochures could continue. Because many Argentine women are Catholic and prefer to use only the rhythm method, one faculty had students make Cycle Bead bracelets to help the women follow the method.

By 2004, we were aware that much could be done within the community to help prevent some of the complications encountered in the hospital. If we could expand clinical experiences to the community, more students could be involved and would be able to interact with the families they had known only in the hospital. Several students and a community health nursing instructor visited a very poor area of the city of Tucuman, called Las Tipas. We had a meeting with a local sanatoria, a lay health promotion worker, to learn about the needs of the area and to discuss possibilities for student involvement. One major theme was identified: malnutrition. In an effort to combat the problem, government and humanitarian aid organizations provided meals to children via comedors, small, often outdoor, kitchens that served only one meal a day. In 2004, we observed how the comedors, run by local volunteers, functioned, and determined that medical students could conduct height and weight screenings of the children to determine risk of malnutrition.

We had gained the trust of the community and devised a plan from our assessment. Students worked in groups of four per each comedor and its surrounding area; they accompanied the sanatoria, conducted home visits, and taught classes. The students conducted community assessments of hemoglobin and height and weight screenings with the sanitorias and medical students, making it a true partnership. In all, 353 children were assessed for height, weight, arm circumference, and hemoglobin. Of these children, 42 were found to be malnourished (12%), according to BMI, and 22 were found to be anemic (12% of the 184 were hemoglobin tested). Students interviewed families and learned about the barriers to proper nutrition, which included lack of knowledge, lack of resources, and nutrition as a low priority. Students also identified several other needs including oral health, lack of running water, and sanitation issues. One group organized a trash clean-up day for their area. Enlisting the children in the area they picked up bags and bags of trash and in the process taught the students the importance of sanitation and community pride.

Students presented their data and findings to the local sanatoria who oversaw the area, as well as the medical doctor from the local health clinic and other civic and religious leaders. All worked together in discussing solutions and ideas. Two students used the principles learned in the community assessment project and applied them in the hospital. After identifying a need on the adolescent postpartum floor, students created nutrition posters for the hospital walls. Two other students worked on independent projects to better identify barriers and increase mothers' knowledge about good nutrition. These data were invaluable in the community project.

We have been able to maintain our relationship with the sanatorias and the comedors and, in 2007, added a local senior center. Height, weight, and hemoglobin screenings were conducted again, this time on older adults as well as the children. In addition, one student conducted a project that looked at the nutritional content of food served at the comedors because we noticed that the meals did not contain all the nutrients children needed. The comedors were meant to supplement what the children ate at home; however, for many children, these meals were the only food. In addition, in some areas where space was limited, children brought their food home, instead of eating it at the comedor. Sanatorias noticed that the food would then be shared with the entire family, decreasing the calories meant for the malnourished child.

In 2007 we also added 24-hour recall food journals for the children and analyzed their meals for iron content. One of the most significant findings was that 54.7% of the beverages (mostly mate, a very important local drink) were found to be iron inhibitors. So although iron was being consumed, the body was not absorbing it. These results, along with recommendations on how to increase iron in the diet, were shared with the local sanatoria workers and doctors. This was also a great learning experience where the students learned about culturally sensitive interventions. The people of Argentina are certainly not going to stop drinking mate, so the students had to provide workable suggestions such as drinking at times other than meals, so as to allow the iron in the meals to be better absorbed.

These experiences helped students broaden their understanding, learn about another culture, and practice important nursing skills. The impact on the students is evident in the following quotes:

"This [community experience] is when I learned that as a nurse, I will have to start small, at the root of health problems and hazards.

I cannot change things overnight and can only give my knowledge to help others."

"Helping others to change does not include giving them hand-outs; true change occurs when we give people the necessary tools so that they can make the change themselves."

BRAZIL
Esther G. Bankert, Joanne Joseph, and Kathleen Sellers

At SUNYIT we proposed the framework of service-based learning for students and faculty to allow them to acquire cultural sensitivities and competencies, and to advance professionally within their chosen discipline. We discovered this can become actualized through recently formed our global partnerships with students and educators who share mutual respect, humility, compassion, and the quest for patient-centered care, innovative exchanges, diversity and change in curricula, and collaboration.

Our recent ventures brought SUNYIT students, faculty, the dean, and staff to Brazil to explore collaborative partnerships where service-based learning projects could be actualized. Three major universities were visited by the dean of nursing, nursing and psychology faculty members, and one graduate and two baccalaureate nursing students to learn of partnering relationships within the disciplines of nursing, psychology, and sociology over a ten-day period. We visited three major universities: One was located in Belo Horizonte (500 miles from Sao Paulo) and two others were separated by a car ride of two hours or approximately 100 miles. Each university we visited provided different educational levels, from pre-licensure to graduate programs; we centered our attention on programs in nursing, psychology, and sociology, which were available in traditional classroom settings and Web-enhanced/online virtual forums as well.

Our first visit was to Isabella Hendricks University (IHU) in Belo Horizonte. This university is rich in tradition, having been founded by Methodist missionaries in the early part of the nineteenth century. Upon entering IHU with our translator, mutual connections and open dialogue began immediately. We met with the university's representative from the vice president and the nurse director; all parties were excited and warmly received, especially considering that service-based opportunities could be actualized with students and faculty from SUNYIT and Brazil.

A visit was also made to a nurse-directed clinic in the city's heart where community services were desperately needed. The clinic's nursing administrator provided us with an overview of their services. We were impressed by the independence these nurses demonstrated while meeting the community's needs and learning to advance in their profession. We actively engaged in discussions and discovered that we could learn much from their work ethic and from collaboration with our student nurses at the baccalaureate and advanced practice levels. We identified service-based opportunities with our Brazilian colleagues, and collaborated to develop an interdisciplinary primary care clinic with nurse and psychology leadership, nursing and psychology students, and community volunteers, all sharing the philosophy of serving impoverished populations. We were delighted to learn that their nursing program's conceptual framework was based on the renowned nurse theorist Dorothea Orem's self-care model, and that this theory was commonly known to nurses in other parts of Brazil.

The clinic and the nursing program had a strong natural sciences core; however, current nursing practices in the clinic focused on what we identified as practices from thirty years past when nursing services included the autoclave and the sterilization of bandages and instruments before treating patients. All supplies were donated by manufacturing companies, but the preparation of kits and folding packages were done by nursing students.

Our shared foundation created opportunities with IHU faculty and students for nursing, psychology, and sociology. With enthusiasm we drafted a plan for forums for exchanging concentrated content areas that cross cultures and yet are meaningful to basic levels of the three disciplines. These forums included workshops on English as a second language; Portuguese for health care professionals; and health assessment skills. These offerings were to be designed to accommodate online or classroom learning based on the school's resources; to include concentrated sessions with hands-on experience; to team Brazilian and U.S. students as peer tutors in language courses; and to combine real time discussions in the classroom with virtual discussions where resources allowed.

Our discussions focused on exploring exchange programs and teaching content in nursing theory. We also included content designed to foster leadership skills within interdisciplinary teams, respectful dialogue within health teams where nurses are often in subservient roles, and supportive skills to foster professional accountability and shared responsibility. Our mutual goal was to enrich studies within nursing, psychology, and sociology programs with both IHU students/faculty with SUNYIT, and SUNYIT students/faculty with IHU. Content areas could be expanded to include critical thinking, evidenced-based practices, and team research projects.

During our visit, the service-based learning project was actualized with two baccalaureate nursing students working with the volunteers at an orphanage in the city of Belo Horizonte for children diagnosed with IIIV. The orphanage provided a rich experience for our nursing students who assisted with basic chores of the orphanage and maintained the facility. Their work focused on teaching children basic hygiene and improving the living environment. They engaged students, faculty, and staff to support the children in using proper hand-washing techniques while applying Nightingale's principles of cleanliness and Pender's model of health promotion. The students studied late that night so they could teach hand washing techniques while singing "Happy Birthday" in Brazil's native language, Portuguese. They explained the twenty-second rule to "stomp out germs." They themselves purchased soap and paper towel dispensers for all orphanage bathrooms to encourage children to continue proper hygiene; these purchases came with the guarantee that supplies would continue to be provided. This service-learning experience with students and faculty working side by side was a collaborative effort with the orphanage's volunteers and older children who would continue modeling the lessons taught.

Research projects also emerged in which the psychology doctoral students and the nurse leadership could work with the SUNYIT faculty. Some examples of interest included obesity in children and stories of breast cancer survivors and their resilience.

Universidade Metodista de Sao Paolo (UNESP) is located outside Sao Paolo, a metropolis of seventeen million people. UNESP does not have a nursing program. However, they do have a robust health psychology program and are interested in collaborating with both the SUNYIT Psychology Department and the School of Nursing and Health Systems in numerous research endeavors. They discussed studies of cross-cultural replication on adverse childhood experiences and its impact on adolescent pregnancy complications and risks, and the resilience of breast cancer survivors.

We met the Vice President for Distance Education who toured us through the distance education offices and labs. UNESP's distance education program is quite complex and fully supported with resources from the Brazilian government to democratize higher education. Distance learning is viewed as a means to bring formal educational opportunities to the vast rural areas of Brazil, thus offering higher education to many who otherwise would not have access to this privilege.

The distance learning platform is an open contract based on a model from the Massachusetts Institute of Technology and, thus, there may be opportunities for online courses between UNESP and SUNYIT. They utilize a team approach for course design. The professor gives a weekly lecture via satellite that is projected to a class of 300 to 400 students. Students are then supported by tutors in groups of eight to facilitate virtual seminars.

Our last visit was to Universidade Metodista de Piracicaba (UNIMEP). This university is located in a more rural area near the small city of Piracicaba. The area resembles upstate New York with fields of sugar cane instead of corn. The region is on the verge of an economic boom as sugar cane is emerging as a source of bio-fuel.

We soon discovered that the nursing program at Universidade Metodista de Piracicaba is very similar to SUNYIT's baccalaureate nursing programs. The collaboration seemed seamless and a perfect fit to employ numerous exchange endeavors and faculty research projects. Discussions of current research with high interests in gerontologic populations seemed to brighten all involved on this trip, with many suggestions to replicate current studies as cross-cultural studies. A validation of Gueldner's well-being picture scale within the Brazilian population was a project many faculty at multiple sites could engage in, with students assisting in the data collection. Plans for research included submitting proposals to the Institutional Review Boards for Human Subjects and starting these projects with IRB approvals. Plans for a "nurse's week" for students was suggested with the possibility of faculty exchanges. The activities could be replicated and offered at both campuses. We are currently dialoguing with SUNYIT faculty to invite our guests during the summer months when our Brazilian friends could be hosted at the college dorms.

Also discovered was high interest in offering an online course in Portuguese for our students, which would be taught by a professor and graduate of SUNY Albany currently working in the Office of International Affairs at UNIMEP, Brazil. This proposed course is being addressed with the School of Arts and Science faculty as a possible distance education course.

Lastly, we designed a multidisciplinary course that is currently under committee review for endorsement. We designed this cross-discipline and cross-cultural course using a team approach. We anticipate that this new course will facilitate inviting our translator as a visiting lecturer, assisting us with teaching the course and speaking at professional forums.

As we continue to develop our university partnerships with the people of Brazil, our service-based learning projects also extend to annual humanitarian missions along the Amazon River. We are embarking on our second humanitarian mission in remote villages of the Amazon to provide health care, social support, and medical supplies, and to make lasting friendships that will forever change who we are. Our partnership with the people of Brazil has put new meaning to "nursing without borders" and has helped us understand we are not very different.

CENTRAL AMERICA
Patricia Kinser and Chris DeWilde

Our bags were packed to the brim. They were not full of clothes or tourist paraphernalia, but with supplies to support our annual week-long trip to establish and operate health clinics in a third-world country. We were taking 8,530 children's vitamins, 1,380 prenatal vitamins, 20 bottles of scabies medication, numerous malnutrition and rehydration packets, 400 doses of parasite medications, and more.

During the previous year, our team prepared to spend spring break in a rural mountainous area of Haiti. Unfortunately, due to a bout of increased political unrest in the Haitian capital, our plans were derailed. As anyone who has done medical mission work in a third-world country knows, flexibility is key. So, with a week before our scheduled departure to Haiti, we scrambled to find another area in need of our health care services, and of course we did.

The 2008 mission team included one nurse practitioner, six nursing students (one of whom is the second author), and two registered nurses. Together we flew to the Dominican Republic, drove five hours up mountain roads to San Juan de la Miguana, and established a base camp at a lovely guesthouse. To our pleasant surprise there were functioning toilets, which contrasted with previous experiences in Haiti. In the rural areas of the Dominican Republic, residents receive minimal to no regular health care; our goal was to expand our team's worldview, expose nursing students to the health needs of another culture, and help students incorporate lessons learned from this setting to the provision of care in the multicultural United States. As service learning, the mission trip would enable students to apply culturally sensitive nursing interventions as they combine the multiple domains of nursing—psychomotor skills, cognition, and compassion.

The annual international mission experience provides an experiential medium for the maturation of our nursing students and faculty as individuals and as professionals. Students, faculty, and alumnae from the Bon Secours Memorial School of Nursing have been participating in outreach mission trips since 2000 to Haiti, the Dominican Republic, and the Eastern Shore of Virginia, offering nursing students an opportunity to learn and practice community health nursing in settings with limited resources. Students' comments, both during and after the mission trips, reveal changes in self-confidence and increased abilities with independent critical thinking. In addition, through the required preparatory course entitled Transcultural Nursing and participation in the trip itself, interpersonal culturally competent skills increase, as students increasingly respect others' differences. The experience gained during these mission trips is difficult to replicate in our developed country. Participants leave one's comfort zone, provide quality nursing care to individuals of a different culture, communicate via translators, and work side-by-side with other nursing students and faculty for one week. These elements weave together to become foundational for personal and professional growth.

Each day we travel in the back of pick-up trucks to different *barrios* (neighborhoods) whose residents had not seen health care providers in years. Our mobile clinics were held anywhere convenient to the people—one day in a church, the next in a community center, another day in someone's home or under a thatched roof by the side of the road. We never quite understood whose thatched roof it was, or why it was there at all, but the people came, and came, and came. They brought chairs for us to use in the clinic while they stood, some for hours at a time in the hot sun, waiting to be seen by our team.

The clinic's layout included an area for intake and triage, three assessment stations, and a pharmacy. The settings afforded minimal privacy, making critical and creative thinking necessary to provide discrete care. The "pharmacy" was a large wooden box filled with medications we stocked each day. We cared for patients who were suffering from hypertension, cough/colds, parasites, amoebas, infected wounds, vaginal infections, headaches, GERD, scabies, dehydration, malnutrition, and more.

Over 1,000 patients were seen in the six days as our small team worked diligently to provide the highest quality of care. It was not feasible to take enough medications to treat everyone for every aspect of needed care; the needs were too great. So, with patient safety in mind, medications were provided for acute conditions and education was provided for chronic illnesses and complication prevention. For example, a patient with symptoms of an active myocardial infarction was given aspirin and quickly driven to the nearest hospital—a journey that would have taken an entire day by foot—whereas a patient previously diagnosed with hypertension was provided with heart-healthy diet education and given a referral to a local clinic to refill their prescription, where the effectiveness of the antihypertensives could be followed more closely. Patients with new diagnoses would leave our clinic with enough medication to either treat their current acute condition or begin a longer-standing regimen. Patients were referred to a local physician for follow-up, if needed, and copies of their charts were provided to the physician to allow for optimum continuation of care.

However, much of what we gave our patients was not about medications. It was teaching, it was time, and it was care. In those clinics we taught hand-washing, hydration, nutrition, and chronic disease prevention to the local residents. We taught them practical, not unrealistic, ways of acquiring clean water to clean infected wounds. Though most patients were not educated, they were certainly bright, and we were not the first to tell them they needed to be using and drinking clean water. But for many, it seemed, we were the first to take the time to learn about the day-to-day experiences of their lives and to educate them about ways of obtaining clean water without disrupting their delicate work/life balance. We taught them ways to ensure that clean water was always on hand, about the best times of day to eat to stave off the debilitating effects of hunger, and how to find hidden nutrition by drinking the stock from boiled vegetables rather than discarding it.

It is enlightening to be the student providing this teaching. In the typical hospital-based clinical setting in nursing school, we are not usually afforded the opportunity to have the real life experience of meeting a patient in his or her home or village and to create a plan of care in such a culturally appropriate manner. As a nursing student, it was an amazing opportunity to personally provide care that included traditional healing practices, education to the patient about recognizing signs and symptoms and how to seek help, and finally, education about the disease itself. No matter how diligently a student has attended class or how conscientiously a student has prepared for tests, none of that compares to the depth of understanding and integration of the subject matter in students' minds when it is applied to humans in their care. It is a powerful teaching tool, even beyond the clinical experience within the hospital setting. Furthermore, I was provided with a sense of personal fulfillment from holding the hand of those in need and demonstrating true compassion through the care I provided.

The preparatory course, Transcultural Nursing, focuses on delivery of culturally competent nursing care. Students develop a self-awareness of their own values and beliefs, as well as analyze major concerns and issues encountered by nurses in various populations. Instead of focusing solely on other cultures, the class enables changes in students' attitudes and knowledge because the class begins with an analysis of their own culture. This process is relevant to prepare for working in a third-world country and to be a culturally competent practitioner in our own country. Students are reminded that a holistic view of patients is important whenever the nurse assesses and develops health promotion interventions. Although the course is sixteen weeks long, it is emphasized that developing cultural competence is a life-long process of cultural awareness, knowledge, skill, and encounters. Students learn that memorizing facts about different cultures is not as important as the ability to challenge presumptions, contemplate personal beliefs, and communicate openly.

While providing health care in a rural area of Haiti, a woman came to the clinic experiencing pain due to a rash on her abdomen. Upon assessment, she was diagnosed immediately with shingles, due to the characteristic unilateral band of fluid-filled blisters on her trunk. She reported that the rash was due to the presence of an evil spirit, so she had been placing a heated spoon on the rash in attempt to burn the evil away.

Our "Western medicine" explanatory model of shingles is that the rash is caused by a viral outbreak of herpes zoster, which cannot necessarily be cured, but the severity of symptoms can be reduced by use of antiviral medications. Belief in the supernatural is widely accepted in many traditional cultures and should be discussed with patients. How would you, as the nurse, provide education to this patient about this virus, when the patient has a completely different explanation for her condition?

Critical thinking through case studies and learning to apply culturally competent caring interventions to the situation help prepare students for situations they may face on their upcoming mission trip and beyond. Through this and other learning activities during the Transcultural Nursing course, students report that they enjoy exploring "feelings about certain kinds of patients that we will all come in contact with sometime during our nursing career" and "this course is greatly enlightening and has changed how I view the world and the people I will be caring for."

In addition to expanding views on culturally focused nursing practice, the Transcultural Nursing course offers an opportunity for team-building and for learning about the culture where we will provide care. Students and faculty work together to plan for the trip, from studying key phrases of the local language to learning about typical medical conditions that would be faced, to discussing ways to provide appropriate health education and medications to the local residents. With knowledge that the mission trip's goal is to support self-sustainability of the community, students are reminded of the importance of health-promotion teaching that enables residents to help themselves achieve a better quality of life.

During the Transcultural Nursing course, students and faculty work hand-in-hand on fundraising efforts. By running school- and community-based fundraising activities, we not only raise the necessary financial support, but also raise awareness throughout our school and community about the value of community outreach. Other students, faculty, and staff witness the passion and commitment of our mission team; often, this encourages them to undertake local or international community work themselves.

While our trips to the Dominican Republic and Haiti have an immediate impact on the health of the people we served, our hope is that the impact runs deeper. A short-term mission trip is not necessarily the solution to a problem, but rather the opportunity to embrace others and enhance the community's health. By showing that we care, by providing nursing presence, by holding the hand of the hurt and sick, we spread a sense of hope to our patients and empower them to care for themselves and each other. The success of a mission trip is difficult to measure—Is it the number of medications that were distributed? Is it the number of patients that were seen? Or the personal impact on the team members?

As nurse educators, it is relevant to consider the impact of mission trips on our students and ourselves. There are a multitude of reasons that students report to explain their interest in a nursing mission trip. Most often, the various drives for participating include the desire for hands-on experience in providing care, giving back to a community in need, improving critical thinking skills, spiritual fulfillment, and personal education, among others. In addition, educators may have similarly diverse reasons for leading trips. Certainly, my greatest satisfaction comes from seeing the growth of my students, both as individuals and as nurses. I am able to provide them with an avenue for improving their nursing skills without the added pressure of thinking about grades; I am able also to give them hands-on experience in another culture and facilitate learning experiences in a short but continuous period of time.

The work required to prepare for and lead a mission trip is considerably greater and more demanding than that required for a classroom teaching role. Considering this is my third year leading our annual mission trip, there must be something even deeper than the personal satisfaction provided to me when I see the growth in my students. Indeed, I gain significant personal fulfillment when I am able to work first-hand with populations in great need. There is a natural amount of selfishness related to mission trips—while I am able to give an education to my students and health care to our patients, I also am able to truly receive the gift of deepening my practice, increasing my knowledge, and improving my abilities to teach. In a setting where our daily needs are taken care of by our local guides, I am able to focus more on my students and our patients. I do not have the distractions of committee meetings, lesson planning, and research. Rather, in a beautiful setting, with a group of talented women and men, I relax and apply my knowledge for the betterment of my students, our patients, and myself. So, as a nurse educator, it does always come back to education—the education of my students, our patients, and myself.

When students and faculty return from the mission trips, we all experience a sense of urgency to continue supporting the health and wellness of the community we served. After a recent mission trip to Haiti, it became readily apparent that setting up an educational partnership between our school and a nursing school in that country would be of great benefit to the health of Haitians and to our students. Realizing that our week-long work in the clinics can have limited long-term effects, discussions were initiated with the dean of the only baccalaureate nursing school in Haiti. After electronic discussions and one face-to-face meeting, our school began to provide numerous resources for this nursing school, such as textbooks, practice glucometers, and catheter kits. Equipment that would be considered out-of-date and unusable in the United States has found new life in assisting Haitian nursing students with their education. We recognize that enabling long-term change to occur in Haiti requires enhancing the health-related infrastructure and availability of nurses. Our school plans to continue working closely with the Haitian nursing school and other organizations within Haiti regarding resource exchange, lecture "swapping" (via video feeds), and potential exchange programs. Similarly, during our next mission trip in 2009 to the Dominican Republic, we hope to establish partnerships with schools and clinics for which we can provide additional support that goes beyond our yearly visits.

As a nurse educator, I feel privileged to have had these opportunities to work with numerous students in the Transcultural Nursing class and in our outreach to Haiti and the Dominican Republic. Taking students out of their own (and my) comfort zone provides invaluable opportunities for transformative nursing education and personal growth. In every instance, I witness tremendous progress in their assessment skills, critical thinking, management abilities, and communication patterns. Even more importantly, students develop a passion for learning from their patients, instead of endeavoring to simply jump in and provide cures for an illness. Indeed, students learn about teamwork, cross-cultural communication, and provision of nursing care with limited resources; yet, through this immersion experience, they gain a truer sense of self and clarity of vision regarding the meaning of nursing. In conclusion, the words of one student captured the essence of her experience: "The Dominican Republic changed my life. I knew that the work we were doing was special, and I knew that it would indeed require long hours of fundraising, planning, and organizing. I knew that all of us were serving a cause much greater than ourselves. What I did not know was that the sum of what we were all offering as individuals would grow into a life-altering call to service, and that the care we were providing would create a spiritual connection with the people we were helping, as well as with one another. It is this call to service and spiritual connectedness that has helped shape my goals as a health care provider and deepen my passion for providing humanitarian aid."

ECUADOR
Kim Curry

The University of Tampa is a private, comprehensive university with a student body of about 5,800 undergraduate and graduate students. The Department of Nursing consists of three degree programs: a baccalaureate program, an RN to BSN transition program, and an MSN program offering family health or adult health nurse practitioner tracks. The university maintains an active quality-enhancement program that, for the past five years, has focused on international education. To support these efforts, the university has an office of international programs to assist faculty and students in experiencing international travel and gaining skills specific to major areas of study and scholarship.

Until 2005, the Department of Nursing did not offer international experiences specific to nursing students. The reasons for this included the limited number of faculty (eight full-time faculty), the busy classroom and clinical schedules of the students with limited time availability, few existing programs tailored to the nursing curriculum, and the complexities of setting up and initiating this type of travel course.

The nursing department director and faculty were contacted in 2005 by a local community college to discuss a collaborative international course. An existing troika experience was presented as a possible collaborative effort. We pursued this opportunity because it overcame several obstacles we faced in creating our own course. Working with faculty from other schools, we were provided with additional faculty to accompany students. Because course arrangements were handled through Community Colleges for International Development (CCID), travel and in-country arrangements were already in place. Finally, the course's focus was critically important. The emphasis was on transcultural nursing involving numerous experiences in direct patient care and community health nursing. We agreed to participate in the summer 2006 troika program.

By definition, troika experience involves three schools traveling together. For purposes of bus travel within the country, there is a limit on trip numbers to no more than twenty to twenty-five people, including one or two faculty per school. One University of Tampa faculty member and two students attended the inaugural trip. No scholarship money was available to the University of Tampa nursing students to subsidize trip expenses. However, one undergraduate and one graduate student asked to participate and were selected.

A didactic course, including an introduction to the country, health statistics, and basic Spanish words, was offered online to all students and faculty. This course helped prepare students for arrival in Ecuador. For example, few Ecuadorian citizens, including almost all medical professionals, speak English. Translators and bilingual students and faculty were necessary for successful service and learning. Ecuador converted to the United States dollar as currency in 2000, so exchanging money was not necessary but understanding coin and bill references in Spanish was a challenge for some.

The in-country experience consists of one week in Quito, Ecuador's capital, and one week in the Napo province, a rural rainforest region on the east side of the Andes Mountains, a part of the country known as the oriente. When this course was originally developed, the founding faculty member had experience as a missionary in Ecuador through a religious organization and had established some in-country contacts. The Central University of Ecuador School of Nursing agreed to an annual collaboration with the University of Tampa. In addition, a missionary with several decades of experience in Ecuador agreed to coordinate the in-country arrangements. Finally, faculty from Arizona State University, which maintains an educational camp in the Napo region, coordinated rural field experiences.

While in Ecuador, students were exposed to South American medical practices, hospitals and other medical facilities to deliver patient care, and the Quechua Indian culture in the Napo region. Early in the trip, students spent a day at the Central University nursing school in Quito and received instruction about Ecuadorian nursing education. The baccalaureate degree is the minimum preparation for a nursing license. However, no nursing doctoral programs exist and advanced practice and specialization are very uncommon. Most nursing faculty are at the master of science level.

Faculty from the United States nursing programs accompanied students and participated in all experiences as well. Some faculty served additionally as translators. Faculty were responsible for ensuring student safety and monitoring practice. Students and faculty wore professional nursing attire to all patient care experiences. Examples of specific medical and cultural learning experiences included:

1. Visits, guided tours, and patient care in a major public hospital, private hospital, chronic psychiatric facility, and children's hospital
2. Interviews with Ecuadorian nursing students
3. A tour of the Museum of Nursing History at the School of Nursing in Quito
4. Discussion of medical insurance coverage and professional liability differences between the United States and Ecuador
5. A visit to the town of Tena to conduct a windshield assessment of health facilities
6. A lecture on herbal medicine and a herbal plant hike
7. Discussion of Quechuan health beliefs and childbirth practices
8. Work with local public health departments in the community.

To date, fourteen students have participated, representing the university's three nursing programs. A written evaluation is completed at the trip's conclusion. Student comments and evaluations have been overwhelmingly positive. The trip is popular with students, who now independently seek other opportunities for international medical work. In addition, the student applications have increased annually. In 2008, twenty students applied for five available seats, despite the trip's expense. For the past two years, an alumna's family contributed $4,000 per year toward partial student scholarships. We were notified that this amount increased for 2009. Students who receive the scholarship communicate with the donor family individually before and after the trip, sharing travel results and photographs.

Ecuadorian faculty members have traveled to Tampa to visit the two nursing schools participating in the troika experience. This occurred despite considerable resistance from the Ecuadorian government to grant international travel visas to nurses. The faculty visits enabled us to exchange further information about associate and baccalaureate educational preparation, and the growing number of doctoral programs. Many Ecuadorian nursing faculty expressed a desire for doctoral preparation.

In the future, we hope to arrange opportunities for their educational experiences.

A few of our powerful take-home messages were:

- One cannot understand a country's health care system and beliefs without understanding something of that country's history and politics.
- Insight into your own culture is gained by expanding your knowledge of other cultures. Without this knowledge, there is nothing to compare and contrast, creating a cultural blindness.
- The European-based, illness-oriented medical system practiced in the United States is not necessarily the best method for solving all health problems.

Organizing and implementing international experiences of this complexity involve months of planning, preparation, and education. While it is never possible to feel adequately prepared for a trip of this magnitude, students are provided with detailed lists of recommended travel items including clothing, food, medications, mosquito protection, and toiletries.

Difficult to convey to students are the cultural differences that they will experience. Also, the trip is physically demanding with considerable physical activity and several daily planned experiences. Ecuadorians tend to be more physically active than their U.S. counterparts. In addition, there is little unscheduled time. This may be the most difficult aspect for some students. The physical and emotional shock, a true culture shock, results in occasional emotionally wrenching experiences for some participants.

Faculty members have discussed this situation and have developed appropriate student and faculty screening mechanisms. These incorporate both specific information about the trip (you will see very large bugs, you will walk several miles each day, etc.) and questions related to the student's background, including travel history, dietary habits, need for schedule adherence, and related items. This tool is refined each year and helps in selecting students who are a match for this course.

Joining an existing travel experience is an invaluable opportunity to learn from experienced faculty. To date, the University of Tampa's Nursing Department has offered three summer trips to Ecuador. Using student evaluations, we have considered requests for formal Spanish language instruction and plan an international experience in Mexico. Students receive Spanish health care training as well as community and cultural health experiences. We are excited about our international experiences in Latin America.

GUATEMALA
Deborah Bell and Debbie Mahoney

We first visited San Raymundo, Guatemala, in June of 2000. We were struck by the overwhelming need of the poor of Guatemala. Many of the poor have no access to health care. The infant and child mortality rate is among the highest in Latin America. Safe drinking water is not available in most areas of the country. The literacy rate is low. Guatemala has the highest perinatal mortality rate in Central America. In addition, this small but populous country ranks sixth in the world in terms of malnutrition among children. Guatemala had a thirty-six year civil war that ended in 1996 that devastated the country, resulting in virtually no infrastructure to provide and maintain essentials such as roads, schools, and hospitals. Guatemala has also experienced numerous natural disasters such as hurricanes, earthquakes, floods, and mudslides.

On that first trip, many of us treated patients suffering from giardia, a water-borne illness. One particular infant was treated for dehydration and touched us deeply. Deborah Bell wrote: "When he cried, there were no tears; his mouth was parched as he lay in his mother's arms, limp. When he cried, it was a quiet weak cry, not what you would expect from a 9-month-old baby boy. When he cried, his mother would put him to her breast to feed him, but he would soon lose interest and cry out, seeming to be in pain. When he cried, his eyes would roll back in his head and his head would drop back as if he didn't have the strength to hold it up any longer." This child had parasites. He was "wormed" and given intravenous fluids. He would soon be able to drink from the same water source that caused the illness and the likelihood of survival is grim. There are many such children seen at each clinic.

Within two years, Deborah Bell co-founded Refuge International, a nongovernmental, nonprofit organization. The mission statement reads, "Refuge International is dedicated to the goal of improving the lives of families and individuals through the collaborative development of sustainable programs in areas where health care, adequate nutrition, clean water, and education are lacking or nonexistent. We believe that all of humanity is of equal worth and should have their essential needs met without regard to culture, ideology, or religion. When people reach out to meet a need, those who choose to help benefit as do those who are in need."

Initial efforts focused on health care. Texas nurses and physicians held clinics in aldeas or villages in Guatemala. Patients were seen, and life-saving surgeries were performed. The first clinical site was in San Raymundo, which is about one and one-half hours from the Guatemala City airport. Another clinical site, Sarstun, was added. Sarstun is a more remote location on the eastern coast of Guatemala and is inaccessible by roads. Traveling to Sarstun entails a five-hour ride from the airport, an overnight stay in the port city of Porto Barrios, then a two-hour boat ride. With the help of partners in Guatemala and the United States, a clinic/hospital was constructed in Sarstun. There is now a Guatemalan

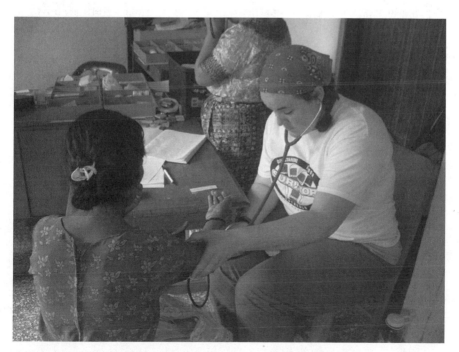

Morgan Booth, a nursing student at Harding University, treating a patient at a mission surgical clinic in Guatemala.

physician, supported by Refuge International, who is providing care to 12,000 people in an area where there was previously no access to health care. One of the women told a Refuge volunteer, "Before Refuge came to Sarstun, our children were dying. Now, our children don't die anymore." A third Guatemalan clinical site, Chocola, was added in July of 2008.

It quickly became apparent that the lack of clean drinking water was the cause of much illness and mortality. Deborah Bell and other volunteers attended drilling school. A portable drill was purchased and wells were drilled, providing clean drinking water for entire villages in San Raymundo, Sarstun, San Juan, and Alta Vera Paz. Efforts to drill more wells are ongoing.

In 2005, Hurricane Stan devastated the western coastal areas of Guatemala, causing landslides that buried entire villages. Crops were lost and starvation was imminent. Through collaborative efforts with USAID and another nongovernment agency, containers of dehydrated food were distributed to the hardest hit areas.

Malnutrition remains the principal health problem in Guatemala. As in all developing countries, those most affected are children under the age of five. One Guatemalan woman, working with Refuge, tells the story of entering a family's home where the father was eating three eggs along with some beans and corn tortillas. The four children in the family were allowed to eat the tortillas dipped in the beans but nothing else. The situation's reality is that the father had to have enough to eat to continue working. There are many such stories in Guatemala.

When they initially arrived in the Sarstun area, health care volunteers were struck by the degree of malnourished children. They had bloated bellies, stringy hair, and open sores on their upper and lower extremities. Parasites are quite common in Guatemala. Food is scarce and what little nutrition the children received was being robbed by intestinal parasites. Initial de-worming efforts consisted of administering Albendazole to patients presenting at the clinic for medical care. At the next visit to the Sarstun area, it was noted anecdotally that the children appeared much healthier. The open sores were healed, their hair was shiny, and the bellies were normal in contour.

Early in 2006, Mary Ann Brown, a Refuge Board member; Dr. William Sorensen, a University of Texas at Tyler faculty member; and Deborah Bell began working on a research proposal involving the eradication of parasites in Guatemalan children. The objective was to determine how often children in developing countries needed treatment for parasites. There was no definitive published information regarding the use of worm medication and how often it should be given. In reviewing the literature, the researchers knew of a particular test for fecal parasites. However, they could not locate a source to purchase for these kits. Mary Ann called researchers who used the test kits in their parasite research at Yale University's infectious disease department. A joint research study was initiated with the University of Texas at Tyler and Yale University to study the prevalence of parasitic infections of school-age children in eleven villages. A high prevalence of infection was found and many of the children had infections with multiple parasites. "Adios lombrices" or "Goodbye worms," a campaign to eliminate parasitic infections, was begun. The education system was utilized to distribute the medications. Funding sources were explored. Through collaborative efforts with several organizations and key people in Guatemala, one million children have now received three doses of Albendazole, a medication known to significantly reduce the parasite burden in infected individuals. In October of 2006, the initial data were presented at the American Society of Tropical Medicine and Hygiene. A second research project with Yale and the University of Texas at Tyler regarding malaria on the eastern coast of Guatemala is in the data analysis phase.

Access to education was another factor observed as a hindrance to the well-being of Guatemalan people. Refuge International assisted in building a school in Sarstun as well as paying teachers' salaries. Student enrollment increased from 45 to 168 children within two years. Generous supporters continue to contribute school supplies for schools throughout the Sarstun area.

Dr. Debbie Mahoney invited nurse practitioner students to Guatemala. Four graduate nurse practitioner students went to San Raymundo and experienced invaluable clinical opportunities for professional as well as personal growth. Dr. Mahoney presented slides of the trip to the Nurse's Christian Fellowship organization at University of Texas at Tyler. Undergraduate students asked if they could also go. That began involvement of both undergraduate and graduate nursing students and faculty in international relief. Students at University of Texas at Tyler who were unable to travel to Guatemala volunteered to put hygiene packs together, which contained basic items such as a toothbrush, toothpaste, washcloth, soap, shampoo, etc. These packs are distributed to patients presenting at clinic sites in Guatemala and quickly became very popular. Hundreds are taken on nearly every trip. Undergraduate students produced a video tape on basic hygiene and dental care that was shown to the Guatemalan people who came to the clinic.

Additional students, both undergraduate and graduate level, from Case Western Reserve have been active participants in the work Refuge International is doing in Guatemala. Through Sigma Theta Tau, Margaret Bobonich, a nurse practitioner who was a participant in Survivor Guatemala, was contacted regarding Refuge International. She created a keen interest among the students and faculty at Case Western and brought three groups of nurse practitioner students along with another faculty member, Carol Sarvin, to provide care for the Guatemalan people. In addition, a group of students aspiring to go to medical school have participated in health care mission trips.

The Saul project began when children with health problems that cannot be adequately addressed in Guatemala were seen in clinic. In Hebrew, Saul means "asked." Saul was the first child discovered in a remote area of Guatemala with significantly deformed feet from uncorrected congenital club feet. He had never worn a pair of shoes. He could not attend school because it was too difficult for him to walk to school. In developing countries, children such as Saul receive less food and fewer clothes than those children who can actively participate in helping the family survive, and Saul was no exception. After several surgeries and months of rehabilitation, Saul walked home and took several pairs of shoes with him. Refuge International brought three young children to the United States, two for treatment of club feet and one for a nonarticulating femoral fracture. An old farmhouse was designated as living quarters for one of the children visiting with his father in order to receive surgery from Scottish Rite Hospital in Dallas. University of Texas at Tyler students and faculty, along with Refuge volunteers, gave up a Saturday to prepare this house with much love for the Guatemalan guests. The house was thoroughly cleaned. Furniture, kitchen items, and linens were donated. Two of the students with decorating talent placed pictures on the walls and arranged knick-knacks so that a cozy home-away-from-home awaited the family. Each of the surgeries performed by the talented staff at Scottish Rite Hospital has changed the lives of the treated children.

Believing in the value of international collaboration including faculty and student exchanges, Dr. Susan Yarbrough, Associate Dean of Graduate Nursing Programs at University of Texas at Tyler, initiated a relationship with Lic Rutilia Herrera Acahabon, the Directora of the Escuela Nacional De Enfermeria, and the national nursing program in

Guatemala City. Soon after, Dr. Yarbrough, accompanied by Tyler faculty members, Dr. Barbara Haas, Dr. Gayle Varnell, and Dr. Debbie Mahoney, visited the school along with an undergraduate student, Allison Green. The group was impressed by the beauty of the school and grounds, as well as by the generosity, humility, passion, and dedication of the faculty and students. The group left with a renewed respect for our Central American counterparts and what they were able to accomplish with severely limited resources. The group was shown a computer lab that had carrels, chairs, etc., everything needed for a computer lab except the computers. It was built with the hope that computers would become available. The library had only a few stacks of books, most of which were published in the 1970s. The books showed signs of extreme wear and many were taped together. Because of the critical scarcity of textbooks and the inability of students to afford to buy books, students shared the few books that were available.

After hearing of the deplorable situation, Iota Nu, University of Texas at Tyler's chapter of Sigma Theta Tau, the Honor Society of Nursing, adopted the Guatemala School of Nursing as one of its major projects. Goals were established that included providing computers and books to the Guatemala school. The chapter worked tirelessly through that year to raise funds and solicit donations. It was with great excitement that we visited the school again in February of 2007. At this time, two computers and printers were presented for the computer lab and approximately fifty new Spanish textbooks were donated for their library in collaboration with Elsevier Publishing. A scholarly exchange was also started when Dr. Yarbrough made a presentation on evidence-based practice to an audience consisting of Guatemalan faculty and students, as well as Tyler faculty and students. Karen Torres, a current Sigma Theta Tau member, has spearheaded this project and plans to continue contributing resources to the nursing program in Guatemala City.

There was another major event that took place during this trip. One faculty, Otilia Arguita Dominquez, and two students from the Escuela Nacionale worked for a week with their American counterparts in the clinic at San Raymundo. This was a valuable experience in sharing cultural perspectives and health care information. This was a first step toward what we hope to do more often, that is, student and faculty exchanges.

Two University of Texas at Tyler faculty, Dr. Susan Yarbrough and Dr. Cheryl Cooper, conducted a research study focusing on health-related conditions in several small villages in rural Guatemala. The aim of this study was to explore the nature of health concerns as perceived by the comadronas (traditional birth attendants) that live and work in highland villages north of Guatemala City in the area of San Raymundo. The midwives were given disposable cameras and asked to document the needs they find in their practice. The photos introduced new ideas and ways to study some of the issues that emerged—child labor and its health implications, aging and how the elderly are cared for, mental illness and developmental disabilities, and how males might perceive health in their villages and how their photos might compare to those taken by women.

Anecdotal findings of advanced cervical cancer led to a Pap smear program, which was supported by the Guatemalan government. Pap smears were collected by Refuge team members and read by the Guatemalan Health Department's personnel. This program has led to the discovery and treatment of numerous cases of early cervical cancer. Dr. Debra Mahoney and Deborah Bell have done a descriptive study of the prevalence of abnormal cervical cytology in two Guatemalan villages and presented their data at numerous advanced nursing conferences.

There have been several years of collaboration between the University of Texas at Tyler and Refuge International. This synergistic relationship has proven to be a valuable experience for undergraduate and graduate students and faculty. Over sixty graduate and undergraduate students have traveled to Guatemala for intercultural learning experiences. Health care services, health education, educational supplies, clean water, and hygiene supplies have been provided to the poor of Guatemala by Tyler students and faculty. Several research studies involving Tyler faculty and students have been conducted regarding health issues in Guatemala. The efforts of University of Texas at Tyler's faculty and staff have had a positive effect on the Guatemalan people.

GUATEMALA
Kim Larson and Melissa Ott

We climbed an active volcano, shopped at the most famous Mayan market in the world, and enjoyed one night in a wonderful eco-resort. But it was not all fun and games. In May of 2008, after a year of planning, thirteen East Carolina University nursing students and two nursing faculty traveled to Guatemala to live, work, and learn with the Mayan and Ladino (Spanish and Mayan mix) cultures. Based on previous international work in Peru, Honduras, and Guatemala, Dr. Kim Larson, East Carolina University nursing faculty in the Undergraduate Department of Nursing Science, and Melissa Ott, family nurse practitioner faculty in the Graduate Department of Nursing Science, developed a cultural immersion course offered in Guatemala for East Carolina University nursing students. The course's goal was to establish a partnership between East Carolina University's College of Nursing and an indigenous Mayan community to ensure ongoing community health outreach projects and to sensitize future nurses to the cultural ways and needs of one of the many Latino populations living in the United States.

Between 1990 and 2000, the Spanish-speaking Latino population in North Carolina increased by almost 400%, giving North Carolina the fastest growing Latino population in the nation. During this same period, research reports highlighted disparities among Latino communities in areas such as education, health care, and social services. In 2006, the North Carolina Department of Health and Human Services adopted the Cultural and Linguistic Competency Action Plan that requires all health care providers serving populations that receive public health and social services to increase their cultural competency. In this Action Plan, health care providers are urged to improve communication through linguistic competence, demonstrate outreach initiatives to the Hispanic/Latino population, and increase research efforts that address the elimination of health disparities among Latino immigrants in particular.

As academicians, we are faced with the new and growing challenge to grow students who are culturally competent. In addition, the Carnegie Foundation for the Advancement of Teaching has set forth guidelines for community engagement in higher education teaching. As nurses, this mandate in educational preparation seems critical as we prepare others to care for patients in the diverse communities in which we live and practice nationwide. The Carnegie Foundation further recommends that these courses involve voluntary, not mandatory, service learning and community partnerships, in which electives are offered to engage students who choose this route of learning to be above and beyond their normal curriculum mandates. Our course was offered as an elective that preceded the community health course held in the final semester of their four-year nursing baccalaureate degree. This was planned so that approval was obtained for our students to "bank" twenty hours of clinical time that they earned while in Guatemala to use as partial credit toward earning their community health course credit. It made sense to keep these students in one clinical group following the Guatemala experience, as they would have the ability to complete their community health clinical requirements twenty hours sooner than their classmates.

The East Carolina University College of Nursing houses a very large undergraduate nursing program, as well as many graduate programs including a doctorate in nursing program. Many East Carolina University nursing students have not traveled outside North Carolina. As the population of eastern North Carolina continues to grow and become ever more culturally diverse, the age-old problems of racism, stereotyping, and ignorance continue to plague our communities. It even can be said that within our communities and within our classrooms, a sense of segregation can be felt as our citizens tend to separate themselves into groups of like-cultural background. This is most certainly driven by the basic human need for safety and security in feeling a part of a community with similar attributes, but nonetheless is a major barrier to increased understanding between cultures of people who are living in the same communities. One important point to consider is that university and college students across the United States score well below their counterparts in other advanced countries on indicators of international knowledge. Further, one major barrier to nursing students becoming involved in study-abroad coursework is the rigorous and inflexible nature of some baccalaureate nursing curriculum designs. They are often excluded from study-abroad opportunities as the experiences coincide with the scheduling required for clinical progression within their programs. This necessitates that programs in nursing become tailored to the nursing students' schedules for them to participate. Consideration of this dilemma was factored into this course opportunity. It is also true that many nursing faculty are unable to travel with their students due to the nature of teaching assignments in nursing education. Another phenomenon that remained a barrier for many students to participate is that, even with the course offering taking place between mandatory curriculum course work, the majority of nursing students need to work to earn money during their course-free periods.

Guatemala is most famous for the indigenous Mayan culture and ruins of Tikal and Coban. The country has four major ethnic groups:

Mayan, Ladino (Spanish and Mayan mix), Xinca, and Garifuna. Most of the country is mountainous with numerous active volcanoes. While its 12.7 million people have a per-capita annual income of $5,000, approximately 7.1 million Guatemalans live below the country's poverty level. Since the Peace Accord of 1997, signed by then-President Clinton, Guatemala has benefitted from a more stable government with improved international relations.

In preparation for the trip, we held weekly one-hour lunch meetings called "*mesa* (table) Latina" to practice Spanish vocabulary. These informal meetings also lowered the students' anticipatory anxiety by addressing pertinent questions. Our students also benefitted from meeting and befriending a fellow classmate who had emigrated from Guatemala at the age of thirteen. This classmate attended our mesa Latina and shared his experience of learning English as a second language and navigating his way through a U.S. education and into an American university nursing education. Students also read numerous articles about international health care, medical outreach, and the impact of immigration on families and communities.

It was critical that we prepare students for the hardships that they would inevitably encounter. We held information sessions for interested students to explain course objectives and an immersion experience, and that they would be temporarily removed from the luxuries of their American lives. We prepared them to prevent illness related to *Escherichia coli* infection, and asked them to examine their own abilities to embark on an experience that required personal hardiness.

Students were housed in pairs with a Guatemalan family, selected by the host organization, La Union Centro Linguistico. La Union is owned and operated by a Guatemalan family who run this Spanish language school with a civic mindedness that includes offering partnership in charitable outreach and service-learning projects with visiting groups from many nations. Juan Carlos Martinez, president of La Union, has had Peace Corps experience and integrates his desire to promote sensitivity to indigenous Guatemalan people's culture with a desire to promote international collaboration aimed at meeting communities' needs while preserving their ancient cultural practices. La Union introduces international visitors to volunteer work in a local hospital that houses many children and elderly with physical and intellectual disabilities who could not be cared for in their rural communities. While not part of our original goal to work in rural villages, students discussed the impact of this experience in comparison to the U.S. health care that they take for granted. They recognized the effect of poverty and the lack of access to state-of-the-art health care that exists in a third-world country.

La Union identified major health problems that existed in communities with which we would visit and work. Three areas were sanitation, oral hygiene, and nutrition, which were greatly impacted by the lack of potable water, a problem that ultimately makes every health promotion and improvement effort more difficult. For each outreach project there was a need to carry bottled water and a sense that the lack of sanitary drinking water was an intense barrier to making an impact on the community's health. Students learned that daily bathing was a luxury for many people in rural pueblos.

Every morning after breakfast with their host family, students attended Spanish language class at La Union, and in the afternoon they were involved in clinical outreach and community service projects. At the end of each day, students returned to their host family to discuss their work, eat supper, and help the family clean up. Students worked in groups to complete their community service projects. In Santa Maria de Jesus, students provided children with a nutritious snack and created a bingo game to facilitate learning about how certain foods strengthen different parts of the body. In Alotenango, students developed and taught a song about toothbrushing to another group of children, providing each child with toothbrushes, toothpaste, and other school supplies. At this school, the East Carolina University team spent the rest of the afternoon painting walls with a needed coat of paint. The children responded with a specially prepared song of thanks for the visit.

For students to understand traditional healing beliefs of some Latin American peoples' culture, one afternoon was spent learning about natural healing practices from Tijol, a Mayan *curandero*. He described the practices as a combination of spiritual and herbal treatments. His explanation of medicinal plants and their healing properties included plants such as geranium, basil, sage, and white lilies. These plants, along with candles, spices, incense, liquor, and tobacco, contribute to removing negative energy and evil spirits in people who seek care. On a table inside the room where he worked, Tijol introduced us to *Maximon* (pronounced mosh-ee-mon), a small mannequin-like figure of a man. This pagan god is considered the protector of evil and negative energy, and assists Tijol in his healing practice. He readily admits that the Catholic Church does not approve of this aspect of his work. One student was not feeling well on the day we visited and asked if she could receive a *limpia*, a natural cleansing treatment. Tijol invited her to take a seat near *Maximon* and gave her a whole lime slightly cut open and a handful of tiny candles to hold. He took the medicinal plants and circled them around her head numerous times and down both arms and legs. He did the same with the lime and candles. Throughout, Tijol chanted, prayed, and tossed the used plants, candles, and spices into a small fire causing the room to fill with plumes of smoke. He then sprinkled the student's head, arms, and legs with plant extract followed by a clear liquor. Out of respect and awe, the group silently watched Tijol practice his art. Minutes later the student emerged from the room feeling better and two other students requested and received a *limpia* that afternoon.

As our community partner organization, La Union helped us schedule a medical outreach clinic in Vuelta Grande, a mountainous rural pueblo with limited access to health care. Barriers that existed included severe poverty and lack of transportation from remote areas to the cities with health care resources. Furthermore, men in these pueblos are more reluctant than women to seek health care. Here, our East Carolina University team was joined by Dr. Sonia Patricia Gaitan de Cuyun, a Guatemalan physician known for her work with *Echinacea* in reducing newborn infections. The clinic took place in a modest, cinder-block building with limited medical supplies, an examination table, privacy screen, desk, and chair. This clinic was a ground-breaking endeavor to establish assessments of the community's most prominent health care needs.

In preparation for the clinic, students went to local pharmacies to purchase necessary medicines and supplies. By negotiating with local pharmacists, students practiced Spanish language skills while learning about the availability and cost of medical care in rural Guatemalan villages. During the clinic, while some students gathered health histories from Spanish-speaking mothers and grandmothers, others wrote instructions as medications were prescribed. As families passed through the clinic, students engaged in communication to overcome their language barriers, played with children while mothers had time alone with health care providers, and comforted children to demonstrate their caring attitudes and desire to help.

As faculty we were aware of the need to develop a sustainable partnership for our future work, and to research and document the outcomes and impact of our interventions with the communities. Returning to Guatemala meant the opportunity to nurture old friendships and establish new ones in the familiar cities of Antigua, Ciudad Vieja, and San Miguel Escobar. For the students, the trip meant a chance to shape the future. Plans were made to return to the Mayan pueblos of Vuelta Grande and Alotenango to begin community health outreach projects to benefit each unique community. During the medical outreach clinic, several serious problems were identified among women and children such as a complicated cardiac condition, hepatitis A, and hearing loss. However, most health problems could be addressed with appropriate prevention and primary care if access to resources were available. Annual course trips by future East Carolina University students to implement health education programs will result in a collaborative, trusting, and sustained program of health care.

It is obvious that our mission needs to explore partnerships with other disciplines to best benefit the communities we serve. One idea to pursue is that of enlisting the aid of those with an engineering background to build sanitary wells to bring much needed water to the people. There is a considerable amount of work to be done.

HONDURAS
Teri Kaul

As I reflect upon my "giving through teaching" over the past twelve years as a nurse educator, many of the traditional activities related to the educator role come to mind. One of the most profound ways in which I have been able to participate in this program was my role in designing and developing a course called Global Perspectives in Healthcare. I had the privilege twelve years ago to design and develop this global educational course for our graduate nursing students.

Because advanced practice nurses care for people from diverse cultures, the need for cultural competence is important. This experience is designed to expose students to a cultural setting different from their own. The students examine their own cultural beliefs and values and become more aware of what constitutes culture. Many cultures were examined by students including African American, Hmong, Amish, American Indian, Hispanic, Latino, Mexican, Honduran, and Indian. However, the cultural experience associated with this course that is most reflective of my giving through teaching was the faculty-led medical–spiritual mission trips to countries like Mexico, Honduras, and India.

The very first medical–spiritual mission trip that I organized was to Honduras and occurred eleven years ago. Twelve students and four faculty members were invited to be part of a forty-two–member medical/dental team to provide care to a small village in Honduras about six hours from San Pedro Sul. The population was extremely poor, undereducated Hondurans who were not afforded routine medical or dental care except when teams like ours arrived. The team spent seven, very long, hot days providing much needed care to about 4,000 patients in a cement-framed school. This was my first experience leading a medical–spiritual mission outside of the United States and was the impetus for my continued desire to lead more of them. To date I have led six teams of students and faculty to Honduras, Juarez, Mexico, and Baha, CA Mexico.

The impact of these trips on the students and faculty continues well past the week-long experience in the foreign countries. Many students, once graduated, continue this service attitude within their own communities and some have returned to accompany us on other trips. As well, these trips allow me to *give through my teaching* to both patients and graduate nursing students in a way I am never afforded in my day-to-day traditional nurse educator role. I am able to develop a bond with students simply by sharing this personal service experience with them. Although we all feel vulnerable outside the confines of the traditional educational setting, once the experience begins, the students and faculty open hearts and minds to this life-changing event.

The spiritual dimension, although minimized initially by some, to me is the key to the trip's success. As nurses we espouse nursing care that attends to the individual's body, mind, and spirit. However, in our everyday experience in health care work, the reality is that we care for the body and sometimes the mind, but leave the spiritual aspect to others like chaplains. In contrast, while in the small villages in Mexico or Honduras, seeing those beautiful people's faces and wanting to meet their needs, the reality is that we can't always do much for the body or the mind, but we can always attend to the spirit. Initially, students are uncomfortable with spiritual care because it is not something they had in their studies or they are afraid of offending someone. However, it doesn't take them long to see that spiritual care is much more than just religion. In fact, I would contend, it plays an important, if not the most important, role in healing and caring for patients, especially when there appears to be loneliness, loss of hope, or a feeling of despair.

In summary, although this example of my giving through teaching may not have made a colossal impact on the world at large, I do believe it made an enormous impact on my students and faculty at this small Lutheran university. In fact, many students who apply to our program have commented in their admission essays that they have heard about these trips and want to know how they can be a part of them. It is obvious that students want these experiences, and so I will continue to advocate for them. I am also blessed to work in an environment that supports my personal beliefs and values, and completely supports this program of study.

HONDURAS
Dorothy A. Otto

Following my presentation on international nursing and the opportunities that are available to volunteers with specific projects, two young enthusiastic students asked, "Do you take students to Honduras?" To which I replied: "It's never been done (with a pause), but I will make it happen." Since its inception in 2001, I have been a participant in an eight-day mission project in the western Honduras mountains that is sponsored by First Presbyterian Church, Houston, Texas. Previously I took six generic baccalaureate students to Germany in 1990 in an exchange program with Agnes Karll Krankenhaus School of Nursing. In 2006, seven RN-BSN students accompanied me to England for an eight-day observation of the historical and contemporary health care system for their course in Role Transition. However, creating an international Community Health clinical practicum for the first time gave me new challenges.

The Community Health practicum requires 135 contact hours for three-credit hours. I discussed the international project with the lead teacher who was supportive in using two semester credits of the required three hours for this medical mission project. The remaining one hour was completed in a local community health setting upon return from Honduras.

Approval for students' participation was from the Legal Affairs Office, the Associate Dean of Academic Affairs, Chair of the Nursing Systems Department, and the Coordinator of International Programs. Students were required to use personal funds, participate as volunteers, and receive course credit for completing the project. I functioned as volunteer faculty using personal funding and vacation days to facilitate this learning experience. Requirements included liability waivers from the church and university, evacuation insurance, and health insurance and immunizations. Each student received a scholarship from the university's Committee on the Status of Women to partially cover airfare.

My travel considerations for Honduras, including various costs, airfare, hotel accommodations, meals/bottled water, transportation, sanitation needs, money exchange, and Mayan cultural site visits, enhanced their preparation for international travel. Travel by air from Houston to San Pedro Sula, a large business city, and then by bus for three and one-half hours through the mountains to Copan gave the students a view of the fascinating contrasts of Honduran life.

Course objectives were appropriate to providing primary health care to indigenous Chorti Indians in Otuta and surrounding barrios near Copan. Students met course objectives by my progress evaluation and their journal descriptions. They were required to write a daily journal describing activities related to their clinical practice and to cultural experiences.

Team members travelled to Otuta to prepare two school rooms, one as a "farmaceia" and the other for a physicians' area. Students also interacted with nearby children who were mesmerized by us and followed us everywhere, laughing, giggling," and calling us "gringos!" The children were very dirty and each one told us their name. The "clinica" was a six-mile trip from the hotel. The road was filled with large pot holes from the fall monsoon season. The students delighted in standing in the truck bed like the Hondurans.

On arrival, the team and our translators, high school boys with their leaders from the Micah Project, formed a circle for a prayer either in Spanish or English. All persons waiting to be seen participated. Many villagers, mostly infants, children, and women of varying ages, walked miles to be seen. We learned that many men and boys worked picking coffee beans to be dried and exported. One fact became evident—we all smile in the same language.

The day's activities depended on patients' ailments. One student wrote that she was "amazed at the relatively good health of the infants; especially when you think about the condition of the homes, the lack of sanitation, the hygiene of the people...." The most common health concerns among adults were pain (muscular, arthritic, and carpal tunnel), headaches, ear aches, gastritis, asthma, and insomnia. The children usually had similar conditions, scabies, and parasites. Many houses had open, wood burning, brick ovens and no chimney or any other ventilation, except a door to the outside; this resulted in chronic respiratory conditions. One journal entry read: "We got to meet the 'doula' (aka midwife) of the village who said she is 104! She has delivered countless babies. We are wondering how she cut the umbilical cord, and she is coming back to the clinic; so we plan to find out tomorrow."

One afternoon, a physician, some students, and a translator walked a mountainous terrain to reach a patient. The students observed a cholecystectomy surgical incision infection that was cleansed and the patient given an oral antibiotic and pain medication. "Her house consisted of two rooms—one a kitchen and the other room with a hammock. There were chickens, cornhusks piled everywhere and it was very dark and smoky. The best part...was to see the living conditions."

"Giving treatment instructions was a daily challenge. Even the Micah boys had some difficulty interpreting the Chortis dialect. How do you explain to a mother with as many as six children about applying a scabicide solution to the infant and the older children for a specific period of time (minutes to all night)? It was not easy and we trusted that the translator explained timing to the mother." Another journal description read: "One mother [came] with her four children. The mother and each child were prescribed two or three medications and each had different instructions on when and how to take it. It would have been complicated for even a *health care* provider to track. I can imagine how difficult it would be for the mother...she cannot read and has to track all [the] children and their health needs."

Given the illiteracy among adults, the farmaceia team made medication cards for drug administration that were coded with a rising sun, a mid-day full sun, an afternoon setting sun, and stars to help indicate the time to take a medication. Spanish words of instruction told the amount of the liquid or tablet to take at one time. With several children per family, we used a different colored yarn tied around a bottle or a spoon for each child, and then trusted the mother or older children with instructions provided by the translator. Surprisingly, we learned that patients were in a healthy state related to satisfactory blood pressure readings and hemoglobin results. The team purchased most of the medications and brought them in large plastic crates to the clinic. Unused medications were given to the new clinic in Copan for distribution to patients.

"Rotten teeth" were encountered by the dentist who performed multiple extractions. His sterilizer consisted of his family's pressure cooker placed on a stove burner run by a rented electric generator. He brought his own instruments. Even though some patients were left edentulous following extractions, they were pleased to be rid of the "bad teeth."

A key concept learned by students was the cultural influence on one's health status that was defined by an individual's ethno-cultural group. Ethnocentricity is not to be imposed on others of a different ethnic population. The diversity among the Chorti Indians from different barrios/villages provided an opportunity to observe culture woven throughout health practices. Maintaining cultural traditions influenced patients' responses to the team's care and teaching.

Departure time from the clinic varied due to weather, lighting, and the number of patients to be seen. "On the way home from the clinic we stopped at a maternity clinic; it was a small clinic where women in labor usually had their baby while there and left within one-half to one day. They only paid 10 limpiras (about 50 cents) and the government reimbursed the clinic for the rest of the cost. It was a great experience."

As the "nurse educator" who facilitated the students' learning experiences, the initial challenges and the rewards provided indelible memories for the two nursing students and myself. Perhaps this student stated it best: "What a week this has been... one that I will remember and hold near and dear to my heart, always. It was wonderful to have been included on this trip and it has been a privilege to share this experience with an amazing group of Christian servants and I am proud of the work that we were able to bring to the people of Otuta."

HONDURAS
Eileen M. Smit and Mary Jane Tremethick

We developed and offered an interdisciplinary cultural immersion/academic service learning course in Honduras for the past two years. While our course is an interdisciplinary course that encompasses nursing and health education interventions, our work was guided by research conducted by nurse researchers. Little published research exists related to health education, cultural immersion, and service learning courses.

The need for diversity in educational experiences is recognized by universities that are undergoing a shift to international programming. Our university was no exception. This shift facilitated development of a cultural immersion course. We received internal grant funding for a Spanish Immersion course at a nearby college to develop our Spanish-speaking ability and for software to maintain our newly developed Spanish-language skills. We also used internal grant funding to pay for initial course development costs, such as travel to Honduras to explore and develop an in-country network, critical to the success of a cultural immersion course. Developing a network includes finding and developing relationships with in-country professionals who fit with students' needs. We began by exploring international contacts, which led to a partnership with the Yojoa International Medical Center.

One challenge was to fit our interdisciplinary course with the immersion site's needs, including clinical sites and an area where students provide basic health education. Honduras is one of the poorest countries in the Western Hemisphere. Our specific location, Santa Cruz de Yojoa, in the Department of Cortez, is a rural area where services such as ours were most needed. Honduras provided a diverse cultural experience for our students in a safe setting.

Another challenge was to obtain an experience within the price range for students. Honduras had relatively low flight costs and an inexpensive cost of living, approximately $10.00 per day for safe room and board. We currently have the least expensive campus immersion course. We ate most meals at a nearby home where students watched and sometimes assisted with meal preparation. Students also built rapport with family members as they interacted in the home setting.

Our biggest challenge was the language barrier. We encouraged students to review their Spanish-speaking skills prior to travel. We also utilized interpreters. We networked with Peace Corps workers who provided interpretation services. In the future we may list Spanish-speaking skills as a criterion for student acceptance into the program.

Ours is an interdisciplinary course taught by a professor from the Nursing Department and a professor from the Health Education Department. It is cross-listed as a nursing and a health education course. We welcome students from all majors. All students participate in general activities and community education. Student nurses have an opportunity to work in clinical sites.

During the semester prior to the immersion, students complete self-directed learning using online PowerPoint presentations and online discussions focused on the cultural traditions in Honduras, the primary causes of morbidity and mortality, and information about the immersion site. The concept of cultural relativism is explored and the students learn about the need to observe and learn through the norms and values of the Honduran culture. We also have three face-to-face meetings for students to develop friendships and cohesiveness. Assignments prior to departure include identifying unmet learning needs, and the resources necessary to meet those needs.

A primary focus for service learning is meeting current needs. Honduras lacks many basic health resources. Prior to departure, students explored potential health education topics and identified related resources for the trip. While in Honduras, students completed an informal primary needs assessment and delivered programs to meet these needs. We provided basic hygiene education in elementary schools about the importance of brushing teeth and hand washing. Each child received a toothbrush, toothpaste, and soap. While basic to us, a recent study found that only 5% of Hondurans acknowledged the importance of proper hand and oral hygiene in maintaining good health. We provided similar educational experiences in an orphanage. We also treated numerous children for head lice and provided basic hygiene products to a group of women and their children in a domestic violence shelter.

Students solicited donations from businesses, families, and friends to purchase needed health care items. They brought items ranging from disposable gloves to toothbrushes and soap. Students provided some basic services such as taking vital signs and assisting with intravenous infusions in clinics.

We believe it is critical for students to understand capacity building and take part in capacity-building activities. To achieve this, we teamed with professionals from the Yojoa International Medical Center Committee headed by a local physician, Dr. Milton Mendoza. The committee members are health care professionals, educators, architects, and business men and women with a common goal of building a medical center to provide for the health care needs of rural Hondurans. While in Honduras, students were advocates for the Yojoa International Medical

Center Committee, and took part in activities to facilitate this project. Students participated in meetings with government officials explaining the need for this facility as well as the development plans. Students viewed interactions between community leaders promoting the medical center concept and governmental officials. They were active in a strategic planning session and discussed how the class activities contributed to development. Our participation strengthened their community's ability to address local health care needs.

Three students returned to Honduras independently to continue work on this project. One student, presently in Honduras, is collaborating with a professor from our university's business department to develop a website, in both English and Spanish. The website will provide information about the proposed medical center, and will also allow online credit card payment for donations for building of the center. Such ongoing commitment is evidence of the impact this experience had on students' lives. An added benefit with former students in Honduras has been continued development of our in-country network.

Through all the service learning activities, students interacted daily with Hondurans in their home communities. This interaction provided students with many opportunities for cultural learning. Reflection activities were woven into each day's activities. At the end of each day, students and professors met to reflect on the day's experiences, some of which were new and at times disturbing. Reflection enables understanding the norms and values of the Honduran culture and how to place these into perspective.

Students were often struck by the contrast between poverty and the apparent joy of the Honduran people, and learned how wealth is measured in family connections and support. One student commented, "As our bus traveled down the winding roads, I gazed out the window at impoverished houses and felt saddened and useless next to such a devastating sight...we stopped and visited a family living in a small, wooden hut with nothing but tarps for doors and soil carpets. The small children had dirt smudged on their faces and were clothed in no more than underpants, yet greeted us with smiles and curiosity."

Students saw the happiness of living in a community where family is more important than possessions.

Our global education partnership with a community in rural Honduras was a mutually beneficial experience for everyone involved in the project. The graciousness and hospitality of the community has left a lasting impression on the students, and several have made career decisions based on their experiences. As professors, we have grown in our appreciation of the gifts and talents of our Honduran hosts and our students. We have all learned together.

HONDURAS
Sarah M. Ware

Three members of a Baptist church's Health Ministry participated in a mission program to San Pedro Sula in Honduras. One was an RN that I call Cookie, a phlebotomist and dialysis technician I called Rose, and myself, a university nurse educator. The fifty-seven–member mission team represented Baptist, Presbyterian, and Methodist congregations from several Southern towns and a Northeastern city. The support from our church and pastor made this mission a reality. This was our first trip to a lesser-developed country. The church treasury and several fundraisers financed our trip. All expenses, including passports, immunizations, travel, lodging, and meals, were paid.

Following several planning months, all of us departed for San Pedro Sula for a week-long mission. The mission leaders were well organized and all aspects went smoothly. After everyone arrived, we boarded an American yellow school bus with no air conditioning; it was very hot. Three young, Hispanic women greeted us as we entered the bus. They were translators, important for our trip.

It was a long, hot ride to the hotel, even with the bus windows down. We rode about two hours. In area, Honduras is slightly larger than the state of Tennessee. The climate is subtropical in the lowlands and temperate in the mountains. The terrain is mostly mountainous in the interior with narrow coastal plains. The population is 7,639,327 with Spanish and Amerindian dialects. Tegucigalpa is its capital. Honduras is the second poorest country in Central America and one of the poorest countries in the Western Hemisphere, with 50.4% of the population living below the poverty line. Industries consist of sugar, coffee, textiles, clothing, and wood products. Agricultural products include bananas, coffee, citrus, beef, timber, shrimp, tilapia, lobster, corn, and African palm. Bacterial diarrhea, hepatitis A, and typhoid fever are common food- or waterborne diseases.

Our hotel consisted of cabins in the middle of a coffee plantation under the auspices of the Honduran Ministry. Coffee plants, banana trees, and beautiful ginger plants were abundant. On the grounds was a zoo with small animals and a medical clinic that had state-of-the-art dental equipment.

Cookie, Rose, and I shared a cabin, the first in a row of ten. Each cabin had two large steps and a porch with a big chair and a hammock. There were three other cabin rows. We entered an air-conditioned room. Although disappointed in our living accommodations, we ate dinner in the hotel restaurant and meals were buffet style. Fruit juices (including watermelon juice), soft drinks, tea, and water were served. Everything was fresh and delicious. The fruit was sweeter than in the United States. A Guatemalan interpreter said that fruit is sweeter because it is vine ripened.

Our mission teams participated in various projects to improve the quality of life for villagers surrounding San Pedro Sula, and many members served on previous missions . Mission projects included building two houses, a kitchen for a school, a fence around a kindergarten, a water sanitation system, and a gardening project. There was a dental clinic and an eye clinic on the grounds.

For four days the medical team went into surrounding villages and provided health care. We brought four large trunks of medication (one for each day); most were purchased by the mission team and some were donated. We traveled to various clinic sites such as a school site in mountainous Los Andes, a church in San Vuena Ventura, a school in El Jarah, and a school in Aqua Sula. The team was interdisciplinary with U.S. and Honduras physicians and nurses, staff, pre-med students, a dialysis technician, and myself, a nurse educator.

A typical day was laborious yet rewarding. We loaded the bus and obtained medicines and supplies before heading to villages. The people were in long lines waiting for us, often standing in the hot sun. They were patient and tolerant and greeted us with smiles, hugs, and handshakes, and frequently we were greeted by local dignitaries. Sometimes children sang for us as we established pharmacy and medical stations.

There was an organized system in order to receive care from the team. First, a demographic data card was completed; then patients were triaged by Honduran nurses. Next they saw a doctor, who sometimes would work with four or five family members at a time. Those working the pharmacy filled prescriptions and the interpreters gave villagers their instructions and answered their questions. We saw an average of 200 to 250 villagers per day.

Villagers had numerous health care needs. We treated scabies, lice, malnutrition, gastric reflux, indigestion, hypertension, diabetes, arthritis, asthma, and various infections. There was a high incidence of parasites. There were pregnant women who needed prenatal vitamins. Some of the medications used were analgesics, antihypertensives, antidiabetics, antibiotics, antihistamines, allergy medications, asthma medications, gastrointestinal medications, topicals, prenatal and children's vitamins, medications for eye infections and irritation, and worm medications. Some were dispensed, while others were administered on site. On Sunday afternoon, several team members delivered food to needy families. Many described their sadness for the people they served, as there was much poverty and many needs.

During the mission trip we had two occasions to worship with the villagers. And each spiritual service was uplifting. On Sunday night, the mission team worshipped together on the clinic grounds of Honduran Ministry. It was inspirational for different religious denominations who worked together to worship together.

The next to the last day, the mission team dedicated the work we completed. We had a ceremony for the two houses, the water sanitation system, the fence around the kindergarten, and the kitchen built for the school. Many villagers were present, especially the children. Families were appreciative of our efforts.

I felt frustrated with communications as I did not speak the language, but I felt blessed improving the people's quality of life and receiving Hondurans' love and warmth. I noticed that dogs accompany people in villages when they are in public. They seem to blend with the people. No one shoos dogs away. Children are not accompanied by adults as often and as closely as they are in the United States. Education is free until the child is in the sixth grade, then they pay $20 per month. If they cannot pay, they cannot attend school. Some mission team members "adopted" some of the children and send $20 per month so that they can go to school. The school children wear uniforms that consist of white shirts and navy pants or skirts.

American yellow school buses were used for public transportation. Uniformed police rode in pick-up trucks. Some guards were in camouflage and carrying shotguns. There was considerable poverty, one-room houses with curtains as the door and windows, and houses with dirt floors. There were no window panes, screens, or shutters. Living conditions were healthier in the "new part of town."

My experience was challenging and rewarding and the culture fascinated me. I learned tolerance from our living accommodations and working in the heat; I learned patience from the people who waited for us. We could not drink tap water or rinse our mouths with it. We could only use bottled water for these purposes. The restaurant water was safe. My spirituality was enhanced through morning devotions, the fellowship with team members, and the people who worshiped with us. I made a revelation; I realized that this was more than a personal goal; it was what God wanted me to do. I eagerly anticipate another opportunity to serve.

LATIN AMERICA
Martha J. Morrow

I was given an opportunity through my employer, Shenandoah University, to fulfill part of their mission and philosophy as a Methodist-based university. They offered a spring-break mission trip in Hispanic countries. It was a life-changing experience. I was part of a team of faculty, students, and staff that volunteered for construction projects in the Caribbean and Mexico.

We worked side by side with the local people—eating, sharing stories, laughing, praying—and helped stimulate the local economy, more commonly known as shopping. We had a glimpse of the culture and what it was like to live in a country that did not have the resources we had in the United States. We laughed with each other at our attempt to deal without some amenities we thought we could never live without. We mixed concrete with hoes and shovels on the bare dirt. We built sidewalks and driveways to allow the elderly and handicapped to navigate between church and rectory. On another site, the kindergarten and first grade classroom was a dirt floor and it had a corrugated tin roof and cardboard sides. When it rained, the floor was muddy. When the wind blew, the children sat huddled together to stay warm. They needed another classroom for the small children. We dug a 7-foot deep by 4-foot wide trench for the 20-by-30 square foot foundation in one week. The local people could not believe we did it, but we were determined to complete our mission. They did not have the personnel or the tools to start the project, or the resources to haul the dirt away. We dug out the foundation, then shoveled the dirt pile into trucks, and paid for tools and hauling. We left a big hole and numerous shovels, hoes, and picks to be given to parishioners so they could work and earn a living in construction. In another area, the church was building a house and rectory for the minister and his family. The house was nearly complete, but the tile work and painting were slow—tile, paint, and tools were expensive. A group of twenty-five students, faculty, and staff arrived on Saturday, prayed on Sunday, and by the next Friday had completed the painting, tiled the entire second floor and stairs, and finished the project the community had been working on for years.

We came with unskilled hands and learned and worked with the people of the community. We purchased the materials to complete the work and left the tools and materials for the parish to give to members who could not afford their own tools to work. Tools meant permanent work and food on the table. We attended their services and they marveled that we were Christians and non-Christians working, living, and praying together with them. All the communities fed us, provided transportation, and showed us their communities. We experienced a rainforest and a fish hatchery where we got to pick out our lunch and watch it being prepared. We experienced a Mariachi festival, and the wonders of past civilizations. They took pride in their country and heritage, and were excited to share it with us. We experienced the hardships that they endure routinely in one community... a once-in-a-lifetime experience for most of us.

I loved the construction work, b ut I yearned to help with the skills I knew best, health care and health education. I saw the consequences of lack of health care education, medication, and medical care on the people with whom we worked in these communities. So I approached the chaplain of the university. Many of the student volunteers for these mission trips came from our health professions programs, and yearned to experience health care abroad. On one trip we arranged for several students to spend the day with local health care workers. They witnessed a live birth in one home with family present and a midwife in attendance. The students were thrilled, and I wished for more.

With the chaplain, we searched for other experiences to provide health care through the Methodist missions. Finally, we chose a community in Mexico; we have worked there now for three years in a variety of health care and educational roles with and for the community.

At first, we worked with a local physician in those clinics that needed help most and where we identified several needs: preventive education, screening, and medicines. We organized a team of nurses, nurse practitioners, a doctor, pharmacist, and students from nursing, nurse practitioner, physician assistant, pharmacy, physical therapy, and occupational therapy programs. In fact, we created three teams with the local doctor. One team was headed by an American physician who saw patients at walk-in clinics. The team would assess, diagnose, and treat anyone who came through the door. We brought with us medications, vitamins, and medical supplies, either donated or purchased by the teams.

I, as nurse practitioner, headed the second team. As women's care was in great need, we performed breast examinations and Pap smears. The local physician had arranged with a local laboratory to do all the Pap smears we could do in that week for $5 each. We provided the supplies and paid for the laboratory studies. We were assured that if one was positive, follow-up care through the government health program was available. Many of the women were too poor to pay for the tests, and the clinic was too poor to provide it free. The staff consisted of volunteers. So we provided Pap smears and breast exams to the staff as well. We also educated them on monthly breast self-exams and when to follow up with the physician if they discovered a lump.

The third team went to a local elderly group facility, organized and run by the local physician's sister, also a physician. Having an office in a poor area, she had noticed several elderly and handicapped people living on the streets. This was quite an unusual situation as the elderly and infirm are commonly cared for by their own families in their own homes. Nursing homes are not a part of this culture. However, when the family was gone, the spouse had died, and there were no children to care for aging parents, the elderly were unable to maintain a home financially and ended up on the street; a similar scenario applies to handicapped children who had lost their parents.

As a result, this local physician purchased a facility to house the indigent in a dormitory setting and accepted local volunteers to help care for, feed, prepare meals, clean the facility, do the laundry, and bathe the residents. Still, these volunteers had no nursing skills, and the residents had no health care.

In response, nursing students on the team would assess patients for conditions that may need attention by the physician who came once per week to provide medications and treatment plans. In the first year, we experienced two significant events with lasting impact on the facility.

First, as part of community outreach, we attended a church service mid-week. At that service, we were joined by a group of students from another U.S. university who were also in the area on their spring break mission trip. They provided a mime theatrical production on the Christian principles of the teaching of Jesus Christ. No words, just dance and music. The narration was simple and in both English and Spanish, the production impressive and moving. Afterward, the students had the opportunity to share what each group was doing. The students from the nursing home facility expressed their frustration that the residents needed to walk and the facility had a great outdoor area but that because of trash and overgrowth, it was dangerous for the elderly and handicapped to go outside. Many of the residents had not been outdoors in months. The students who put on the production said they were a group of over 500 students from their university who were doing many different services. They would see what they could do. The next day, twelve of these students arrived with trucks, garbage bags, and gardening tools and they worked for two days to clear the debris from the grounds. On the second day, the residents were able to walk outside and sit in the sun.

The second experience involved the team who, on their first day, were met with suspicion and anger from caretakers. The students were devastated. They had not expected this type of reaction to their willingness to provide service. But it was an opportunity for students to examine themselves and how others may view them as volunteers. Often, we are viewed as thinking we are better than the locals and that our way is better. That evening we discussed the students' feelings, and explored reasons why they met with resistance. We strategized a plan for the next day; we would ask the caretakers to help us understand and know each resident and their particular uniqueness. The caretakers had taken very good care of these residents and the students would be sure to mention that. There was also a language barrier, since many of the students did not speak Spanish. So a fluent interpreter was sent with them on the second day. The sharing session that second evening was the total opposite of the first day. The caretakers expressed concern that the students did not value what they were doing. They thought the students were going to take away the opportunity for them to serve these people they had grown to love and care for. The students assured them they were there to help them in caring for the residents, to provide medical resources we had brought, and hopefully to help them to understand some simple basic care to keep the residents functional. The caretakers were eager to learn. Both groups learned to overcome the language barrier with a common goal and purpose—to care for those who were less fortunate.

The second year we discovered a new resident in the facility, an amputee woman who had lost her spouse and thus could no longer live by herself. She was depressed and angry. She could not accept that she was dependent on charity. She was not able to walk and was bedridden. The students assessed that she was still in good physical condition and could use a walker. We obtained a walker from the local community, worked on strengthening exercises, and by the end of the week she was able to walk across the room. She cried; she had not been outside her room since she had come to live there. She knew now that if she could walk, she could work and perhaps be able to live unassisted. The following year, we found out she had moved out to live on her own in a home in the community where she cared for herself and did charity work in the community and at the facility.

All teams also did screening for hypertension and diabetes, two major problems in the Hispanic population. We discussed meal planning and healthy eating options that they could accommodate in their culture and with their finances. We played with the children and taught them about eating healthy, dental care, exercise, and hygiene. We brought toothbrushes and toothpaste, crayons, coloring books, and school supplies. We brought toys and played with them; we taught them English and they taught us Spanish.

We worked with paid and volunteer staff in the clinics and learned of the struggles of the people of this culture. We learned of the politics, of the Maquiladora, the struggles of the "dump" people, and the work of one woman physician trying to improve the lives of her patients. The dump clinic is literally on a dump, a landfill. Years ago the landfill grew and the government hired caretakers for the landfill to help bury the trash. These caretakers worked long, hard hours for very little pay. They were allowed to bring their families and lived on the flat land around the dump. Once the landfill was full, the government leveled it off and then divided the landed into 20-by-20 square foot plots and began to sell them to individuals and families that worked on the landfill or who could afford the purchase price. There is no sanitation or electricity. The early homes were made of cardboard and tin. The temperature fluctuation during the year was from

10 degrees to 110 degrees Fahrenheit. The landfill contained wastes of all kinds—chemical, medical, human, residential, and industrial.

When approximately 3,000 families were living on the landfill, the government approached a local physician who volunteered in the community to create a clinic to attend to the health care needs, and injuries, of the residents and workers of the dump community. The community had grown and included people who did not work for the landfill but were relatives of the workers, or poor who worked in the sweatshops and could not afford land or decent housing. They saved up the $100 that was needed to purchase the plot of land and brought their families. The physician agreed and the first "dump" clinic opened. Her goal was to educate the people, particularly the women and Maquiladoras, to fight for their rights and dignity. Over the years two more dump clinics have developed to serve over 9,000 families living on the landfill. The physician is now branching out to fight for the rights to health care of the indigenous Indian population who are discriminated against.

Some of the experiences with these clinics are hard to take in. One example is mothers bringing their newborns wrapped in a plastic shopping bag. The mothers cannot afford clothing for the infant, and the plastic bag provides protection from the wastes abundant on the landfill. The plastic bag also provides more warmth than wrapping the infant in paper or newspapers, which is the next most common wrapping. Students have begun a layette collection project and we will take a large amount of donated items with us on the next trip.

Other experiences are amazing to us. These people with very little often offer a penny to the physician in payment for her care. The physician is paid a small stipend from the government. The patients are proud and wish to pay the physician—s ometimes with produce or a product, sometimes with a service like cleaning or painting. Most of the clinic's staff are volunteers, learning a trade they can then use to earn a living, but they still find time to volunteer at the clinic. The physician has asked us also to collect scrubs and lab coats for her staff so that when they get a paying job they will have the appropriate clothing. Also, having scrubs or a lab coat is important to them and is an issue of pride in what they are doing.

The university has expanded its mission trips to offer a wide variety of experiences for students, faculty, and staff—in our own community, in other parts of the United States, and in various countries around the world. Locally we work with Habitat for Humanity building houses, the SPCA caring for sheltered animals in the wetlands to clean it up and preserve it, and gleaning orchards and farms for the homeless and hungry. In the United States, we travel to the New Orleans area to help in the Katarina aftermath each year since the disaster. Abroad, there are two mission trips, the one I coordinate in Mexico described above, and one in the poor areas of Nicaragua providing health care to hundreds of people. These are examples of educators delivering care, educating the future caretakers and educators, and educators being role models for students as giving, caring individuals attending to the needs of our global community, whether at home or abroad.

My participation in the mission trip has exceeded my expectations. I feel blessed to be able to give my talents and services to those in need, and feel that I have been more than blessed by meeting these wonderful people.

PERU
Kathleen C. Ashton

Our team traveled to Peru to deliver health care, medicines, and humanitarian aid to some of the poorest individuals in a country struggling to meet the needs of its people. The nursing shortage in Peru reached critical proportions, with some areas reporting one nurse to one hundred patients. Personnel, supplies, and medications all were in short supply.

The people of Peru are descended from the Inca rulers and other pre-Colombian indigenous people and speak mainly Spanish, the language of the conquistadors, as well as Quechua and Aymara. The indigenous people live in extreme poverty amid vast mineral deposits and dwindling resources. Many indigenous people migrate to Lima from the jungles and mountains to find work and a better life for their children. Frequently, they become part of the shantytowns and struggle as street vendors, laundry women, and construction workers in a city where most people are unemployed or underemployed, and only 23% of the country's population has health insurance.

The Ministry of Health and the Social Security Health Institute (ESSALUD) provides the majority of health care for the people of Peru through twenty-four geopolitical departments or regions. Respiratory and cardiovascular problems are the leading causes of death, in part as a result of the heavy pollution. Infectious diseases are also prevalent and many people die from accidents and injuries. Acute respiratory infections, especially pneumonia, are the leading cause of death among children and young adults.

When I was given the opportunity to join a medical campaign to Peru, I immediately signed on. The team consists of approximately 140 individuals from all walks of life who wish to be of service to people in need. Together with physicians, dentists, pharmacists, teachers, nurses, cooks, engineers, and opticians, I have served in both Lima and Ica, bringing health care to individuals for whom it is unavailable or inaccessible. The annual eight-day campaign commences with the set up of the clinic boundaries—a school, municipal building, or sometimes bamboo sheeting erected in an open space—in one of the poorest areas of Lima or in the neighborhood of Parcona in Ica.

The local Peruvians join with the "gringos" to do whatever is needed to help those less fortunate. The line outside the boundary starts forming as soon as word gets out that we are in town. Each day of the campaign sees individuals coming in from surrounding areas earlier and earlier until toward the end of the week, whole families may come the night before and camp to wait their turn to be seen. They wait patiently until, even on the last day at closing time, they are there, and they will remain hopeful until the bus rolls out of sight. Several patients now return each year and seek me out to give me an update on how they are drinking more water, or lifting using their legs, or eating less fried foods. Some show off their new baby, or tell of other life milestones with unrestrained joy.

Theirs are lives of hardship coupled with the indomitable spirit of survival. One woman looked around the bamboo enclosure and said, "This is like my home." She was an asthmatic and the dust was everywhere. Without a refuge to protect her, she coped as best she could in that harsh environment. Unfortunately, with our basic medications and resources, there was not much that we could do for an asthmatic living in a house of bamboo sheeting in the middle of a dry and dusty city.

Felix was a young man in his early twenties when his mother practically carried him to the clinic, lethargic and barely conscious. He was about thirty-six hours away from death. The cause? An abscessed tooth in need of penicillin that could be purchased at any pharmacy in Lima for about two dollars. Yet, this was beyond his means, so the infection had spread to his jaw, his neck, and across his shoulder. We lanced the area and about eight ounces of pus gushed out. Using a bag of intravenous fluid, we mixed some powdered penicillin and flushed the area thoroughly. Fortuitously, he had come on the first day of the campaign, so we had him return every day over the next week for flushing and assessment. By the end of the campaign, he was fully coherent and returned to say good-bye with his wife, four-year-old son, and infant daughter. He even returned the following year and asked how he could be of service to others during the campaign.

Many people who are seen during the mission are adept at using local herbs and folk remedies that have been handed down from their ancestors. Through our interpreters and my rudimentary Spanish, I have learned of many practices and remedies that are used with or instead of pharmaceuticals for a host of conditions. At every level, medical missions are ideally about an exchange of ideas and personal growth for everyone involved. An important benefit of working under the conditions imposed by the nature of the mission is that I can take as much time as I need to connect with my patients, listen to their stories, learn about their lives, and gain a wonderful perspective of the similarities and differences among all people.

One value that is shared and made evident is how much the Peruvians love their children. For example, a local boy had a rather serious mishap on his bicycle. A visit to a hospital in Peru entails having the cash to pay not only for the medical care, but any medications or supplies needed. Most hospitals are situated adjacent to pharmacies to allow family members to purchase, in cash, the needed medications and supplies. If there is no cash, there is no treatment. The injured boy required sutures and we were able to serve as an emergency facility and provide care for his injuries. So appreciative was his aunt that she made beaded necklaces for every member of the team, not just those directly involved in his care. She thanked everyone profusely as she personally distributed her handmade gifts.

Gratitude is abundant among the Peruvian people and they give their best gifts from the heart. One young couple had become especially close to a man serving with the team in a maintenance capacity. As we were breaking up camp, the couple brought him a gift that reduced him to tears. They presented him with their wedding photo and insisted that he take it as a token of their gratitude for his service to the people of Peru. The man keeps that photo on his desk.

Epilepsy and mental illness are seen in a different light in many Latin American cultures. Rather than a treatable condition, epilepsy is often viewed as demonic possession and individuals manifesting seizures are avoided and shunned by society. During one mission trip, a pregnant woman suddenly experienced a seizure while waiting in line. We cared for her and made a makeshift table from some blankets. Her husband and father accompanied her and before long both of them also began seizing. Upon further investigation, we realized that none of them had adequate medication to control the disease.

One year, a dermatologist had misgivings about joining the team, thinking he would be of little use. That year, two women came in to the clinic, both of whom had melanomas. One woman in her thirties had a melanoma on her right cheek. Our colleague was able to excise it in a procedure accomplished on a blanket-covered table with one of us holding a flashlight for more direct light and another handing instruments from a pack. More than likely, that young woman's life was saved by a procedure that she would not have been able to afford otherwise. The other woman was an elderly woman with a large growth on her lower eyelid. Due to the position of the melanoma and the likelihood of profuse bleeding, we were not able to operate on her. The dermatologist went on to diagnose a twenty-year-old woman with tuberous sclerosis, a rather rare condition that has dermatological manifestations and can affect several internal organs. Both the woman and her seventeen-year-old sister had the disease that is characterized by dimpling and toughening of the skin of the lower back known as shagreen patches, mental retardation, and the formation of tubers in the nail beds. The dermatologist quickly and adeptly diagnosed the condition and demonstrated what a wonderful asset he was to the team that year.

Many middle-aged individuals have not been able to read for the lack of a pair of reading glasses. Others suffer from various deficits that can be easily corrected with a pair of glasses. Throughout the year, team members collect used eyeglasses and then bring as many pairs as possible to Peru to be distributed by the optician. On one mission a woman had traveled over eight hours to get to the clinic and when she arrived we searched for a pair of glasses that would correct her vision problem. None were left that would be of use to her. Not knowing what else we could do, we searched the table again for an appropriate pair of glasses. Suddenly there was a pair that was just right for her. Had they been there all along? We tried them and she was ecstatic. With tears in her eyes she told us, "I knew you could help me."

While patients are waiting their turn to be seen, teachers and other lay workers hold classes on hand hygiene, toothbrushing, and basic nutrition. Health aids such as soap, shampoo, toothbrushes, and combs are distributed. The children are kept busy with stories, coloring books, and puppet shows that are used to teach basic principles of hygiene.

During each campaign we see more than 2,000 patients, pull hundreds of teeth, dispense thousands of prescriptions, and distribute hundreds of pairs of eyeglasses. One year the Customs held our trailer of medicines until the end of the campaign; we were able to purchase some medications from the local health department and distributed these until they were gone. The upside of this was that we were forced to slow our pace to stretch the supply as long as possible, which allowed ample time to spend with each patient. We now purchase all medications in-country, which results in less variety, but saves the shipping costs and avoids the usual inspections and hassles with Customs.

I am usually the only nurse practitioner on the team and, as the only woman, many female patients prefer to see me rather than one of the male physicians. I have formed a deep friendship with the woman who assists me as an interpreter—with my nursing expertise and her connections to the community, we are able to provide care or obtain services on some level for the patients we see.

I have completed eight mission trips to Peru over the last nine years. On many of the missions I have worked with new nursing graduates or young people interested in a career in nursing. I am actively working to increase those opportunities for the students I teach through mission opportunities and exchange programs in Peru and China. Providing an opportunity for students to experience nursing as part of a mission team entails a great deal of networking and working behind the scenes with key individuals to accomplish the goal. There are lessons to be learned from the experience that simply cannot be taught in the classroom or skills laboratory.

PERU
Nancy Phoenix Bittner

As a nurse educator, creating communities of learning, service, and diversity is foremost in my vision of nursing education. As a faculty where the mission is guided by the Congregation of the Sisters of St. Joseph (CSJ) values, our vision is infused into every level of nursing education. The

CSJ tenets include collaboration with others in identifying and responding to the global community's needs, which undergirds our nursing program's philosophy. The stated goals of Regis College, which flow from the institution's mission, include preparing students as leaders to provide service in the modern world.

There were efforts to connect Regis College nursing programs with global communities. That opportunity came through a service mission planned for students during spring break; the current service mission was developed by the Regis College's Campus Ministry. The mission involved working with a group of youth located in a small parish in Villa El Salvador, Peru, completing small labor projects such as painting, building, and cleaning. This program was an opportunity for nursing students to provide invaluable service to the Villa community. The existing service mission trip had nothing to do with nursing or health.

The story of our community building in Peru began in March of 2007 when I embarked with another nurse educator on a service mission trip for preliminary research. We traveled to Villa El Salvador, Peru, an extremely impoverished, thirty-year-old coastal village of about 400,000 residents located approximately twelve miles southwest of Lima. Prior to departure, months were spent raising money to support the mission and collecting medical supplies and personal care items for the Peruvians. Seventeen suitcases of collected medical supplies and goods were distributed to two health clinics and a nutrition clinic. Health care workers were grateful for the unexpected gifts. The inhabitants lived well below the poverty level on less than one dollar per day. The village children have one school and one daycare center; most children are malnourished and struggle to survive. School supplies, clothes, and other necessities for children were a welcomed surprise.

Our students and faculty cleaned and painted a village sector where most live without running water or plumbing. The medical care systems in place were investigated. In addition, they spent time in clinics and participated in outreach programs, including the community kitchen, nutrition center, daycare center, youth program, and elder care programs. The only hospital had one doctor for 40,000 residents. There was always a line of ill people waiting to be seen. We spent time with the staff and leadership of the two medical clinics. Students, amazed at what they saw, wanted to continue focusing on Peruvian people's needs and helping them.

The trip was a life-changing experience. It was incredible to see people with so little survive. Every day is a struggle to find work, feed their children, and provide an education. The organizers and supporters of this squatter's community, along with the Catholic Church, did an incredible job providing some basic needs. The belief is that teaching Peruvians the skills to combat their poverty is essential to building a new life. Leaders provide education on nutrition, food preparation, cooking, childcare, exercise, health promotion, and disease prevention throughout the community.

Most of the Peruvian health care providers are volunteers who have practices elsewhere and return to give back to those in need. They are well prepared and able to provide basic health care. Peruvian nurses' education level is similar to our associate degree nurse, involving a two- to three-year program. Some have a professional degree, which is a five-year program. There are very few master's prepared nurses in Peru, and they teach in the more prominent and costly nursing programs. In the Villa clinics, there were only technical nurses, including their director.

Following the first Peruvian mission, we submitted a proposal to college administration for an alternative clinical experience during the community health nursing course. Selected faculty and six students from the undergraduate community health course would travel to Peru as part of the March 2008 mission. With requisite approvals and support from the college president, we began planning for the student experience although nearly a year away. Although careful planning is essential, being able to think through situations and improvise as you go along is invaluable. Senior nursing students only were selected based on the following criteria: GPA of 3.0 or better, intermediate Spanish-speaking skills, a nursing faculty recommendation, a personal essay, and an interview. Once selected, weekly preparation sessions began, with students in group meetings with service mission students to begin to acclimate to Peruvian culture, mores, and values. Also reviewed were dress, social practices, and language differences, as well as Peru's rich and tremulous history.

Once in the Peruvian health clinics, students adjusted to the environment quickly, working easily with patients and staff. Their command of Spanish was critical in patient communications. They used their skills in assessment, intervention, and evaluation in this very diverse medical community. The more confident Spanish-speaking students helped the less-confident Spanish speakers. Both faculty and students learned and taught side by side.

Because opportunities to teach important health promotion concepts within the Peruvian culture abound, students completed community clinical experience requirements with faculty at various places in addition to the clinics within Villa El Salvador. The objectives were congruent with course and clinical objectives of the USF community health course. Course and personal objectives were met through clinic work and through extensive home visits.

We visited the Padre Luis Tezza Nursing School of the Ricardo Palma University and were graciously welcomed; we participated in classroom and laboratory experiences with Peruvian students and faculty. The exchange between students and faculty about each program was amazing and ended with an invitation to me, in the same year, to present my research on delegation and omitted care at their International Congress on Patient Safety.

Students who traveled to Peru shared their life-altering experience informally and formally through presentations in the classroom, and clinical and college settings. This experience enhanced their learning and professional development. Students frequently journaled, sharing their sense of awe at the exceptional care that nurses and doctors provided with few resources. They compared practices and interventions, identified the enormous gap in access to quality care, realized their confidence in the skills they applied, and expressed elation with their autonomy level when they gave care in patients' homes. Students expressed pride in their leadership and nursing skills, and described the experience as one of spiritual, personal, and professional growth. Many students were thankful to meet such wonderful, loving, and faith-filled people. Many stay connected to this day and continue to communicate with the youth group members by e-mail.

For me and the other faculty, the Peru experience influenced our teaching and professional development. Now I use examples I learned while working at Villa. My focus is to be vigilant about teaching culturally competent care. I feel the greatest gift I received was that of acceptance and respect for differences. I often need everything perfect and hold others to high levels of expectation. In Villa, working with and caring for people in clinics and homes, it was liberating to not be perfect. Caregivers had little resources and yet they cared for people more effectively than in more developed countries. Their ingenuity and compassion more than makes up for lack of resources. I have tremendous respect for them and the care they give. I continue connecting with my colleagues at the nursing school and within the Villa community. Developed bonds are deep and enriching. Plans are in process to create a two-week exchange program for students and faculty with Padre Luis Tezza and Regis College. Planning also continues for the next community health practice experience.

Knowledge of the site, an understanding of the people's needs, and the resources at the health care site are important. These materials take months to collect, organize, and prepare for transport. Medical and nursing supplies are essential to support many clinics. However, some materials used in the United States are useless in some settings. Generally, gloves, dressing materials, over-the-counter medications, prescription medications, bandages, and cleansers are in need. Quickly, we discovered the need for blood tubes, Petri dishes, and wound care supplies. It is necessary to investigate requirements for bringing goods into a country, as many governments do not permit even philanthropic organizations to bring goods without an imposed tax. Immunizations and health precautions for areas to be visited must be investigated. Passport and visa information should be sought early in the trip planning. If students have passports from countries other than the United States, they may need special visas to travel to certain countries.

Student selection must be carefully planned and consistent. In the second selection, a requirement to converse in Spanish with faculty during the interview was added to ensure the ability to interview the patients. Continuous translation was not practical or efficient in the short clinic visits. Conducting Spanish as a class was not enough to avoid the need for translators.

Students, including the service mission students, participated in discussions about their general expectations of such an experience. Many felt that they will "save the world." It is essential that they realize their contribution, as well as what they will receive in return.

Success is measured in various ways. For nursing students, their growth in leadership and nursing skills, and their contribution to nursing care in a place where there is a need are extraordinary. Many students verbalized personal and spiritual growth that was fostered through the services they attended and the nightly reflection by the group. This was their experience of a lifetime, one that will influence them as a nurse and as a human being. For me, it is a long-awaited opportunity to serve those in need and to provide students with a glimpse of global health with the hope of influencing them by connecting communities.

MULTIPLE SOUTH AND CENTRAL AMERICAN COUNTRIES
Kay Medlin

I began my ministry of international nursing in 1986, when I joined a group called Volunteers in Medical Missions (VIMM), an interdenominational group located in Seneca, South Carolina. VIMM's primary focus areas are Central and South America, although they also go to other areas of the world. They make approximately fifteen trips each year with teams of fifteen to thirty people, including physicians, nurses, dentists, other allied health personnel, and lay volunteers.

Clinics are held in various locations. We give free medicines, vitamins, worm medicine, do some minor surgeries, have a special ministry for children, and give gifts to everyone who comes to the clinic. We also include teaching in hygiene, nutrition, and oral hygiene. We work with local medical doctors while in the country. The governments and the people are very appreciative of the help given them. They are eager to learn how to better provide for themselves.

My first trip with VIMM was to Honduras. After this trip I was challenged to make these trips to developing countries a part of my life each year. Since my first trip, I have made numerous other trips to Honduras, and also trips to other countries. In 1995, I traveled with a team of twelve to mainland China. We traveled to the city of Kunming in southern China, and from there we traveled to a village called Luquan, which is located on what was the Burma Road during World War II. You would assume that a village is small, but this village had a population of 250,000 people. Our clinics were mainly held at the local hospital, where we ministered to several hundred people each day. One day we traveled the Burma Road and into the mountains to minister to the Meow people, who were very hospitable and appreciative of our clinic. We were well received everywhere we went in China. Several Chinese doctors traveled with us each day. They want us to come back to China and do more teaching next time.

In 1996, I went with VIMM to Iquitos, Peru. Iquitos is a city located on the Amazon River, and can only be reached by boat or plane. After spending the night in Iquitos, the next day, we traveled up the Amazon to the Mazan District, which is in the rainforest. The accommodations were primitive, but our team was successful in treating hundreds of Indians, and also performed one rather major surgery. An Indian man had cut his hand with a machete, and had severed the tendons. Two of our doctors worked four hours to sew the tendons back together in his hand. He came back to the clinic each day for six days, and I gave him antibiotic injections. When he came to the clinic on the last day, he could move his fingers, which was a very rewarding experience for everyone on the team. We left him enough antibiotics to finish the healing process. If our team had not been there at that time, he would probably have lost his hand. Even though we had no running water or electricity, and had to sleep on the floor of an old school in sleeping bags, with mosquito netting over us, we had a wonderful trip. We were able to treat approximately 2,000 people during the six days we were there.

In 1997, I traveled to Tanzania, Africa. This country is one of the poorest in Africa. They have virtually no infrastructure. The buses we traveled in were thirty to forty years old, and subject to breaking down. There were sixteen people on this team, three medical doctors, one dentist, one nurse practitioner, five nurses, and the rest were lay-people. One of our doctors did a major surgery while there. A young man in his twenties presented with a huge mass under his chin. At first the doctor thought it was a goiter, but after further examination, he determined it to be a cyst. He deadened the area with local injections, removed the mass, inserted a drain, sutured the area together, gave him injections of antibiotics, and asked him to come back each day for further injections. We were there six days, and he was doing fine at the end of our stay. He was given further antibiotics to take by mouth to complete the healing process. Not many doctors would have attempted the surgery because our clinics were held in a straw hut that the locals had erected for us to use. It was their winter; everything was very dry, and the wind blew red dust through the clinic all day. This was not a very suitable situation for any surgery. The young man was so desperate that the doctor decided to go ahead and trusted God to guide his hands so that the surgery would be successful, and it was. What we were able to accomplish in those six days was a real blessing to the people in that area, which was primarily the Baribaig and Maasi tribes. Several of the men on the team also constructed a small, crude clinic while we were there. This clinic will be a blessing to these people. We have had teams going back periodically, and the clinic is still in operation and ministering to the people in the area.

In 2003, I traveled to Ambato, Ecuador, in South America. While there we ministered to the Quichua Indians. This was a more difficult trip because of the altitude. Some of the team members suffered from altitude sickness, but even with that, we were able to treat in excess of 1,000 people. We also had children's ministries of puppets and games. The children loved that. We visited an orphanage and had a party for them, which they really enjoyed. The Quichua are a timid people, and were not as quick to come to our clinics as other people we have worked with. Even with some obstacles, we felt our trip was a success and that many people were helped by our being there.

Most of my other trips brought me back to the country of Honduras. This is where I have worked the most and love to go. My interest in these trips is primarily the children. Each day on this beautiful planet of ours, over 50,000 children age five and under die of malnutrition-related illnesses. That adds up to over 18,000,000 lives a year. These children are the victims of a moral and political failure to ensure that every person has the basic necessities of life. These trips are one way I can do my part to help alleviate their problems. I fell in love with the people of Honduras, especially the children, from my first trip in 1992, and I hope to continue going back.

A dear friend of mine, who had made several trips with me, was killed in a motor vehicle accident in 1997. My husband and I felt compelled to build a clinic in Honduras in memory of her. She was well known in our community, so we had no problem raising the money for the clinic. Since 1998, we have raised over $50,000 for the clinic. The property for the clinic was donated by a Honduran woman who wanted a clinic built in her community. It is located in the town of Olanchito, which is near the city of Le Cieba. It sits at the base of cloud-covered mountains, and is located on the outskirts of the city. A local taxi service transports people to and from the clinic for a small fee. It serves an area of approximately 100,000 people, and has been very successful. There are three Honduran doctors on staff full time, along with a nurse staff, a pharmacy, a lab, an x-ray room, and an emergency room that is open 'round the clock. They see an average of sixty people each day, and are self-supporting. They are in the process of adding a birthing wing onto the clinic. This clinic provides much better care than the local hospital and has proven to be a real asset to the people in that area.

We have also helped to establish several nutrition clinics in Honduras. Each clinic feeds thirty to fifty children two meals a day, five days a week. The Honduran doctors we work with oversee the clinics and ensure they are operating as they should. Most of these clinics are located in the country where most of the very poor live. Many little children would go hungry were it not for these clinics.

In addition to the medical clinic and the nutrition centers, we are working on property, approximately four acres, that was purchased in 2003 by a VIMM member. There was an existing building on the property, and we are currently in the process of remodeling it. This building will house fifty people, and will be used throughout the year to house medical teams coming into the country. Also, it will be used for teaching seminars for the Hondurans.

I did not become a nurse until I was forty-five years old. My primary purpose for becoming a nurse was to make mission trips to developing countries. This dream has been realized, and it has exceeded my expectations. I have also always been active in my church and community, but as I become older, I feel a greater need to do more in my local community. I am now preparing to start a parish nurse program in my local church, which will help the needy in my community. I am very excited about doing this, as well as continuing my medical mission trips.

Each of us has a unique contribution to make as the history of the world unfolds in our time. As we meet the challenge to treat the desperately poor, we have a tendency to lump them all together and use the term "the poor." But the poor have faces, and they are all unique and different, just as we are. When we look into their faces and respond to their needs, we are blessed. As we give our one loaf and pass it out to the multitudes, it will feed them and return back to us basketfuls.

12

Nurse Educators Who Work in Other Countries

ARMENIA
Salpy Akaragian

My nursing profession expanded beyond the United States in 1991. The first exposure to international colleagues was when a group of Japanese nurses requested to visit UCLA Medical Center and learn about U.S. health care. I was the appointed liaison and educator for the team, and, almost two decades later, we continue to share our knowledge and experience with Japanese nurses as well as many other international colleagues from all continents.

As we continued collaborating with our international colleagues, we also had the opportunity to create and maintain multiple international projects in other countries. One of the countries where we made a considerable impact in nursing and health care is Armenia. In 1995, Armenia's First Lady, L. Ter Petrossian, visited the UCLA School of Nursing with USAID/AIHA representatives. Soon after that visit, UCLA Medical Center, through a grant from USAID/AIHA, developed and implemented the first BSN program in Armenia. Faculty and staff from UCLA taught the first graduates and prepared the new BSN faculty. In June of 1999, in the presence of Armenia's First Lady, the U.S. Ambassador to Armenia, USAID/AIHA representatives, ministers, UCLA Medical Center's Chief of Nursing Heidi Crooks, and other dignitaries from the United States and Armenia, we experienced a historical day when the first BSN class of students graduated. Today, the Erebouni Nursing College continues to educate and prepare BSN students, and now has more than seventy-five graduates.

Some graduates continued on their career paths and received master's degrees in nursing; one of the graduates completed a doctorate degree in the United States. The majority of the graduates are based in Armenia and are leaders in nursing. Graduates took leadership roles in nurse-managed clinics, home health, administration, education, and government. A year after establishment of the BSN program, the Armenian Nurses Association was formed, with our assistance, in Armenia. Today, the Association has over 5,000 members and nursing conferences are held with attendance from around the world. As the BSN program continued, more health care reform projects were developed. For example, under the leadership of Dr. C. Barrett from UCLA, the Neonatal Intensive Care Unit was created at Erebouni Medical Center by Dr. H. Koushkyan, where, for the first time, a premature infant received Surfactant. After intense training of the physicians and nurses, we created a neonatal resuscitation center and because of this project, the infant mortality rate decreased 50% at the Center. Today, this group of physicians and nurses travel to rural areas in the country and educate their colleagues. In addition, we concentrated on improving women's health by training surgeons to perform gynecologic laparoscopic surgeries and they became the pioneers in performing such surgeries in Armenia. We also opened the first ambulatory health care center (ARMA) based on the U.S. model.

As the above-mentioned projects were progressing successfully, USAID/AIHA awarded another five-year grant to begin planning the model for primary health care in Armenia. With the leadership of UCLA Family Medicine's department under Drs. Dowling and Bholat, we started the project in the Lori region, which is two hours away from Yerevan, Armenia's capital. After training the medical doctors, nurses, laboratory personnel, pharmacists, and other health care providers, and purchasing appropriate equipment and developing guidelines, the clinic transformed into a practice very similar to what we have in the United States. We conducted health fairs annually in the region providing services to over 10,000 people and collecting data to better understand the health status of the region's citizens. The program extended to villages and provided special women's health services; Pap smears, breast exams, and ultrasounds were provided to over 200 women each day. Women who had questionable ultrasound results were transported to the ARS-Akhourian Mother and Child Clinic for follow-up mammograms. Women received the results before they returned to the region and those who needed further follow-up were referred to the oncology center in Yerevan.

USAID/AIHA took note of our success in Armenia, evidenced by measurable quality outcomes and success in bridging the practice and education chasm with consistent and continuous education and training. Therefore, they approached us with another initiative, which began our journey to elevate the quality of nursing care in two major hospitals in Yerevan, Armenia, by implementing American Nurse Credentialing Center's Magnet standards and practices. Under the directorship of Dr. Linda Aiken, we launched this project and within two years the hospitals restructured the nursing departments, created policies, developed job descriptions and performance evaluations, began professional development courses, developed and implemented committees, nursing documentation, and care guidelines, and began performance improvement activities, all in line with Magnet standards. It was remarkable to see the nurses learn the process of performance improvement and conduct their prevalence surveys and analyze the data. At the end of the program both hospitals received a special award called Journey to Excellence by the American Nurse Credentialing Center.

While the Magnet project was progressing, another project was being considered in Armenia by the Ministry of Health for Erebouni Medical Center. Dr. Akira Ishiyama, Professor of Head and Neck Surgery at David Geffen UCLA School of Medicine, along with several leaders in the Armenian community, began discussing the possibility of establishing a cochlear implant center in Armenia. After much discussion and planning, as well as establishing the project's infrastructure, the program was launched in 2003. The project marked its success with Armenia becoming the regional center for cochlear implant surgeries. Due to philanthropic and volunteer efforts, over thirty-two children and young adults have received the "gift of hearing" via the cochlear implant surgeries and are now living in mainstream society. The project's success is due to collaborative efforts of the United States' and Armenia's medical teams, as well as the Armenian International Medical Fund, under its founder and chair Salpy Akaragian, for its financial and administrative support. This project is also recognized by the Armenian government as one of its innovative health care projects. In addition to cochlear implant surgeries, plans are underway to begin a neurosurgery project, to establish the Armenian National Ear Center, as well as to continue with the exchange program agreed upon between David Geffen UCLA School of Medicine and Yerevan State Medical University.

Even though much was accomplished in a very short time, I would like to share the following story, which has stayed deep in my heart. In 1997, during one of my trips to Armenia, I was asked to visit a three-year-old girl named Narine in the intensive care unit. Narine was recovering from a splenectomy and was soon to begin chemotherapy for the diagnosis of hystocytosis X. To confirm the diagnosis, I was asked by Dr. S. Avagyan to assist this child by arranging the appropriate consult and proper treatment. After much discussion and fact finding, we obtained blood work from Narine and sent it to major laboratories in the United States. Thanks to a number of volunteer physicians and laboratories in the United States, the child was re-diagnosed with Gaucher disease and thus there was no need for chemotherapy. You can only imagine the mother's happiness when she heard the news that chemotherapy was not indicated. Even though the initial diagnosis was not accurate, the current diagnosis was not treatable in Armenia. With the help of the Armenian Government Ministry of Health, the Armenian Relief Society, and other organizations, Narine flew to Germany and received the treatment necessary to control her health problem. Today, Narine is an adolescent and enjoys life to its fullest. After twenty years, my commitment and dedication continues for people less fortunate than us, and stories like Narine's inspire me daily and fulfill my life.

CAMBODIA
Marietta Bell-Scriber

I arrived at Sihanouk Hospital Center of Hope (SHCH) in Cambodia with teaching materials related to cardiovascular topics, such as cerebral vascular accident, angina, myocardial infarction, and valve disease. Then, Phalla, one of the SHCH nurse educators at SHCH, chose interpretation of electrocardiograms (ECGs) as my teaching topic. Thus, on my first day at the hospital, I began teaching ECG interpretation to Cambodian nurses who came daily to the site.

Teaching in Cambodia was halfway around the world from where I teach nursing at Ferris State University in Big Rapids, Michigan. I traveled alone to this a distant location to teach nurses within another culture. Working in partnership with Health Volunteers Overseas (HVO), sponsored by the American Association of Colleges of Nursing (AACN), there was a mutual agreement that I would teach in Phnom Penh, Cambodia, for two weeks during spring break. The purpose was to educate Cambodian nurses who have barriers and limited access to quality education. E-mail communications with Phalla prior to my arrival were brief and limited. So, although we had agreed on several cardiovascular topics, I arrived not knowing where I should focus for the best learning outcomes. Thus, I compiled and brought with me many teaching materials, hoping that some would be useful for their learning needs.

As I began teaching, I quickly discovered there were a few challenges with the language barriers. I found one of the best teaching methods to be free-hand writing and drawing on a white board. Initially, when I asked the nurses to identify anatomical structures, I often found it difficult to understand their pronunciations of English words. However, after a few sessions, I noticed that nurses were slowly repeating my pronunciations of English words. Every time I said a word, they repeated it. Not only were they learning how to read ECGs but they were also learning English. This was an unexpected learning outcome, indeed!

Teaching presented a further challenge because some of the nurses were more advanced in their ECG-reading skills and spoke better English than others. Therefore, nurses with advanced knowledge and skills would answer my questions. The others who did not understand ECGs or English were silent and struggling. To reach the struggling learners, I wrote most information on the white board. I was surprised to discover that numbers did not always easily translate to another culture. My intention was to emphasize consistent patterns used to interpret rhythms as they reviewed rhythm strips. For example, one pattern is: (1) identify the QRS; (2) determine whether the rate is regular; (3) identify whether there are p waves; and so on. Then, they were to determine abnormal rhythms. Finally, there was interpretation of the rhythm.

After the first week, the nurses entered the classroom and greeted me by saying, "Hello, Teacher!" When they asked me a question, they said, "Teacher, can you explain …?" I cannot fully explain why calling me Teacher was so touching. Perhaps it was the underlying respect and humbleness. It was an honor as these nurses perceived and accepted me as their teacher.

We fell into a comfortable pattern over time: they would listen to me talk, I drew pictures of the heart and wrote words on the white board

to explain what was happening in the heart, then we would review practice rhythm strips, and finally, I would coach them how to interpret the
rhythms. I taught more slowly and they began to ask more questions. I
eventually perceived that they were actually learning useful information
applicable to their practice.

Did I mention how much the Cambodian people smile? As soon as
their eyes met mine, they smiled. I never realized how much I did not
smile until I found myself smiling back, to the point where my cheeks
ached. Here was a developing country whose people struggled in so
many ways, and yet they were always smiling. I still find this demonstration of happiness incredible. This experience made me question what
one truly needs to be happy.

Toward the end of the two-week program, one nurse asked to place
my ECG lectures and practice strips on the hospital's intranet so they
could download them and continue to practice. I was surprised that they
wanted to do this. Revisiting previous learning was a practice very far
removed from my traditional American nursing students who tend to
leave previous learning behind, and to not revisit earlier content.

There were three nurse educators who took leadership in order to
educate nurses at Sihanhouk Hospital and in the provinces. These educators shared an office at the hospital with the nursing supervisors. This
office is also where I spent my time prior to the ECG teaching sessions.
After a few days of my presence, the nurse educators came to me with
questions. I never knew what they were going to ask and, of course, I did
not always know the answer. Examples were, "What does 'altered mental
status' mean?" or "What does it mean when it says 'half-life' (drug)?"
and so on. Thank goodness for the Internet and access to my university's
library, because I located and then explained the answers.

One nurse educator, Rossi, brought me a teaching video related to
human immunodeficiency virus (HIV) infection. It was very complicated:
How the virus invades the cell, the enzymes that work to break down
the cell barriers, how the DNA is transformed, and so on. He wanted
me to translate it into "simple English." No easy job! HIV is a very difficult subject that requires a detailed understanding of how the body
works. Although I wondered whether someone could interpret it for me
so I could interpret it for them, I was able to interpret the HIV video
using a resource I brought with me. Coincidentally (or I should say syn-
chronistically), I was teaching pathophysiology that same semester and
took my pathophysiology book with me to Cambodia. This book enabled

understanding and interpretation. After I completed the interpretation, I told them to circle anything that did not make sense and I would make the interpretation more clear. After reading my interpretation, they said they understood and thanked me for my assistance.

Phalla, the nurse educator with whom I interacted most frequently, discussed her struggles in finding education materials to teach the Cambodian nurses. Although she spoke English, she revealed that she was not always able to interpret the information from textbooks or via the Internet. She described sitting and crying, feeling frustrated as she tried to read and interpret health and nursing information from English to Khmer, their native language. Although it was a gift when nurse educators were sent to Cambodia by Health Volunteers Overseas, she often was scheduled to staff the emergency room and could not attend the teaching sessions. I observed that she only attended a few of my sessions although a male nurse educator, Hong, came to several others. Of course, the ideal is to educate the trainer so the education can continue after the nurse educators leave, but patient care was always a necessary top priority.

I was asked by Phalla to create policies and procedures that were missing from their hospital manual. She requested a section on pericardiocentesis and I selected one on synchronized cardioversion. I was provided with their policies and procedures manual to view the format and I accessed information via my university's library and the Web, and I completed both policies and procedures. This was quite a challenge because I did not know what equipment they had available to them and was aware that best practices might not make sense in this setting due to a lack of resources and could increase their frustration. After I completed the policies and procedures, the nursing supervisor reviewed them to determine if they were appropriate for their resources and this setting.

The male educator, Hong, is their ECG expert who is self-taught by using an old ECG book that he translated from English to Khmer for understanding by the Cambodian nurses. While I was there, he asked me several questions from the book to ensure he was interpreting ECGs correctly. However, the information available to him was limited because there were several pages missing from the book, including an entire section on atrial rhythms. Before I left, I ordered a new ECG book for him to be delivered directly to the hospital. He e-mailed me several months later, thanking me for the book that had finally arrived.

Cambodia has survived decades of civil war launched by the Khmer Rouge and the Pol Pot regime in the 1970s. This war resulted in the genocide of 2.5 million Cambodians, a severely damaged infrastructure, and a broken education and health care system. I was told by the nurse educators that the doctors and nurses who were not killed during this regime fled the country. Thus, Cambodia was left with a severe shortage of health care labor and the expertise needed to rebuild their health care delivery system.

Phalla shared that, at the present time, the nurses received an education perceived as poor quality because of limited resources. She said this is why nurses are excited when nurse educators come from other countries and they can learn from experts in their fields. Some nurses who came to my presentations traveled at their own expense from surrounding areas and provinces. These nurses usually spent a dollar for transportation, which is considerable money for them. Although the nurses are paid better at the Sihanouk Hospital of Hope, the nurses are not paid well in the government-owned hospitals. They may receive only $25 for a month's work. Thus, spending a dollar is like spending a day's wage.

The hospitals nursing care may be less adequate because of limited supplies. If the government-owned hospital obtains supplies, then it must charge a substantial fee to cover costs. Thus, the only hope for many Cambodians, who have little money, is the free care available at Sihanouk. Every morning, these needy people arrive with family and friends, and line up under the hospital's awning, hoping and often begging to receive care. People who are ambulatory line up on the left, people in wheelchairs line up in the middle, and those awaiting surgery line up on the right. If they are not able to receive care after they are triaged, the family returns home, often manually lifting them into a Tuk Tuk (a small carriage with seats pulled by a small one-person moto taxi). They may return the next day and repeat the process again.

Although my purpose for traveling to Cambodia was to improve the education of the Cambodian nurses at the Sihanouk Hospital Center of HOPE through nursing presentations, I decided to write about my experiences in an effort to express what I learned. Because we decided to adopt learner-centered teaching strategies in our nursing program prior to traveling to Cambodia, I decided to connect some of my teaching-learning experiences to this approach. What follows are the lessons I learned.

When the Cambodian nurses selected said that they wanted to learn ECGs, they made a decision about their learning. This power sharing created motivated, confident, and responsible learners excited about learning. As the teacher, I found that their energy drove me to be more of a risk-taker who became more visual and my teaching pace slowed down.

This was a life-changing experience for me. I cannot say any one moment was more powerful than another. Each day touched me differently. Now that I am home, although I remain sad at leaving Sihanouk Hospital Center of Hope and the Cambodian people, I am hopeful that I made a small difference. I know they made a big difference in my personal and professional life. Perhaps my gift to them was hope for a better tomorrow. Their gift to me was an appreciation of our U.S. resources and a deeper understanding about teaching and learning that will be embedded in my practice for years to come.

CAMBODIA
Susan C. Taplin and Sharon W. Dowdy

On April 17, 1975, the Khmer Rouge rolled into the capital city of Phnom Penh and evacuated two million people from their homes, businesses, hospitals, schools, and pagodas into the countryside. Over the next four years, families were separated, schools were closed, and all religious activity was forbidden by the new regime. Saloth Sar (also known as Pol Pot or Brother Number One), influenced by the works of Stalin and Mao, hoped to create a perfect, classless society of peasant workers and farmers. In an effort to meet his goals, he brutally tortured and killed anyone suspected of being a threat to the Angkor organization. Educated people were targeted and killed if three incident reports of crimes against the government were made to the leadership. Targeted occupations were Buddhist monks, teachers, government officials, bankers, business owners, and health care providers, including physicians and nurses. During this reign of terror, without hospitals or clean living conditions, many people died from disease and severe malnutrition. Malaria, typhoid, dysentery, and other grave illness were rampant.

Cambodia lost so many of its educated people. Today, the population has increased to an estimated four million people; many live in villages with no running water or electricity. Poor nutrition and limited access to health care are continuous concerns. The health care system suffered tremendously in terms of destruction of hospitals and loss of workers. Present-day nurses include some who were able to hide during the regime and others who have been trained in nursing, although often without any formal education prior to nursing school.

In 1996, HOPE Worldwide, a charitable faith-based organization that serves the poor, began the Sihanouk Hospital Center of HOPE. The hospital, located in the capitol city of Phnom Penh, was established to provide free post-graduate training to health care professionals while providing high-quality free care to the Cambodian poor. For the past twelve years, the hospital has worked toward the goal of developing Khmer health care professionals to lead and manage the hospital.

For the first ten years of the hospital's existence, expatriate nursing volunteers and hospital staff provided education and training to the nursing staff at HOPE. The first expatriate director of nursing served for seven years followed by two others, one of which was a previous Belmont University nursing instructor who served for two years. The nursing department, the largest in the hospital, was the first to meet the hospital's goal of having a Khmer health care professional lead the department. After several years of leadership and management training of a core group of charge nurses and supervisors, a Khmer director of nursing was chosen from this core group. Intense interviewing was conducted by representatives from human resources and nursing expatriates to choose this person, which was followed by a year of close one-on-one training with the expatriate previous director of nursing. Then, the expatriate nurse stepped back and the local director of nursing led the nursing department.

Following the appointment of a Khmer director of nursing, the next goal was to develop a nursing education department for continuing education of nursing personnel, including the nurses at HOPE and the nursing schools within the country. Another identified goal in the country was for "capacity building," the purpose of which is to strengthen and develop skills and resources of local government hospitals to increase the standard of health care for all Cambodians. Additionally, capacity building projects help form a professional community for sharing knowledge. To accomplish these two goals, four Khmer nursing educators were selected through a stringent interview process that included candidates presenting an assigned educational nursing module in English to a selection committee composed of expatriate nurses and Khmer human resource personnel. This group of nursing educators is now charged with meeting the educational needs of the nursing department, teaching in the local government hospitals, and organizing expatriate nurse volunteers.

Nursing professionals, along with other health care professionals, share several problems in the wake of the Khmer Rouge regime. Many emotional issues continue. Much of the work force includes people directly affected by the genocide; many suffer from post-traumatic stress disorder with little psychological help available in the country. Often due to cultural mores, nurses are promoted based on age and sex rather than job competency, leading to issues of mistrust and jealousy. Considerable time was spent on wielding support for the Khmer director of nursing from the core nursing leadership. Further, education is conducted in English, which may be a second or third language for Cambodian people.

Because of a dream that a faculty member related to the nursing dean at Belmont University had before leaving for Cambodia to act as director of nursing at Sihanouk Hospital Center of HOPE, a study-abroad course to Cambodia began. The dream was based on a desire to provide support and to bridge an educational gap in the HOPE nursing department, while providing an opportunity for nursing students to learn and serve in a developing third-world country. This dream aligned with the university's mission statement, "Belmont University is a student-centered Christian community providing an academically challenging education that empowers men and women of diverse backgrounds to engage and transform the world with disciplined intelligence, compassion, courage and faith." Within five months, the dream turned into a reality with the first student group arriving in Cambodia. The dream has continued with successful trips for the past four years.

The study-abroad course to Cambodia is a three-hour nursing elective. Trips are planned for three weeks, including the time to travel to and from the country. Students experience clinical rotations in the emergency department, triage area, medical and surgical units, outpatient clinics, the operating room, and the chronic care facility that cares for HIV patients. The students have an opportunity to accompany a social worker on home visits to HIV patients, learning about the daily lives of these patients. Village trips (some overnight) are organized for the students to experience life in rural Cambodia while providing needed supplies such as rice, clothing, bicycles, and medical care. Cultural experiences are peppered throughout the trip with opportunities to eat local food and visit museums and temples.

The study-abroad course has evolved over the last four years based on several lessons learned from Belmont students and Cambodian nursing staff. For the first trips, organizational meetings were held a few weeks before departure. Required reading was assigned, but not completed prior to the trip. In our latest rendition, classes are scheduled throughout the spring semester with deadlines and assignments for the readings, allowing time for team building, learning about the culture, preparing for hospital presentations, and understanding course expectations.

Other changes in the course relate to the challenges of students and faculty being together in close quarters for extended periods. The students view the nursing faculty in all aspects of stress and joy, and vice versa. This constant appraisal of one another can lead to added stress. To combat this problem, the faculty have relaxed their stronghold on the students' every move and set boundaries instead. Students are advised of the dangers of being in a foreign country, are given specific perimeters of freedom, and then trusted instead of watched. Student evaluations have reflected satisfaction with this more flexible style of leadership. The faculty members encourage each other with positive feedback and prayer. All persons are advised to spend some time alone.

An important bonding ritual for the group is to share "highs" and "lows" at the end of the day. Students experience events they have never even considered before. For example, the hospital experiences include young patients suffering from congestive heart failure due to an untreated streptococcal infection, diabetics coming into the emergency room in a coma before knowing they have the disease, and patients with wounds treated by traditional medicine by packing with mud and weeds who have subsequently developed gangrene. On the street, they see children sleeping or caring for younger siblings, begging from patron to patron. During visits with the social worker, they see HIV-affected families struggling to survive, with mothers sewing items from discarded rice bags to make enough money for food, school for the children (about $0.25 per day per child), and the $10 monthly rent for the simple dwelling. Sharing their evoked emotions helps the group to bond, show compassion, learn from each other, and grow.

Another lesson learned is how to fund the international study-abroad trips. For the past four years, students approached their families and local church congregations for support monies for the study-abroad programs through Belmont University. This year, two separate funds are being started within the university, one so that support for students' travel can be raised throughout the year through tax-deductible gifts, and the other to provide for the needs of the Cambodian poor. In addition, faculty and staff in the College of Health Sciences were approached this past year to contribute to providing for the needs of the Cambodian poor. Specifically, there was a bicycle fund to buy bicycles for students in one of the villages when they completed sixth grade, allowing them to ride the long distance to the next village and attend high school.

Two more developmental changes have occurred. Based on the dates for the Cambodian king's birthday holiday, during which the hospital is minimally staffed, and the jet lag component, a few days of rest and sightseeing is now scheduled before arriving for work at HOPE Hospital. Further, a "blog" of the trip, including pictures and individual student postings, has been kept for the last two years. The blog has been an invaluable experience for the students as they receive positive comments from friends, family, faculty, and staff. It has also been very enlightening and encouraging to those in the United States. The experience is shared in real time while thoughts and feelings are fresh.

The village trips have also changed over the years. The first year, a trip was made to a village that is known for pottery-making skills. The students spent a few hours learning about the process of making clay pots and firing them with no electricity, baking the pots in the sun. Rice farming was also explained to the students, and they were able to see how rice in rural Cambodia is processed. While this was a good experience, it did not allow the true "lived experience" of rural Cambodia. The following year, the village trip was overnight, allowing the students a more realistic experience of life without running water, electricity, or the comforts of home. It helped the students have a better understanding of lack of access to health care and the issues that contribute to poor health in the country.

This past year, the Belmont University group partnered with another nonprofit organization that is building sustainable schools in rural Cambodia, and spent two days in one of the villages. Students taught basic hand washing and oral hygiene to students and staff of a rural community elementary school. Food-handling principles were shared with the school cooks. Three-fourths of the students, around 200 boys and girls, were assessed by the Belmont group for nutritional deficiencies without the use of laboratory findings. A mini-health clinic was conducted, with students evaluating heights, weights, temperatures, and nutritional needs. One of the Khmer nursing educators from HOPE provided wound care, as well as teaching and translation services. The experience was phenomenal; students and faculty learned lessons in organization, communication, and logistics, as well as serving as a cultural experience for all.

An important aspect of the trip is to build and strengthen the partnership with the nursing department at the Center of HOPE and Belmont University. The two Belmont faculty members provide nursing education to the nursing leadership and staff during each trip. Bedside teaching rounds are conducted, where specific patient cases are discussed and recommendations made for areas of continuing education. For example, it was observed during teaching rounds that nurses were not using draw sheets or proper body mechanics to turn and position patients. Therefore, recommendations were made to the Cambodian nursing leadership to reinforce the importance of turning patients every two hours using proper body mechanics. Cambodian nurses are challenged in critical thinking skills during these nursing rounds and are provided with educational opportunities to understand why they perform the care they do. Cambodian nursing educators and Belmont nursing students also participate in the rounds. It is a lively discussion, which helps to identify reinforcement teaching needs. Additionally, formal classes are taught based on suggestions from the Cambodian nursing leadership in areas of pathophysiology, nursing care, and leadership/management.

The two Belmont faculty members built rapport and mutual trust with the Cambodian nursing educators. Each trip provides mentorship opportunities. Sessions are conducted whereby the two Belmont faculty members listen to and critique lectures developed by the Cambodian nursing educators. The growth seen in the educator group has been amazing over the past three years. The Belmont faculty has helped develop and continue an annual, hospital-wide skills check-off session for the Cambodian nursing staff. Now that the annual session is in place, Belmont students can organize and participate in this process every year. The skills check-offs ensure that each Cambodian nurse has certain competencies for providing basic nursing care, thereby setting a beginning standard of care for the hospital and perhaps, in the future, for all of Cambodia.

Every year has seen growth in the Cambodian nursing leaders' ability to search the literature, organize information, and understand scientific information in another language in order to present up-to-date, continuing education programs to the hospital's nurses. Cambodian nurse educators are involved in grant-funded, capacity-building projects to teach and train nurses and health care providers in government hospitals and clinics in rural Cambodia. They travel to villages and provide assessment, education, and training, thereby helping the country raise health care standards. Local nursing schools also send students to HOPE, where Cambodian nurse educators ensure a meaningful clinical experience.

Another enrichment method for professional development of HOPE nurses is through a journal club. Belmont nursing students choose one or two articles in English about an applicable nursing topic to share with local staff. Students conduct a journal club meeting to help the Cambodian nursing staff increase their reading comprehension skills. The journal club provided Belmont nursing students with opportunities to interact with the Cambodian nursing staff in a fun, meaningful way while helping nurses develop skills in understanding difficult medical terminology in English. Many times, Belmont students have initially expressed apprehension about leading a journal club but find that they feel a sense of reward and accomplishment upon leading the club.

The partnership between Belmont University College of Health Sciences and HOPE Hospital is in the growing stage. In addition to the yearly trip, the HOPE nursing leaders use e-mail to exchange ideas with the two Belmont nursing faculty. Belmont provides textbooks, lab equipment, and other supplies to the HOPE nursing department. Each year, the Cambodian nursing leaders participate in developing the study-abroad trip.

Recently, the Cambodian director of nursing and one of the nursing educators visited Belmont University. This provided an opportunity to meet with Belmont University leadership and strengthen relationships by providing face-to-face interaction. The two nurses from HOPE also met with the faculty and dean of the College of Health Sciences to discuss joint goals and to collaborate in developing a shared vision for the future. For the two Cambodian nurses, it was an opportunity to see and experience a culture different from their own, to deepen relationships, and to strengthen understanding of each other. Upon their return to Cambodia and on reflection of the trip to Nashville, Tennessee, they said in an e-mail, "View of Nashville is green and lovely place for us but coming to Belmont was more interesting and surprising. Tea talk made us feel honored and welcomed by vice president and other professors. We would like to see the nursing students coming to Cambodia to exchange experience with culture and knowledge every year."

Future plans include developing a certification course for the nursing staff that would include online courses to be completed during the year. Testing and evaluations would be done by Belmont faculty during the yearly trip. Plans are underway to include other disciplines within the College of Health Sciences, such as pharmacy, physical therapy, and occupational therapy in the partnership, as well as non-health-related disciplines at Belmont, including business, entrepreneurship, and journalism.

It is difficult to express in words the deep bond that has developed over the years between the Belmont faculty and the nursing department at the Center of HOPE. The opportunities to see the nursing leaders' and staff's growth, as well as changes and learning by Belmont students, are true gifts. The experience continues to be awe-inspiring, faith-building, and educational.

CHINA
Gwen Sherwood and Huaping Liu

China commands fascination as one of the earliest civilizations, with 5,000 years of recorded history. Its enormous land mass is home to 1.3 billion people and 56 ethnic groups—an evident challenge to a rapidly changing health care system. As a result, the past two decades have seen significant revision in the health professions' education, particularly nursing, as much to align with global standards as to launch initial efforts in workforce planning.

Nurse educators have been remarkable pioneers in the evolving history of nursing development in China, most notably in the last two decades of resurgence. The first training programs are recorded in 1835 and the first school in 1888. Some of the earliest baccalaureate nursing education programs were developed in China in the early 1920s; the program at Peking Union Medical College (PUMC) was led by Anna Wolf, later dean of nursing at the Johns Hopkins University School of Nursing (JHUSON) in the United States. Nursing education was awarded formal status in the government education system in 1934.

Nurse pioneers Lin Juying and Wang Xiuying, widely respected throughout China, were among those educators whose commitment to nursing education as the means to advance the profession ensured China's global recognition. Their perseverance brought focus on the need to improve nursing education to match the rapid developments in health care reform and outcome expectations. By 1983, baccalaureate programs had opened in the major medical universities, even with a scarcity of nurses with advanced preparation to lead them. With support from New York's China Medical Board, a philanthropic organization devoted to advancing health in China and neighboring Asian countries, local and international collaborations were formed to build the educational infrastructure that would propel rapid advancement in nursing to parallel developments in medicine. Rather than a prescriptive application from other countries, a multistep plan of partnerships developed well-articulated basic and graduate nursing programs that reflect intrinsic health and cultural expectations.

The first collaborative initiated by the China Medical Board was the Committee on Graduate Nursing Education (COGNE); sixteen nursing faculty from more than a thousand applicants from China's eight leading health universities were selected to attend one of six selected U.S. schools of nursing for two years to obtain master's degrees in nursing. That all of these were successful demonstrated China's readiness for professional advancement in nursing. Although only four are known to have returned to work in China, one of those was later awarded a scholarship to obtain a doctorate from George Mason University, the first Chinese nurse to earn a Ph.D. and return to teach in China.

Seeking a higher retention rate, the China Medical Board again worked with the major medical universities for a new initiative. Although there were some efforts to launch master's-level education in nursing in China as early as 1992, there remained a dearth of prepared faculty to lead from a nursing perspective. In 1993, the China Medical Board convened a group of nurse leaders from China's eight major medical universities for a week-long intensive meeting to develop a cooperative degree program with Chiang Mai University in Thailand. The Program on Higher Nursing Education Development (POHNED) was housed at Xi'an Medical University and admitted 16 students per year for five years, graduating 84 nurses over the program's history. Degrees were awarded by Chiang Mai University, and their experienced faculty helped mentor Chinese faculty for teaching in graduate education. This infusion of qualified nursing faculty thus began a redesign of nursing education in China with a nursing philosophy.

With a growing cadre of master's-prepared nursing faculty, the China Medical Board next supported an intense week-long workshop to develop a new model of baccalaureate nursing curriculum based on a nursing philosophy unique to China. Both authors of this chapter had leadership roles in the workshop. Faculty focus groups at Peking Union Medical College, China's oldest and most developed nursing program, redefined course content, contact hours, curriculum sequence, and learning strategies for each course in a new, visionary, four-year baccalaureate degree, a baccalaureate completion degree, and an associate degree program. These groundbreaking curriculum models received government approval to be adapted across China and helped stimulate curriculum reform, as well as an increasing conversion of secondary programs to baccalaureate programs.

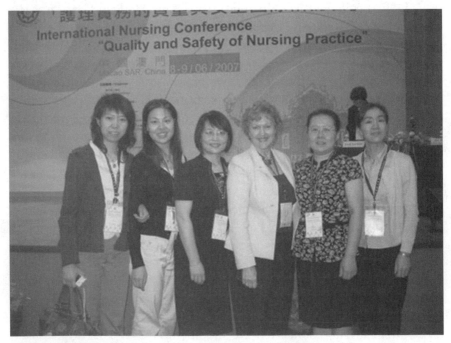

Pictured from left to right at the International Nursing Conference in 2007 are Jing Li (Peking Union Medical College [PUMC] School of Nursing faculty and Visiting Scholar), Ke Xu (PUMC faculty), Huaping Liu (Dean, PUMC, and co-author), Gwen Sherwood (University of North Carolina at Chapel Hill), Zheng Li (PUMC Associate Dean for Research), and Liping Wu (PUMC faculty and former Visiting Scholar).

Program articulation provided educational mobility for nurses and also allowed nurses to participate in continuing education to advance from secondary levels of education to the baccalaureate level. With these program developments, China began to produce an increased pool of master's-prepared nurses, as well as increasing the pool of baccalaureate graduates qualified for graduate school enrollment. This advancement in nursing education greatly expanded the leadership capacity of nurses and influenced clinical practice as well as changes that spread across China.

The first doctoral program was a cooperative agreement between Peking Union Medical College and the Johns Hopkins University in the United States. The three-year program includes six months of study at the Johns Hopkins University School of Nursing. Teaching as well as supervising the research synthesis projects is a joint venture between the Johns Hopkins faculty and PUMC faculty. Fifteen students were admitted during the first three years, and the first group of five graduated in July of 2008. In the meantime, five other schools have launched doctoral programs, although there continues to be a scarcity of nurses with terminal degrees to lead them.

Concurrent with the massive restructuring of nursing education was the necessary development of educational resources to replenish materials lost in the Cultural Revolution. Western China University led a textbook and writing development project, supported by the China Medical Board, but involving all of China's major nursing schools. Nurse educators were commissioned to complete a set of nine contemporary nursing textbooks written in the Chinese language and from Chinese perspectives. These textbooks were standardized for all schools and adopted by the Ministry of Health including Fundamentals, Medical, Surgical, Obstetrics, Pediatrics, Intensive Care, Management, Psychiatry, and Research. Due to the overwhelming success, an additional six have been commissioned.

Nurse educators contributed to the launch of Chinese-language nursing journals to promote knowledge development and dissemination. Nursing journals published in the Chinese language reach across education, research, and practice topics. Further, nurses are increasingly publishing their work in English language journals as well.

Education is foundational to establishing nursing as a scholarly discipline. The collaborative programs pioneered by Chinese nursing leaders offered the educational mobility needed for professional advancement.

China is experiencing the same growing complexity of patient care requiring higher levels of preparation to meet health care needs as in other developed countries. With an increasing cadre of nurses with higher levels of education, baccalaureate programs have increased, middle-level nursing programs decreased, and master's programs have proliferated.

The strategic period of 1996–99 marked significant nursing education reform facilitated by Lin Juying, Wang Xiuying, and Huaping Liu through the Higher Education Reform Committee. Schools across China moved nursing higher education from the traditional medical model to a contemporary nursing model that embraced intrinsic health beliefs with nursing concepts. Remaining true to its history, nursing in China is melding traditional Chinese medicine with principles of Western medicine in a culturally attuned model. The new model for baccalaureate programs is built around concepts based on human body function and needs. The reform initiative reduced program length from five years to four, and integrated classroom and clinical. Combining medical and surgical nursing was based on six organizing concepts: social interaction, activity–rest, nutrition–elimination, oxygenation, reproduction, and cognition–perception. Community health nursing, professional nursing, nursing education, and research are new additions to the curriculum.

There has been an active professional nursing association in China since 1909; still, political constraints prevent membership in the International Council of Nurses. The Chinese Nursing Association, with 334,655 members, is the only professional association for nurses in China. Its goals are to serve members by uniting Chinese nurses, developing the profession, providing professional evaluation, and supporting research. It helps distribute new knowledge and skills in nursing journals and books, as well as providing continuing education programs for members. The association serves a major function by advising and informing major policy makers and communicating information from members to the government, while also seeking to protect the rights of members.

With these professional advancements there is high demand for nurses with clinical and leadership skills. The International Council of Nurses, the World Health Organization, and the Ministry of Health collaborated to host a groundbreaking leadership development program at PUMC from 2007 to 2009, First Leadership for Change™. The ongoing work seeks to prepare nurse leaders to participate effectively in health policy development and decision making. Developing effective leaders and managers in nursing and health services positions ensures that nurses have a role in health care reform. Trends in reform are moving from government provision of care to care that is increasingly privatized. The workshop also sought to help nurses influence appropriate changes in nursing curricula and educational systems.

Another educational program is from the Dreyfus Health Foundation, which worked collaboratively across China to advance critical thinking. Their program, Problem Solving for Better Health™, had a ripple effect as participants apply learned skills to change health care outcomes and work toward evidence-based standards of care.

With advances in education driving practice developments, China's nursing leaders have initiated the first workforce planning efforts to examine nurse staffing, updated position descriptions, workload measurement, and evaluation of nursing development strategies. The data has led to changes in workforce policy. Evidence-based nurse staffing standards match human resources with patient care needs to reduce costs. To address China's nurse shortage, the Ministry of Health used these data and measurement methods to formulate its first nursing work force plan, the Strategy Plan for Nursing Development 2005–2010.

Research in other settings confirms the positive impact of a well-educated nursing work force on care outcomes. Creating an educational system that provides educational mobility and advanced nursing roles will continue to enhance the image of nursing in China and to provide the needed professional growth. Graduate education has provided faculty for schools of nursing, but now a growing interest exists in developing specialty practice for advanced clinical nurses.

Nurses need expertise to establish formal pathways to guide practice for health-oriented populations. This requires specialized knowledge that goes beyond basic nursing education. Nursing education and health care delivery must collaborate, working in tandem to determine roles, education, and desired clinical outcomes in developing appropriate and relevant advanced practice models.

Challenges remain. Even with expansion of baccalaureate programs, 70% of nurses are prepared at the secondary technical level. Nurses need increasing research skills to build an evidence-based practice, to measure nursing quality indicators, and to develop expertise in methods and measurement tools. There is a need for developing community health nursing models to address increasing incidence of AIDS/HIV and other infectious diseases, as well as an aging population. The need for expanding leadership capacity through greater access to higher education and mobility will continue. Accreditation and practice standards are in early developmental stages and will impact future educational development. With China's entry into the market economy and privatization of health care, nurses will need to be informed on issues related to financing, access, and opportunities for professional role development.

Nurse educators in China have sought to develop the profession in a way that maintains its culture by blending Eastern traditional medicine with Western acute care. The goal has been to develop a nursing approach that matches Chinese beliefs and expectations to provide relevant health care. POHNED graduates are playing important roles in nursing education and are becoming leaders across nursing. With advances in education, Chinese nurses will be able to provide the best care for their population.

DOMINICAN REPUBLIC
Charlotte Souers

This innovative Nursing Field Studies course was coordinated through Ohio University's Office of Education Abroad to provide a cultural experience for nursing students in a health care clinic setting. The focus is with an underprivileged population in a developing country. These students were participants of a medical team traveling to the Dominican Republic; their goal was to provide screenings, diagnostic testing and assessments, and limited treatment to the poverty-stricken villages. An additional goal was to provide educational experiences to the volunteer health care leaders in this community, who were called Healers. They are a new group willing to be first responders and to continue providing basic health care needs for their community, which creates an opportunity for continued, although limited, services. As a result, the students gained a sense of professional volunteerism as well as a cultural appreciation for health care in different settings.

I have had previous participation in mission work with multiple non-profit organizations. Some experiences were of a medical or surgical nature; however, participation to date with this organization consisted of building adequate housing for selected families of a mountain village in the Dominican Republic. Through experiences working with the village, it was apparent that the village people's health care was inferior or absent. Basic hygienic needs were not being met, in particular for the children. In fact, the knowledge base to provide hygienic care, as well as the means to provide it, were lacking.

Basic needs such as clean water, skin care, food storage and preparation, sanitation, and animal safety were some of the issues recognized as being deficient. Education regarding growth and development, well-child care, and pregnant woman care was needed. From these observations, a needs assessment was completed by health care professionals serving on the board of the nonprofit humanitarian organization. From gathered information, the medical mission was developed to expand services and recruit medical professionals willing to serve in this capacity. The nursing faculty board member also saw this as an excellent and relevant opportunity for nursing students to participate as part of the medical team; students could develop professionally in a volunteer capacity, enabling them to make a difference professionally in another's life.

The villagers were eager to participate in previous building projects; would they be eager to learn about health-related issues? The organization's director, through a selection process, chose five women from the villages who were eager to learn first aid and basic health care, and to provide continuity of services after the missionaries left. These women became the communities' Healers. Through these efforts, a lasting impact was made by the students who enabled these individuals to provide continued important health services.

This transformed into a Nursing Field Studies course, which was offered to associate degree pre-licensure students, as well as baccalaureate nursing students in an RN to the BSN program. It was a dual-listed course for four hours of academic credit. Faculty members' experiences with previous mission trips were included among the course topics, along with coverage of culturally sensitive health care, nutrition, basic needs, and professionalism.

An information session was held to introduce the course to interested participants and to provide further insight into the learning experience. A slide presentation, depicting photos of areas where the clinical trip would occur, was shown. Other details such as a course description, dates, fees, and other expenses for immunizations were discussed. Topics regarding housing, safety, food and water, and cultural communication were presented. Application packets were distributed.

Just as with any nursing course, a traditional syllabus was developed. However, these objectives also included the concept of professional volunteerism and developing cultural adaptability to a diverse population, issues important to this experiential learning.

The syllabus described the evaluation methods and class and clinical requirements and activities. The clinical requirements included the nine-day mission trip, individualized according to the student's academic level. For example, the RN to BSN students functioned in an RN capacity during the clinics. Students were to demonstrate commitment in providing health care to the underserved.

There were class and clinical requirements for the Nursing Field Studies course. The class activities consisted of pre-departure sessions and activities. A pre-departure session was an orientation held by the faculty member for the nursing students interested in enrolling in the course. This was held approximately three months prior to the clinical trip. This time interval allowed students to become more informed regarding the mission work and primitive conditions in which the group would be living.

Three weeks prior to leaving, a joint-session meeting was held with all participants—students (both nursing and medical), community health care professionals (nurses, nurse practitioners, and physicians), and faculty. This was an opportunity for members to meet and get acquainted prior to departure. Also, pre-departure details were explained to foster a comfort level, camaraderie, and teamwork during the experience.

About two weeks prior to departure, a third pre-departure class activity was to attend a campus class consisting of completing a self-assessment using a Cultural Learning Strategies Inventory. The students assessed their cultural tolerance, adaptability, and openness to discuss cultural differences. Students had no awareness of how their attitudes and openness would be directly influenced by a different culture; they expressed their gratefulness after the activity for the opportunity to discuss cultural aspects in preparation for the cultural immersion and unexpected cultural adaptation when returning home. We also reviewed a PowerPoint presentation on Medicine in a Third World Culture.

After returning from the course, an optional class activity was a Summary Session, and students' families were also invited to attend. Pictures were gathered and shared digitally at this time. Families were able to experience the cohesiveness achieved by the group. They also gained an appreciation for and understanding of the stories they were hearing and the newly formed friendships. Another post-trip class activity was to give a presentation about the mission trip for the purposes of sharing experiences and of fostering an interest in developing professionals' volunteerism and service. Some presentations were information sessions about community activities and potential opportunities for involvement.

Clinical activities consisted primarily of clinic participation in the remote mountain villages. During the second year of implementation, an additional focus was to provide educational sessions to the Healers. The students presented a pre-assigned topic during the educational session (discussed later in this narrative). The other activity was journaling, a significant activity for reflection of experiences gained during traveling. Guidelines for journaling were distributed, and completed; journals were due at the experience's conclusion. Keeping a personal journal was encouraged for private thoughts. Journal sections included their personal and professional goals and their thoughts about volunteerism. Students also maintained a daily activities log with descriptive content regarding their observations of cultural habits, people, group dynamics throughout the activity, and their adaptation to experiences. The "reflective upon return" section encouraged students, upon re-entry to their country, to reflect on how they changed, what they learned, and what they wanted to share with others, and how they planned to use their learning in their future professional practice. Self-evaluation was a significant aspect.

The students were informed of planned activities for the clinical experience, with the caveat of being flexible, as plans and clinics may be adjusted regarding location and transportation availability and use of the villages' shelters. This course has been implemented twice. During the first year, there were two interdisciplinary teams consisting of physicians, nurses, and medical and nursing students. The nursing students were supervised by nurses, and their roles included registering people, taking vital signs, gathering basic lab values, and assisting wherever there was a need such as the planning or waiting areas. Each student rotated among roles, allowing student experiences to vary.

Following evaluations, two teams traveled at different times the second year with each team having a primary focus, as well as providing clinics for poverty-stricken people. The Nursing Field Studies course consisted of a physician, a nurse practitioner, nurses, and nursing students for a total of thirteen participants. Most days students were in clinics with similar experiences each day.

The makeshift clinics were created by the teams in the communities being served. Areas such as schools, churches, and community buildings were used. Students provided community-based care for an underserved population in a very basic setting. Through this experience, the students observed the diversity of living conditions, as well as results of extreme poverty.

Interpreters assisted with communication between students and the local people. Medical history cards were initiated and parasite medications were given to most of the villagers. Following explanations of the procedures, temperature, heart rate, respiration rate, blood pressure, and oxygen saturation measurements were taken and documented on the card. Next was the visit to the lab workstation. Glucose checks, hemoglobin checks, and urine dipsticks (in a private facility) were completed per standing orders from the physicians. The nurses completed a brief, focused history, concentrating on the chief complaint, and assessed the patient accordingly. This documentation accompanied the patient to the physician/nurse practitioner visit. Patients then visited the pharmacy when applicable.

During the second year, the students also presented educational sessions for the local Healers. These consisted of proper hand washing concepts and techniques, CPR, taking and initial interpretation of vital signs, obtaining lab work and their meanings, wound care/bandaging, well-child/-infant care and safety, care of the pregnant women, and basic medication administration. Students prepared handouts in English and Spanish. Each Healer received a notebook to store materials. At completion of these sessions, a certificate and gifts were presented during a time of celebration.

Evaluation was an ongoing process, as suggestions arose to improve the clinic's traffic flow and use of the local Healers and other village helpers. A debriefing session was held on our last day in the Dominican Republic to evaluate the experience and make constructive suggestions for future missions. Students suggested that more time be devoted to educational sessions with the local Healers, as well as to the clinics instead of the cultural activities designed as entertainment to tour the surrounding area. The teams collated the data gathered from completed medical cards and included gender, age, and diagnostic groups such as musculoskeletal issues, cardiovascular conditions, and skin disorders.

The nursing students participated in a course evaluation and an evaluation from the Office of Education Abroad. Results showed positive course outcomes. Accompanying comments included, "This made the first three difficult quarters of nursing worth it," "This was an experience of a lifetime," "Thank you for the opportunity to complete this type of mission work, I learned so much about myself in the process," "I walked away with a more open mind and more respect for another culture and feel that I am a better person," "I really want to come back next year and do this as a nurse, thanks for the opportunity of a lifetime."

From the reflective journals came insights regarding their experiences, such as the mission group's teamwork and the bond between the community and the group. Students repeatedly spoke of their humbleness and their increased awareness of cultural diversity and the importance of accepting others' practices. Some students spoke of their need to re-evaluate their life's goals. One student gave these highlights, "A personal high for me was becoming so close to the Healers. It was as if our hearts...connected through our work. A professional high was working in the pharmacy. It was a confidence booster by being amazed at how much [I knew] about the medications." She also stated that she "... has changed so much from this experience...a different perspective, different priorities...intensified my drive to stay actively involved in my community searching for more volunteer opportunities." Another student wrote, "I don't think I have ever done anything so rewarding....Part of me wants to stay and help these wonderful people....I felt our group made a big impact on the Healers." The cultural impact of the experience was felt by another student who wrote, "This experience provided a more positive insight as to how different systems work....I hope someday to go back and learn more and to help more." The students commented that it was a life-changing experience for them, both personally and professionally. The knowledge of skills, the intensity of collaboration, the gentle touch of compassion during assessment, the giving of knowledge, and the receiving of unconditional and genuine kindness were experiences felt by all participants.

The Healers were appreciative of the team's efforts. They were responsive to educational sessions and strove to perform the skills accurately and to understand the results. They enjoyed the opportunity to learn the skill as well as to demonstrate it back to the students. At the presentation of certificates, one Healer spoke in appreciation of our efforts by saying that, "The group was like angels from Heaven coming to teach us." Many Healers asked the team if they could return next year. Nurses are energized by these simple acts of appreciation. The faculty also found it gratifying to oversee students contributing to a community's education and health areas. The concept of professional volunteerism was developed from the seed previously planted in the classroom and by example, and many vowed to continue serving others in a similar capacity. The idea of respecting other cultures was now a reality, not an obvious practice seen in their previous clinical experiences.

The partnership of a university's School of Nursing and a medical team traveling to a developing country to provide basic medical health care made a difference to the people of that culture. However, another important aspect was the impact that the experience had on the nursing students and their learning. Not only did the students gain valuable knowledge of adapting clinical experience to a diverse population, but also they worked collaboratively and closely with a team to determine appropriate interventions.

HAITI
Pamela Cone

General education in Haiti has not included the principles of health and hygiene, and there is little difference in knowledge and understanding of these concerns between those who have had a primary and secondary education and those who have not. Nine years ago, I co-led a health care provider group from Azusa Pacific University in Greater Los Angeles. We traveled to northern Haiti to conduct mobile health clinics, to distribute appropriate medicines gathered in the United States through donations, and to teach health and hygiene in remote villages with minimal health care access. It became apparent that the people of Haiti had no knowledge of germs; in fact, there was no word in Krayol (Haitian Creole) for microorganisms. This led to a shift in emphasis from health/illness care to health teaching and promotion, and to a plan for an ongoing educational process over a number of years. It also resulted in some exciting experiences and changes in rural north Haiti.

Although the northern city of Cap Haitian has almost one-half million people and several other large cities and towns are scattered across the north, most of northern Haiti is mountainous with many remote rural areas where many people have no access to health care. Christian University of North Haiti is a small, private Christian university that is making a difference in the lives and futures of Haitian young people and local villagers. Haitian students are raised knowing Krayol, are taught using French at school, and learn English during their first two years at Christian University of North Haiti. This makes them ideal translators when non-Krayol speakers provide health care to villagers or give educational presentations to local groups.

In the summer of 1999, my team leader, Dr. Aja Lesh, Dean of the Azusa Pacific University School of Nursing, and I went to Haiti for three weeks to conduct mobile clinics in villages near Christian University of North Haiti and to obtain English speakers as translators. This gave students a work scholarship opportunity, and it exposed them to health education and training, something that they had never had. Haitian village people are polite to foreigners, but they do not trust what is said unless someone they trust provides a stamp of approval on the activity. So, we decided to use the local village's house church structure to gain access to villagers and to establish rapport and trust in what we hoped to accomplish. The plan was successful, and we were able to introduce concepts of health, illness, germs, and the relationship of germs to health and illness. It was an aggressive agenda, but one that had long been needed.

During the onsite planning at Christian University of North Haiti, a discussion arose among health care providers and local university student translators about the lack of a word for germs in the Krayol language. This led to coining the French term "mikwob" for "microbe" so that we could teach about the causes of waterborne illnesses and other types of infections. Many words in Krayol are taken from French, so it was within the language construction to adapt the French word for our teaching use. This was an important step facilitated by the university students who spoke French and Krayol. As a Krayol speaker, I offered to teach patient groups. In collaboration with student translators, nurses provided problem-focused teaching based on individualized needs, while my group, teaching in Krayol, addressed germs, hygiene, and health promotion. It was a challenge to discuss the phenomenon of bacteria with a people who had little or no formal education.

We visited nine villages that summer, one of which was in the crater of an ancient volcano, where people are born, live, and die without ever leaving that remote valley. The drive to the mountainside took two hours,

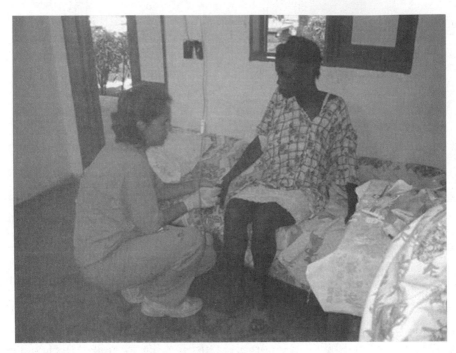

Rural clinic nurses must be creative. Here makeshift IV setups are devised when traditional equipment is scarce.

so we left Christian University of North Haiti before daybreak. Then we began the arduous climb up an old, rocky mountain track that had more holes than rocks. Several times we dismounted with our supplies to allow the vehicle to ease over large rocks without hurting the undercarriage. After climbing the outside of the mountain, our jeep literally drove along a crest that was as wide as the jeep itself before we found a trail that led into the valley. That was a hair-raising ride, but worth it to provide the much-needed health care and education. The people were grateful for our interest and genuine care, and for making such a long and arduous journey; they insisted on providing lunch made by the village's women. Several group members were sad to see the rooster we had just been listening to sitting on our plates, but the graciousness of the village folks was touching. One home visit provided an opportunity to teach care of an elderly woman who had suffered a stroke, which was helpful to her family.

We followed the Limbe River almost to its head waters where there was a remote, but quite large, community. We had a small Toyota pick-up to take our medical supplies upriver a short distance to the place where we would begin a four-mile hike to the village. After driving the trail leading to the first crossing, we searched to find a shallow water bed over which the truck could be driven without getting its motor too wet. Of course, that meant removing our shoes, since we did not want to do the long hike in wet tennis shoes. After crossing the water, we drove along its track to the next river crossing. Did I mention that the river snaked back and forth as it wound its way through the valley? During one crossing, I took the wheel and maneuvered the truck from a sand trap while the stronger members of our team pushed. They got a bit of a shower. We had three river crossings before the trail became too narrow between riverside gardens to allow further driving. There were thirteen crossings in all, and it was quite a funny sight to see us walk the trail, stop to remove our shoes, cross barefoot, dry our feet on our shirts, put our shoes on, walk to the next crossing, remove our shoes again, and so on until we reached the village.

The villagers at all sites were avid listeners, and since the Haitian culture places a high value on knowledge as power, they listened with respect, as we were perceived as powerful (knowledgeable). The plan was to use the local house church structure to access villagers and to gain their rapport and trust. Villagers gathered from curiosity and remained because they perceived our work as beneficial. The discussion required long explanations of how germs could be present without being seen and how these unseen enemies could negatively affect them. Their religious background of voodooism prepared them for a belief in the concept of unseen enemies, so they readily accepted that idea and wanted to know what to do to prevent the unseen "mikwob" from causing harm to them and their children. At the end of my teaching session, I discussed how to purify water through boiling, as well as when to use boiled water, which gave them some tools for health promotion and disease prevention.

We developed a system of health referrals. I told one woman with a softball-sized, seemingly encapsulated tumor on her right breast to talk with the local house church's lay leader, who would take her to the mother church's pastor. This pastor would take her by bus to the Cap Haitian church convention office that had a vehicle to transport her to the Sacred Heart Hospital. A team of surgeons from the United States travels there annually to conduct operations. This method of referral used the village's power structure, but it was the first time such a strategy was used in the villages. A letter of introduction of myself and my credentials, including my evaluation of the patient's problem and the family's lack of health care access, was to accompany the woman as a means of accessing the hospital. I spoke with the lay preacher and church pastor about helping this family access the hospital where surgery was done free of charge. Another family had an eighteen-month-old girl with a cleft lip and pallet who had a lower-than-average weight due to feeding difficulties. Their grief over their daughter's problem was heart wrenching, so I followed the same referral procedure and hoped for the best.

That same summer, we taught the very first CPR and Basic First Aid course in northern Haiti for any and all university students who wished to attend. We had ninety-nine attendees at that class! These students were eager to learn, and by speaking Krayol, I was able to connect with their "heart language" where deepest learning occurs. The students asked meaningful questions and practiced, to a limited extent since we had no mannequin, the CPR procedures. They particularly enjoyed the Heimlich maneuver. To them, it was an exciting new thought that you might be able to save a life using this method. When we discussed wounds and wound care as well as emergency procedures, they asked about self-protection. They were aware of HIV-AIDS and were concerned about how to help without harming themselves. We discussed protective measures during all types of first aid and CPR. They received the information with enthusiasm and asked that we return next year for more teaching.

This health teaching continued each summer from 1999 to 2003, followed by several years of hiatus due to political turmoil, and then a renewal of annual summer teaching sessions in 2007 and 2008. In 2000, another group of nurses and nursing students from Azusa Pacific University attended an annual Music Camp offered at Christian University of North Haiti. During this ten-day camp, young people learn about church music and choral conducting, among other things, as they prepare to serve as musicians and leaders in their home churches. The older students are usually lay leaders in their churches, so they are already respected. This provided them with a platform for health promotion and education. We made a plan to teach the campers at music camp as well as operating the rural mobile clinics. Again, the teaching of Basic First Aid and CPR was well received, and the students were excited about taking their new-found knowledge home. They were from all over Haiti, not just the north, so this educational endeavour had a more pervasive application than the training completed with the university students. Teaching the same information year after year was a way to reinforce learning. This is particularly important in an oral culture where most learning is done by rote throughout primary and early secondary education, and those who have not attended school learn by hearing and repeating what is taught. Teaching occurs through repetition, so this was an effective method to use with students and villagers.

We were excited about the numerous changes we saw in individual lives and the village people. The first change we noticed in the second year was village people in the area around Christian University of North Haiti using the word "mikwob" to discuss health problems and to ask if these unseen enemies were responsible for their health problem. By the third year, the term was quite pervasive, and now it is used all over Haiti, thanks to the university students, campers, and village leaders who spread the word. With this understanding of germs came another interesting new word. On my second visit to a particular village, I presented my concern about the use of pure water to make juice for babies and small children. One mother told me that she tries to use "dlo kouligann" because she knows it's pure. I asked what kind of water that was, and she told me that an American company sells water in small plastic bags that are not very expensive. The people know the water is pure, so they have gradually started calling pure water "dlo kouligann" even when it is not bagged or bottled water from that company. Culligan Water Company representatives would be gratified to know the people of rural north Haiti have coined a term using their brand name as synonymous with pure water!

Another change was related to my referral strategy. On my fourth trip, I visited the Sacred Heart Hospital and had a tour of their facility. When I mentioned my name, they immediately recognized it as the one who had referred several patients for surgery. They told me about the woman with the breast tumor and said that it was successfully removed and was completely encapsulated with no evidence of additional cancer. That was a huge encouragement to me and to the lay leaders who had activated the referral system.

That same summer, we found the first two people I sent by referral to the surgery center at Sacred Heart Hospital. After doing my group teaching and seeing patients, I met a timid couple with a four-year-old girl in tow. I asked what they needed, and they said "Nothing," and then asked if I recognized the child, and I admitted that I did not. They had come to thank me for the life of their little girl and for her beautiful smile! I noticed a very fine scar on her upper lip and realized that this was the child with a cleft pallet. Some amazing American surgeon in a Haitian operating theatre did a beautiful surgical repair. Our team's intervention had started this child on a normal life path!

In 2007, we completed important health teaching on mental health and on human sexuality and sexually transmitted infections. The last is a taboo area not discussed with young people. However, with the high prevalence of HIV-AIDS, it needed to be addressed. We were fortunate to have the Music Camp director as the translator for this sensitive session. Dr. Louima Lilite is a product of the Music Camp, having been brought there by his brother at the age of 13 and discovered to be a prodigy. Prof. Laurel Casseus founded the Music Camp thirty-one years ago and gave Dr. Lilite his first piano lesson. He was a child singer and could read music through the French Solfege system. He learned to play scales and to master finger exercises in one week and advanced three years in one. After being tutored and prepared for a U.S. college, Dr. Lilite received his bachelor's degree in Piano and Voice from Biola University, his master's in Voice Pedagogy from Penn State University, and his doctorate in Voice from the Eastman School of Music in Rochester, New York. This achievement earned him respect as a person of great knowledge. He translated the HIV-AIDS teaching and the campers' questions and answers in separate women's and men's classes, which gave accurate information while dispelling Haitian myths about HIV-AIDS. Since the taboo was broken at the Music Camp, there will be greater acceptance in future teaching.

Another Music Camp outcome was the first teaching of small children about health, hygiene, and dental hygiene. One mother told me that her daughter came home with a toothbrush and informed her that she was to brush her teeth in five places, upper teeth, pallet, lower teeth, tongue, and all her gums! The mother realized that her child learned an important life lesson. Dental problems are common and severe in Haiti, and this child now has a healthy start. The children will be seen as knowledgeable by nonliterate parents, who will listen and learn from them.

Teaching health and hygiene began less than ten years ago, but it will go on. The annual teaching and mobile clinics will continue, and more young people will learn about health, hygiene, and health promotion. Hopefully, children and young people will become more knowledgeable and pass this knowledge on to others. Health promotion and disease prevention through education now has a foothold in northern Haiti, and

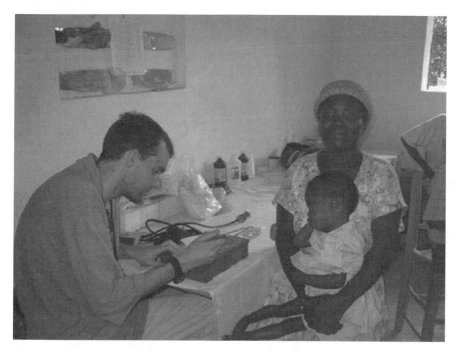

Mobile clinics require portable services and supplies to be set up in any village home with space for consulting.

the many changes that have already occurred are making a difference in many lives. It is amazing what three weeks of sustained service each summer does to change a site and elevate the desire to learn. Actually, mutual change was experienced; the team members' lives were forever changed by their experiences in Haiti. While this is an unfinished story, it is one of positive change where new words, new ways of thinking, and new ways of living are being practiced because some people dared to be agents of change and to bring hope to northern Haitian villagers' lives.

HAITI
Beth Weaver

I served as a missionary nurse while helping my husband build the first solar-powered FM radio station in a town without electricity as part of a nationwide network of local stations. We were invited by a group of forty-two area churches to provide theological education by extension and to install a sixth local station as part of the Radio Lumiere network. The larger church association (Mission Evangelique Baptist de Sud d'Haiti, MEBSH, with more than 270 churches throughout the southern peninsula) had specifically invited us as an engineer-turned-Bible teacher and a registered nurse to begin a medical clinic.

The town of Dame-Marie is located on Haiti's southern peninsula tip in the department or state of Haiti called Grande Anse. Its capitol is Jeremie. Upon arrival to the area, I took my RN license to the Chief Doctor for the Department in Jeremie. He was courteous and appreciative of my visit. Showing all due respect, I sought his permission to start a clinic in Dame-Marie and showed him the church association's letter for a desire to have a church-related clinic. With regret he was unable to grant permission for another clinic, because a Catholic clinic existed there. He offered a site in nearby towns that had no clinic. He suggested doing health education in communities and schools associated with churches, and also using the radio station. He believed that more lasting health consequences and effects would result.

I was disappointed, but within a few weeks I met other missionary medical personnel and we formed the first Haiti Health Fellowship. Dr. Jean Morehead, a visiting public health specialist, challenged and encouraged me to view the situation as a beginning of something bigger and better than a clinic. Her advice was life changing: "It's discouraging running a clinic and treating the same conditions over and over again; sicknesses that could be avoided if you took the time to teach people how to prevent these illnesses." She related the story of Dr. David Hilton, an African missionary physician who trained illiterate health promoters to teach people preventive measures against malaria, tetanus, typhoid, and malnutrition using storytelling and songs. The health situation in his area of influence changed positively, and the government requested that he spread the informal education approach to the rest of the country.

Surely this storytelling could work in Grande Anse as well as in Africa, for Haitians loved to transmit their history and values through oral stories and proverbs. I researched the main causes of death in Haiti and confirmed my list with the World Health Organization's statistics. The vast majority of Haitians believed that one vaccine was all a person needed. They pointed to the scar on their right upper arm, the standard site for giving the BCG against tuberculosis. I realized that a vaccination story emphasizing "getting the shots" would be the best way to reduce epidemics of whooping cough and tetanus. A vaccination story emerged and was about a woman who tried to cook her food in a pot over an open fire using just one rock. Of course the pot fell over and she lost the family meal. Gradually she realized that three rocks were needed to make a safer cooking pot. In addition, a related song was broadcast via radio at least three times a day. Listeners memorized words while singing songs with vaccine names, doses, and schedules.

With guidance from local educators to ensure cultural appropriateness, we also wrote a story for each major cause of death. I was sent by Radio Lumiere to Great Britain to take the Cambridge Radio Course. For my final project I presented a learning application plan to promote preventive health in a rural, largely illiterate Haitian population.

I realized that we faced cultural taboos and animism-fueled fatalism allowing abnormal scenarios to be accepted as normal. For example, I trained local granny midwives about normal postpartum blood loss by pouring 500 cc of ketchup water on a white sheet; they disagreed. They explained that a mother needed to bleed following deliveries because she had nine months of menstrual periods now considered bad blood that she needed to remove. I explained that God placed all blood in the placenta to nourish the child as it grew. When the baby no longer needed blood nourishment, the placenta was delivered right after the child was born. I demonstrated fundal massage and encouraged them to place the baby to the breast because nursing helped contract the uterus to slow bleeding. Soon word would spread that these new mommies were stronger and recuperated more quickly because of quality granny midwives.

My friends, the midwives, changed the subject to clarify colostrum. Mothers could not give first milk because it was thick and oily; it needed to be expressed and discarded. After the baby passed meconium stool, the mother could begin breast feeding. A veteran midwife told me that it was important to first give the baby a concoction of dried cockroach and castor bean oil so the baby passed meconium stool. I explained that God designed the first milk "colostrum" as a special concoction with stored protective ingredients to give the baby protection from the world and to help pass black tarry stool.

They agreed that babies usually died more easily from illness than older children. Fortunately, several granny midwives started the new ideas and were amazed with the results. At the same time, the vaccination story and song were broadcast in every home and village; people took action. The vaccination song is a ballad about a mother whose child died. In the chorus, she laments that if only she knew about vaccines, her child would have lived. Each verse describes a specific vaccine along with schedule and doses. The listeners of Radio Lumiere/Dame-Marie began to talk. Listeners acted upon the new information. Never did I imagine change would happen so quickly, as media experts had indicated that it usually took about six months for people to own a new idea shared through a musical ditty or advertisement.

"We have a big problem that you've caused and we need your help in resolving it," said the Roman Catholic Sister responsible for their Dame-Marie, Haiti, medical clinic. "What exactly is the problem and how can I help?" I replied. The sisters and I had enjoyed a great relationship up to this time.

A Haitian nurse and I dramatized some health stories for broadcasting and recorded some songs to accompany them. "Your vaccination story and song on Radio Lumiere (Radio of Light) the past couple of weeks have everyone around here in an uproar!" the sister exclaimed. "Normally we have about thirty women who attend the Friday Vaccination Day and we give them what is needed, provided they know their baby's age," she continued. "But now we have about 300 women with their babies and they not only know the vaccine names but how many doses are needed. They want their children vaccinated as soon as possible. The regional government that supplies vaccines doesn't believe that we could suddenly have a need for mega vaccine amounts and thus will not release the supply," she said looking defeated. I empathized with her, apologized, and offered help. I then traveled by motorcycle for an hour and a half to see the region's government doctor.

Unfortunately the chief doctor was not available, but an office woman sat spellbound as I told the story and the desperate need for more vaccines. She and other staff convinced the hierarchy in Port-au-Prince's Public Health Department that it was no mistake; Dame-Marie did need ten times more vaccine than normal.

In a few days, the head doctor stepped onto our porch. He saw the Catholic sisters and then came to tell me that he delivered a large quantity of vaccine and wanted to thank me. They desired more information about the local radio station and the other health education projects in process. I told them that I planned to train more non-paid and service-oriented people. We agreed to a list of qualifications for these people. These Health Promoters needed to be people who were respected for their honesty and integrity. I trained these promoters in the fundamentals of successful storytelling. This consisted of asking leading questions to spark subject interest and ask what people already knew. Then tell the story followed by questions. The listener was requested to repeat the story and to ask the audience to help him by answering the same questions. Then they choose several volunteers to dramatize the story. At the end, everyone could answer the questions. I found that the formula of repeating three times and in three different modes was the secret to ensuring that no critical details were omitted and learning was retained.

Later, on-the-job training began; each Health Promoter and I travelled to their village by jeep or motorcycle. I helped them hold "well-baby" clinics in any of the communities that were at least an hour's walk from our town. We weighed babies and each received a Road to Health Chart that was color-coded with green being the normal health road. The yellow to orange to red would be the "ditch of destruction," leading to malnutrition as the child falls off the "road to health." Each Health Promoter had the appropriate and affordable technology of a color-coded string that corresponded with the Road to Health Chart colors. They measured the upper arm of all children in their area and if they were in the "ditch of destruction," they encouraged attendance at Well-Baby Day to learn how children returned to the "road to health."

While mothers waited with children to be seen by the Health Promoters, they listened to a continuous looping cassette that repeatedly played songs and stories about breast milk, malnutrition, tetanus, vaccines, etc. While they waited, we gave vaccines and vitamin A drops to prevent eye problems, weighed babies, and provided worm treatments.

The government doctor encouraged me to field test the songs and stories in several other areas of Haiti and to publish a training manual for Health Promoters to be used throughout the country. At a subsequent Haiti Health Fellowship annual meeting I distributed copies of the songs and stories. Later I was invited by the Mennonite Central Committee to the Central Plateau where the songs and stories were successfully tested.

Two years later, the training manual awaited publication as the Haitian Government Public Health Department decided which written Creole version was to be used. A mission printer prepared the first edition, *Chan Ak Istwa Pu Edukasyon Sante (Songs and Stories for Health Education)*, which sold out quickly. Helen Welle, a colleague who helped prepare the manuscript, and I were driven to use a professional publisher to print a larger volume of the manual more quickly.

During our sojourn in Haiti, swine cholera was destroying nearly every Haitian's savings account, the family pig. These pigs were usually sold when there was a dire need like a hospitalization. Realizing that more epidemics of malnutrition were soon to follow, I decided to introduce a new source of protein, and we invited town officials to our home for a rabbit dinner. Of course I had a top local cook use all the best local spices; everyone agreed it was delicious and asked where they could they get rabbits.

I reminded them of the failure of a prior chicken project that I had started when a hurricane destroyed all corn and chicken feed brought by boat from the capital was not affordable. But rabbits were fed with many items grown locally, were easy to raise, and multiplied rapidly. Several wanted to be among the first to get rabbits.

Many took a short, practical, hands-on rabbit-raising course and had hutches built and inspected for occupancy. All that remained was to sign a contract agreeing to give back a pair of rabbits once theirs reproduced. I remember saying that we will know we've succeeded if someday, years from now, we came back and found rabbit meat sold in markets. On a return visit twenty years later, we found rabbit meat regularly sold in the market!

At the end of eight years in Haiti we worked ourselves out of a job. Radio Lumiere/Dame-Marie was successfully operated by the group of eighteen local program operators and one technician. Each had other day jobs; the radio ministry was their volunteer service to the community. A local nurse took over all the health programming. It was 1986 when we left Dame-Marie and to this day, the station continues providing local news and other education programs, often making personal and public announcements where few have electricity, much less telephones or televisions. Within the first three years of listener-supported Lumiere/Dame-Marie's health programs, combined with the excellent job by the twelve Health Promoters, Haiti's epidemics of diphtheria and pertussis and tetanus were eliminated. Unfortunately, political and natural disasters continue to plague Haiti, but volunteerism is alive and working well in the poorest country in the Western hemisphere.

HAITI
Dawn Michelle Mabry

She squatted on a concrete block above blood that pooled on the floor of the Mission of Hope church building. Her eyes were rolled back in an inner world of pain. Her exhausted body was being propped up by a young man straining to remain calm. A small group of concerned onlookers spoke ominously in Creole. "She's been like this since yesterday" was the interpreted message.

I was in Haiti on my fourth mission trip with a medical and construction team from a church in Fort Wayne, Indiana. A few doctors, nurses, and assistants were providing basic health care to as many Haitians as we could help in one week's time. The clinic had a waiting room, pharmacy, and a few unequipped exam rooms. Patients sat in chairs for their examinations. A recent, welcomed addition was a bathroom with a functional toilet. The medical clinic was staffed only when mission teams arrived. Our doctors gave patients a three-month supply of medication in the hope that we would return before the medicine ran out. The future goal is to staff the clinic with its own physician year round.

The temperature that morning was already hot, very hot. There were no time and temperature signs in Haiti. We didn't know how hot it was, but the hot, dry air was making it more difficult to notice dehydration as we worked. We had to watch out for each other, and encourage and remind our fellow teammates to drink the purified water we all carried to prevent heat exhaustion and dehydration. Just the day before, as I worked in the triage area, my vision went a little fuzzy. I thought I was going to pass out before making my way into the pharmacy to lay down with my feet up. Dr. Rich, our cardiologist, gave me a quick look and told me to keep drinking as he entered the pharmacy to retrieve a certain blood pressure medication for a patient in his treatment room.

Our work at Hope Mission is not only a physical challenge, but it pulls our emotional cords as well. We see infants with extreme hydrocephalus, which makes their heads grotesquely huge. We see malnutrition so severe that black hair is turned an orange color and growth is retarded. Hope Mission has over thirty orphans living there. My heart is overwhelmed by the complete lack of resources. Our mission team members are hardworking, well-educated, experienced, prayerful, and strong individuals. We are able to meet some of the needs, but we alone cannot solve most of the problems we see in Haiti. The problems seem impossible to overcome, but I believe it is just the kind of situation our God uses to display His power and one day Haiti will be a beautiful and healthy nation.

There are dangers in Haiti. One danger is riding the bus to the clinic. It is probably the most risky thing we do. There are no rules on the road. Chaos reigns. The primary piece of optional equipment on a vehicle is a horn. Horns blare out as trucks and buses pass on the right or left. There are no lines on the roads or speed limit signs; there are no traffic signals, no rules. Haiti's taxis are called tap-taps. When you want to get off the brightly painted, small converted pick-up truck, you just tap-tap on the side and the driver will stop to let you off. These tap-taps sometimes carry up to two dozen riders who hang off the sides or ride on the roof top. After arriving at our destination, I always feel like I just survived a near-miss fatal accident. Praying for Joslyn, our bus driver, was something we never forgot to do before we "hit the road." Thanking God for a safe ride was spontaneous once we arrived.

On this day, June 27, I had been looking for a birthday verse for a special friend of mine. He, along with many others, was providing financial and prayer support for this trip. I like to find birthday verses in the Bible by using the number of the month as a chapter and the day as the verse number. Daniel 6:27 seemed perfect. It states, "He rescues and He saves. He performs signs and miracles in the heavens and on earth. He saved Daniel from the mouth of the lion." I started that day happy to have found a good verse, and I was looking forward to seeing God at work.

Haitians are beautifully laid back and polite people. They always greet you with "bonjour" and a smile. They are respectful. They wear their best clothes and manners to the church and clinic. Their soft-spoken Creole language is warmly shared by the Haitian interpreters. They kindly and patiently translate the same set of questions we ask our patients over and over all day long. They make funny little expressions when we try to speak Creole. Without them, the clinic work would come to a screeching halt. My interpreter became my very best friend for the week. I laughed a little myself when I heard them try to pronounce my name Dawn. It just doesn't roll off the French-based, Creole tongue easily. Another funny name-thing happened with my nurse friend Jean. In Creole it is pronounced more like John and is a common male surname. You should have seen the faces when this beautiful, tall blonde woman's name tag was read by Haitians.

As we pulled into the gated and guarded entrance of Hope Mission, someone caught our attention by running to the bus doors and knocking excitedly. Joslyn, our bus driver, turned around and said, "A lady is having a baby in the church." God's plan for the day was unfolding. Dr. Terry Frederick, Nurse Lynn Huett, and I ran from the bus and followed the interpreter into the open air church. We were told that she had been in labor since yesterday. Obviously, the membranes were ruptured and our patient was losing strength. The big guys on our construction team carried this laboring woman by her four limbs into the bus. As we made our way up to the clinic, Dr. Frederick informed us that all we had there was a clamp. The mission team carried all our supplies into Haiti in the suitcases we were allowed to bring on the airplane. The Hope Mission clinic was only stocked with the meager supplies we had left on the previous trip. We all began to pray.

The pregnant woman was again lifted by her arms and legs and, as gently as possible, laid on a table. We shut the door and went to work. Because the temperature in the tiny room was well over 100 degrees, we joked that we didn't need an incubator. Dr. Terry had delivered a baby in this situation before; he and Lynn had helped deliver a baby at the clinic a year ago. However, this was not going to be a routine delivery. The baby's head was presented but rather dry. We tried pushing. The embarrassed male interpreter did his best to help. She pushed. I pushed from the top of the fundus. We pushed harder. Our scrubs were so heavy with perspiration that Dr. Terry, up to his elbows in blood, had to ask someone to pull up his pants. Somehow a pair of scissors was found, with a bulb and suture. Some needles and lidocaine were produced. We prepared to perform an episiotomy. Others gathered outside the room to pray. The door was opened so we could breathe and someone was asked to hold a flashlight as I continued to give my best reassuring and comforting support to this desperate woman. During the hours in that room, different people came in to assist. Most of them fainted. "Catch her," Dr. Terry shouted as a volunteer fell to the floor. Another volunteer came in to assist and she too sank to the floor. A third decided to leave before she passed out. One of the helpers was a young woman who was considering becoming a nurse. "This will make her or break her," I thought. The three of us stood for hours laboring with our patient. We did not take a break or a drink, but I felt an undeniable inner strength. When just the day before I had to lay down, there was not a hint of weakness in my body. I was completely engaged in trying to save the life of this woman and her baby. Her strength was gone and she could no longer push. The episiotomy opened the way for meconium, an ominous sign, and the discovery that the umbilical cord was wrapped tightly around the baby's neck. After unsuccessful attempts to slip the cord around the head, Dr. Frederick decided to cut it. He warned us, "We'll have to deliver this baby immediately after I make the cut." As we held our breath, a full-term, lifeless baby girl was delivered. There was silence. She was grayish in color and did not move as she lay on the blood- and stool-stained towel. We tapped her, and then spanked her without response. I raised my head to the questioning faces at the door and mouthed the word "pray"—please God rescue her. "Come on baby, breathe," I pleaded. Brave Lynn was the first to give mouth-to-mouth respiration. I compressed her tiny chest over the heart. Dr. Terry gave some breaths while I continued to rapidly compress. Dr. Rich, the cardiologist, walked in to see if help was needed. The baby's right foot moved slightly. She took a breath! Oh the joy of relief. We held her up for all to see the miracle. We took a picture, then she quickly turned blue again. CPR was resumed. "Oh no. Please, God, help," I prayed aloud. More quickly this time, she began to breathe. We wrapped her up and I held the baby close to the exhausted mother. Dr. Terry began the task of sewing. He stood without a dry thread, and Lynn beamed as she assisted with the lengthy suturing procedure. When it was complete, Dr. Terry asked me to stay with the mom and baby while he and Lynn went to their exam room to help see some of the three hundred other patients waiting at the clinic that day.

I assessed vital signs and bathed Nadege, the new mother, and her baby girl. Someone found a clean dress for mom and a diaper and blanket for the baby. Someone else brought us each a tall glass bottle of cold Coke. We drank the sweet refreshing syrup as I sang lullabies to Nadege and her daughter. I had memorized the Creole version of "Jesus Loves the Little Children" and sang it now with more meaning than I had ever felt or realized.

At the end of that long day, Nadege and her baby left with the young father. Joslyn drove them home with all the things we could find that might be helpful. We sent some pads, dressings, and gauze. Watching them lug down the dirt road that wound through Hope Mission, I was in some kind of surreal state as I began to realize what I had just witnessed. I fervently prayed that the little new family would survive the night.

Although leaving the secure grounds of the mission was not recommended, we had to check on our patients. The wife of the Mission Director, her body guard, an American translator, and I made a house call to the village where Nadege lived to check on her and the baby. In a small, smelly, tight concrete block room we found a resting mom and baby. I performed a postpartum check while Nadege lay on a mattress on the floor. I held that wonderful, beautiful baby. Beth the interpreter asked what they had named the baby. She said they wanted to name her after me! I thought the translation was incorrect. "Please don't name her Dawn. No one can say it very well here. But if you'd like to use my middle name Michelle, I would be honored," I said. They named her Michelle Jean. And her birthday verse is Daniel 6:27 which reads, "He rescues and He saves. He performs signs and wonders in the heavens and on earth."

God rescued and saved Nadege and her baby. He performed a miracle in having our bus arrive at the right place at the right time. He kept Dr. Terry, Lynn, and I on our feet. He inspired a young woman to become a nurse. He is at work in Haiti and in my heart.

Two years later, after helping to build a Service Learning course at the University of Saint Francis in Fort Wayne, I returned to Haiti with four nursing students. One of these students was the young lady who witnessed the miracle birth and decided to become a nurse. We saw Nadege and the happy, healthy, two-year-old Michelle. I am not sure why God allowed me to see and feel what He did that day in June. I do know, however, that God still works wonders and there is hope for Haiti.

MEXICO
Lisa A. Quinn, Karen A. Lumia, Pamela A. Mead, and Sharon J. Thompson

The Mission de Amistad—the Mission of Friendship—was established in 1971, when Archbishop Manuel Ruiz Castro, the Archbishop of the Yucatan diocese in Mexico, and Bishop Alfred M. Watson, the Bishop of the Erie diocese in the United States, established a relationship of cooperation and support between the two dioceses. Gannon University, located in Erie, Pennsylvania, was involved in this relationship from the very beginning. Gannon is a Catholic, Diocesan, student-centered university, which provides for the holistic development of undergraduate and graduate students in the Judeo-Christian tradition. It offers students teaching and a value-centered education in liberal arts and professional specializations. Faculty of Gannon's Villa Maria School of Nursing wanted to develop a Mexico mission experience for nursing students.

Following discussions with staff associated with the Mexico mission, our goals were an excellent match to the Mission of Friendship's goals. They conducted small-group cultural exchanges between the

Archdiocese of Yucatan and the Diocese of Erie. Each group took part in service projects. To include the nurse's role, their traditional mission experience was combined with one that was focused on health care. So far, we have completed three mission trips. Students focus on health care that includes the role of the nurse, sharing the human experience, and identifying the sameness of human needs within the uniqueness of cultural differences.

To participate, students engage in a rigorous selection process. They submit an essay identifying their reasons to participate, and finalists are interviewed by participating faculty and community members. Selected students attend an intensive orientation session. Topics discussed include cultural differences and students' expectations. Two cultural differences are always discussed. The daily siesta is a cultural phenomenon across Mexico and South America, but can easily be attributed to high heat and humidity experienced there. Another is timing of the daily main meal. Americans usually eat their biggest meal in the evening, while Mexicans eat their main meal in the afternoon.

The Mission of Friendship has a small staff in Mexico. Members live at the mission house, located in Merida, and serve as guides and interpreters. Across the street are dormitory-style units where we are housed for our stay in Mexico. We are responsible for making our own breakfast each day, but the refrigerator and kitchen are well-stocked. After breakfast, we gather in the courtyard area with staff for morning prayers and reflection. Each faculty and student is assigned a specific day and a part of this ritual.

Tailoring the mission experience for nursing students includes opportunities for health education and physical assessments. On each trip, we accompany a physician to a village on one of his or her regular visits. Students conduct physical examinations. Because students have completed junior- or senior-level nursing courses, they are excited to assist in this way.

Entering the village, about twenty miles from Merida, is like entering another world or another time. The villagers' homes are thatch-roofed huts. Many village women are outside, cooking over open fires. In front of the church where the clinic will be held, a line of people are already at the door waiting to be seen.

We organized ourselves into working groups, with students and faculty working side-by-side. Throughout the clinic, students conducted physical examinations on people across the lifespan. The villagers were grateful for our help and were excited to have us there. One of the examined newborns was jaundiced, and we referred the mom and her baby to the doctor. He advised her to expose the baby undressed to sunlight as much as possible. We learned that Mayan women generally keep babies wrapped snugly in a blanket and hold the wrapped baby close to them. This mother opened the blankets while she was with us, but as she walked away from the church, she was seen rewrapping the baby with the blanket. Students also completed physical assessments at the mission-operated Day Care Center—Los Amiguetos. One child complained of a sore throat. We suggested Popsicles to ease the discomfort, but we were faced with another cultural difference! Sore throats are not treated with cold substances in Mexico, they are treated with warm substances. Students were excited to use their physical assessment skills and excited to learn about Mayan customs and traditions.

A special place that we visit on each trip is Nueva Vida (New Life), a shelter for girls. Many girls live there and are provided with the opportunity to attend school. Our students love this experience, and the shelter girls are delighted to interact with college girls. Nursing students prepared education sessions related to health issues and self-esteem. It is a reciprocal learning experience for all girls. When we revisit, the shelter girls who once lived there return to see us and show us how they have grown.

We tour the O'Horan Hospital, the city hospital in Merida dedicated to the care of the poor. Much of their medical equipment is outdated. Our students saw Mexican nursing students during clinical rotations of hospital units. We were told that when patients are discharged, they must find a relative or a friend to donate blood to the hospital before they are released.

Near O'Horan Hospital is a hospice run by a Catholic Sisters order. If discharged people live too far away or are dying, they stay here. Their family can also stay, but they must help with hospice patients' care and other duties to pay for their stay. We saw women in the courtyard making tortillas, and women cleaning and doing laundry. One service day was spent helping the hospice sisters by cleaning rooms and reorganizing supplies.

We also visited San Vicente Albergue, a nursing home. Mission staff members visit the nursing home frequently to interact with residents, who love our visits. When we go, we help each person to the dining room where we play a rousing game of bingo. The residents enjoy winning.

Gannon nursing students are always excited to visit the School of Nursing in Merida. We are given a tour of the classrooms and laboratories. The school has undergone renovations and remodeling, and our students were impressed at how similar the facilities were to our own. In addition, our students come away knowing that, wherever you are, wherever you practice, nurses are doing the same work, with the same compassion for people.

One of the most fulfilling experiences is the home visits with mission staff to mission-sponsored families. Families are sponsored through Amigos, a specific program of Mission de Amistad. An entire family is sponsored for just a few dollars a month. A community member of the mission trip sponsors a family, and we visit this family when we travel to Merida. Another Mexican custom was that when you enter the home, people stand and give you their chair, even if it is the only chair in the home. One woman sent her son to the store for soda because she wanted to give us something. The homes were generally only one room in size. Most had traditional hammocks for sleeping. If the family was fortunate, they had a cement floor, but most were earthen.

Much of our service involves more than providing health care or health teaching. The most enjoyed service project is also the most labor intensive: On each trip to Merida, we provide a cement floor in the home of a mission-sponsored family. The first floor we installed was at a soup kitchen run by the mission nuns. The temperature reached 100° F by 11:00 A.M. and none of us had ever mixed cement before. The job was finished, and later we revisited the soup kitchen. Families were eating lunch and we enjoyed a "job well done." We wrote the words Gannon University in the wet cement and were overwhelmed to think of how many people over the years will benefit from our efforts.

An important part of each mission trip is learning about Mexican culture. Merida is a large city rich in culture and history. We always have the opportunity to explore the city, including a downtown shopping excursion. One day of the trip includes a visit to the Mayan ruins of Uxmal, Chichen Itza Tulum, which is an excellent opportunity to reflect on the deep cultural age and heritage of the people we met.

This trip to another country and another culture provides faculty and students with many memories and reflective moments. One overarching agreement by those fortunate enough to make the journey—we are all more alike than we are different!

MEXICO
Kathie Lasater

The sky was as dark as my thoughts that chilly December morning. Sitting next to the window on a plane from Portland, Oregon, bound for Los Angeles and then on to Oaxaca, Mexico, I felt a weight in my spirit. Loneliness, a growing uneasiness, and the cold of that December dawn washed over me. I could see, in my mind's eye, my husband returning from the airport to rouse our two daughters, still snug in their beds, trying to maneuver his way through that most unfamiliar room, the kitchen, to get them fed before he went to work. Oh, my girls were actually well on their way to independence at ages ten and twelve, and probably at times relished the thought of not having their mother hover over them. Still, it was the holiday season, and I would be gone for two weeks in an unfamiliar place, working with a health care team I had never before met, and caring for Mexican children and adults, whose language I didn't speak.

Christmas in our family was always a month-long event, starting with my husband's birthday on November 30. That day was the symbolic start of the holiday, ripe with a multitude of carefully contrived traditions. There was the advent calendar, the Cinnamon Bear breakfast, the trip downtown to see the lights and to window shop, school and church programs, tree chopping and decorating, the stocking hanging, on and on. I had carefully prepared the advent calendar, filling each pocket with special notes of love and fun activities. As a family, we had negotiated which Christmas traditions would occur while I was away and which could be saved for my return. Being the chief coordinator of such activities, I found it difficult to give up involvement in even one event.

As the plane sped through the darkness, I at least felt comforted by the fact that I had tried to anticipate every contingency. Yet that same nagging loneliness increased in proportion to my distance from home. I knew why I had decided to make the trip. My husband, a pediatrician, had gone in November the year before and had insisted that I go this year. I can still remember his arrival home, just before Thanksgiving. After twenty-five years of knowing this man, I could tell, just by perusing his face and body language, that the trip had wrought a compelling life change. Late that night after two weeks of separation, he began to tell me of his treks through the Sierra Madres with the mournful wind whistling through his tent at night. He described the malnutrition and diarrheal illnesses that made infants and toddlers ill to the point of death, the chronic illnesses affecting elders, which would be easily managed in our country but had to be endured in the isolated regions of the mountains. He told of the incredibly generous hospitality of impossibly poor people and of their unabashed gratitude for his coming to help them. With great emotion, he conveyed the details of their overwhelmingly difficult yet simple lives, their sometimes hopeless medical conditions, and their humble acceptance of what had been dealt them.

So I knew I had to go. I had to see for myself, to experience the culture, to help the people who were actually grateful for the carefully honed medical/nursing skills of the American doctors and nurses. So anxious was I for this experience that when I agreed to this schedule, I didn't seem to remember that December was the holiday season, that our family was always together during the month and did special things every day, even if it was just a cup of cocoa together in front of the Christmas tree. I forgot that I had never been away from my girls for more than a week and that only once, the year before, had my husband and I been separated for more than a week. It was a providential nudge that made me forget. But on that plane I questioned why I felt so generous with my time in December. Who would, in her right mind, leave cherished family and friends during the most blessed and special season of the year? I thought to myself that it was too great a sacrifice.

After ten incredible days in Oaxaca, we had just a day or two more to perform the surgical miracles in the renovated old moving van. During the time we were there, the plastic surgeon from Alaska had transformed numbers of children and adults from being severely deformed with cleft lips and palates to normal-appearing individuals with the hope of bright futures. Coming from the makeshift operating room, they arrived in my recovery room, which was furnished with simple chaise lounges that we had at home on our patio. At the end of the day, once fully awake, they would leave with carefully given instructions for the care of their incisions. Various family members and friends came to take them home; for one adult patient, the village mayor came, speaking his thanks to the entire surgical team, talking about the pariahs our patients would be in their villages without the surgical correction. They would never have jobs, spouses, or children, little hope for happiness, or any kind of normalcy. They would be burdens on their families and communities.

As we saw outcome after outcome, we concluded that there was no doubt we had done some wonderful work that would have long-lasting outcomes for many people. Nearing the end of our stay, my uneasiness had long since disappeared, but the nagging question remained, why December?

Then late one afternoon, just as we were getting ready to send everyone on their way, a young boy, seven or eight years old, and his father arrived at the clinic. They were both dressed in white shirts and long pants. Their skin was the color of café au lait, with black hair and eyes. They seemed weary though the father was only carrying one small, tattered gym bag. The young boy was especially attractive with huge, round eyes, fringed by sweeping black lashes. He also had one of the most severe defects we had seen in nearly two weeks. I learned he and his father were going to sleep at the clinic that night, and we would correct the defect in the morning.

The next morning dawned, just as every morning in Mexico had. The reddish-gold of the sun crept over the city, settled centuries before by the Spaniards. Their legacy had been stately Moorish edifices with beautifully crafted architectural details. The plaza slowly filled with people as the polite, but persistent, little children went from table to table at the outdoor restaurants, hawking their newspapers and their omnipresent Chiclets. They didn't seem to understand that I couldn't read their newspapers and that my jaw didn't allow me to chew gum. Their imploring eyes and bright smiles turned me to mush, and I bought both anyway. We hurried through breakfast to get to the clinic to start our next-to-last day.

Candido was ready for the surgery and as he slipped into the old moving van, I noticed a tear slide down his father's cheek before his boy disappeared for the two-hour surgery. When a very groggy Candido was carried into my makeshift recovery room, I could see that once again a miraculous transformation had begun. Before the surgery, he cautiously explored our faces for signs of the rejection he was undoubtedly used to. He shyly lowered those great paintbrush lashes when we tried to engage him in a bit of horribly spoken Spanish conversation. But now, because of the advances in the technology, his scar and the evidences of his former deformity would be minimal. He was *muy guapo*!

Shortly after my initial assessment of my young patient resting comfortably in his chaise lounge recovery bed, his father crept quietly into the room. As he gazed at his son, he silently began to weep with joy at the miracle before him. When Candido awoke, we handed him a mirror. I wondered if he had ever seen himself before, if he even knew how deformed he was. Certainly, it was a functional annoyance to eat and talk with a hole in his lip and palate. As he looked in the mirror, his huge, coal-black eyes widened until I thought they would pop; his face broke into the best grin he could manage. I knew then that surely he had seen himself before and understood the enormity of the transformation. Again, his father and all of us shed tears of joy.

As Candido and his father prepared to return home, someone told me his story. Some months before, a wandering medic, perhaps even my husband, had been in Candido's village. The doctor, noting Candido's deformity, told his parents that in December, a team of doctors and nurses from the United States would be in Oaxaca to fix people's faces. Living high in the Sierra Madres with no conveniences, such as a phone or mail service, and having no more information than that, Candido and his father ventured out toward Oaxaca. It was a dusty eight-hour walk for this young boy and his father, followed by a less-than-comfortable eight-hour bus ride for them to reach us, to see if we even had an opening in our very busy schedule.

I tried to imagine the worry that Candido's mother must have felt, staying in their village with their other children, as she sent her young son and husband so far away. Perhaps she too was orchestrating and preparing Christmas activities for her family. She must have had hope and, yes, the faith, that there was good reason for such a trip. I could only imagine her standing at the door of their meager dwelling, watching the two of them disappear over the horizon, carrying the little tattered gym bag, lovingly packed with what food and supplies she could spare so they could be gone for four or five days.

Suddenly, the waves of realization washed over me. With shame, I thought back to my feelings that my sacrifice was too big, leaving my perfectly formed children in their cozy, warm house, with all sorts of goodies tucked in the overflowing refrigerator. The "sacrifice" of flying to Mexico in a comfortable airplane, arriving within hours of my departure, seemed stupid and miniscule by comparison to Candido and his family's act of faith. Then I remembered two other December travelers who long ago left the familiar surroundings of their village, knowing they would experience discomfort and pain with the birth of a child in a strange place.

Within days of meeting Candido, I was once again home with my husband and children. We were walking in the crisp air of downtown Portland, enjoying the familiar sights and sounds of the Christmas season. My husband put an arm around my shoulders and gave me a squeeze, "So what do you want for Christmas?" I looked deep into his eyes and just smiled; we both knew that I had already received my Christmas gift.

NEW ZEALAND
Kenneth J. Wysocki

I was invited to join the teaching faculty in the School of Nursing at Otago Polytechnic in Dunedin, New Zealand, due to my many years of clinical practice and innovative teaching. I initially accepted a six-month contract to assist in developing a postgraduate nurse practitioner program at Otago Polytechnic and to help nurse practitioner students become certified. At that time, there were fourteen nurse practitioners in the entire country. In May of 2005, I packed my bags, well aware that I was leaving the Arizona desert summer and 110°F to arrive in the middle of New Zealand's winter, just following a winter storm from Antarctica. Little did I know that my contract would increase to eighteen months in New Zealand and another seven months teaching online when I returned to the United States.

New Zealand comprises primarily individuals of British, Irish, indigenous M ori, and Asian descent. Imagine a country slightly smaller than England or California, with a population of approximately 4.2 million, of which about 24% live on the larger South Island. More than 90% of the South Island was considered rural. Rural health nurses were the main primary care providers for communities, with a traveling doctor who was available in the clinic a few days week or by phone for consultation. My job was to pair nurse practitioner course objectives with the mandates from the Ministry of Health to promote advanced nurse education and nurse practitioner certification as a way to meet the health needs for primary care providers in rural settings. I spent the first month visiting different health care clinics and hospitals in Dunedin and rural communities south of Dunedin. I spoke with nurses and physicians about health policy, health care needs, practice issues, and the political climate for nurses to obtain advance practice degrees, nurse practitioner certification, and prescribing authority.

In September of 2004, the New Zealand Parliament authorized the title of Nurse Practitioner. In September 2005 the Parliament passed new medicines regulations, which included prescriptive authority for nurse practitioners. The 2005 regulation was seen as a timely policy change before national elections, but the Ministry of Health and the nursing profession also saw it as access to primary health care. The regulation's passage was a call to institutions of higher learning to develop programs. Otago Polytechnic campus was considered an institution of tertiary education and training education, similar to U.S. community colleges, and was one of the first to implement nurse education programs as hospital-based education centers closed.

I worked closely with Alison Dixon, Jean Ross, and Alison Stewart at Otago Polytechnic School of Nursing to add two postgraduate nurse program courses: One course focused on pharmacology and prescribing drugs, and another capstone course was embedded in a comprehensive practicum. With other postgraduate core curriculum courses such as advanced health assessment, these courses completed the requirements for the nurse practitioner program.

Aarti Patel, from the School of Pharmacy, who had experience prescribing in South Africa, and I, with ten years of family nurse practitioner and teaching experience in the United States, created a fresh approach to working within the public health care environment for the pharmacology course. The framework was a learner-centered approach in a blended online and teleconference format that included two immersion sessions at the school of nursing, and a clinical practicum in the students' community and professional setting. We built patient case scenarios that could be worked through a modified guideline of the 1994 World Health Organization's Essential Drugs and Medicines policy. I made clinical practicum visits to evaluate the practice settings and learning opportunities; I evaluated student interactions with patients and application of knowledge learned, and used the opportunity for reviewing, teaching course content, and discussing professionalism from an advance practice nurse perspective. The intent of these visits was also to meet with clinical associates (e.g., physician preceptors) to answer questions about course requirements, discuss the evaluation instrument to be completed by the clinical associate, and strengthen working relationships. Mandates by the Ministry of Health requiring cultural sensitivity and health care initiatives were incorporated into this course. Treatments included prescription and nonprescription medications, complementary and alternative medicines, allopathic and naturopathic treatments, and physiologic and alternative treatment interventions. All physician clinical associates and nurse colleagues at these clinical settings were supportive of the advanced practice nurse role. Even while engaging in casual conversation with locals at the café or hotel, I saw that people were supportive of their local nurse continuing to serve in their community and moving toward nurse practitioner status with prescriptive authority.

The second developed course was a capstone course to cover professional issues, evidence-based practice, portfolio development, and preparation for submission of nurse practitioner certification with the Nursing Council of New Zealand. Again, I used a learner-centered teaching approach, including online presentation and discussion of course content, two immersion sessions at the school of nursing, and a clinical practicum in the students' community and professional setting. Evaluation methods included written papers, clinical evaluation by the instructor and preceptor, and portfolio development.

Because courses were a blend of online work, immersion sessions, and a clinical practicum, I worked from home on some of the rainy days. The disadvantage with an online program is that boundaries are blurred, making it easy to spend long hours on the computer. As I was not native to New Zealand and did not obtain my nurse education there, I challenged myself to learn about different health care guidelines, Ministry of Health programs, available medications and herbal products, New Zealand health websites, New Zealand health care resources and publications, the difference in spelling (especially health terms), and cultural differences in approaches to health care utilization.

Aarti Patel and I, after completion of our research study, reported positive outcomes of this learner-centered teaching design and presented our outcomes in a poster at the 2006 conference of the U.S. National Organization of Nurse Practitioner Faculties. The study methods included flexibility of two classroom study blocks (e.g., immersion sessions), online modules with simple and complex diagnostic scenarios, and teleconferences. The classroom study blocks, consisting of three days for each, were provided at the beginning and near the end of the semester. Innovative case modules used a framework of Subjective, Objective, Assessment, Plan/Treatment (SOAP) with modified guidelines of the

WHO Essential Drugs and Medicines policy. Points were awarded on a pre- and post-course evaluation.

We provided students with a scenario, evaluation criteria, and parameters of the scenario, including identifying definitive nonpharmacologic and pharmacologic therapies of choice, and determining the suitability of selected drugs and treatments. Observational assessments of student progress in teleconference and clinical practice assessments indicated their increased competence and confidence with prescribing drugs and appropriate application of the modified WHO principles. This conclusion was further supported by the research. T-test statistical analysis exhibited statistically significant ($p < 0.001$) improvement in prescribing skills from pre-course to post-course evaluations. Students applied their prescribing skills with disease topics and diagnoses not covered in the course. The mean score on these new applications were better than mean scores in the pre-course evaluation. The conclusion was that this approach to teaching provided a vehicle for students to strengthen their diagnostic skills, engage in evidence-based practice, and enhance their ability to defend their treatment choice by involvement in this flexible teaching approach.

I observed the active engagement by the Ministry of Health in health promotion and health care campaigns. A strong public heath department reached out with awareness and education. Notably, during an epidemic of meningococcal B, there was a national campaign for immunization that used all media forms. Secondary health care (e.g., nurse home health visits and health maintenance) had a vibrant community presence. I worked with nurse practitioner students and rural health nurse colleagues in preparation for a possible avian flu epidemic. I also participated in the rural health network by presenting a seminar via teleconferencing on asthma assessment and treatment.

I witnessed large discrepancies in nurse salaries. Nurses in nursing care facilities (nursing homes) earned approximately 50% less than their hospital-based counterparts who worked the same shift. New Zealand nurses worked well both in grassroots efforts and professional organizations to shape health care policy, sort out pay disparity, and address nursing shortages. During my travels I met with hospital nurse executives, members of district health boards, rural nurses who were considering entering the nurse practitioner program, and other nurse leaders in the community and professional organizations. I was well received in all communities and invited to speak and participate at the Ministry of Health, Nurse Practitioner Employment and Development Working Party Sector Consultation Day, in February of 2006. This working meeting, well attended by leaders from all sectors of the health care industry, served as an opportunity for me to speak to national policy makers. In my role as health and professional advocate, I wrote articles for the *New Zealand Doctor* magazine, highlighting patient access to health care and nurse practitioner professional issues.

While employed with Otago Polytechnic I participated in graduate and undergraduate curriculum meetings and course development. I also met with nurse colleagues at different universities to discuss issues of concern in advanced practice education and to nurse practitioner professionals. I also assisted in postgraduate advanced health assessment courses at Otago Polytechnic and the University of Otago, and served in the undergraduate community health practicum faculty.

There were some tough times. The government cut funding to Otago Polytechnic to support more university academic programs. After much deliberation, the postgraduate nursing program was scheduled for closure to reduce costs while the undergraduate nursing program would remain open. This meant an end to an era and a program that educated future nurse leaders across the country. Planning ensured that program students finished their program and then program faculty and staff positions were cut. Later, the University of Otago School of Nursing was given authority to begin postgraduate studies. Discussion ensued to assist transitions for more nursing postgraduate courses and certifications, especially for those living in South Island.

I decided that although the nurse practitioner movement may not have met critical mass, convening the nation's first nurse practitioner conference, open to nurse practitioners and nurse practitioner students across the country, would inject a new spirit and renewed energy in advanced practice nursing in the wake of a postgraduate program closure. The setting would be Dunedin, and the host institution would be Otago Polytechnic. Together with Jean Ross, I worked to secure a grant and other financial resources to underwrite conference expenses. Exhibitors included pharmaceutical companies, textbook publishers, and other health care groups. Leaders in health care were invited to the November 2006 inaugural event. The Minister of Health, Pete Hodgson, and the Nurse Practitioner Registration Manager of Nursing Council New Zealand, Barry Ayling, gave welcoming comments. Education sessions were held throughout the day, with a poster session during breaks.

The conference highlighted advance practice in a variety of settings, and nurse practitioners from across the country were speakers. The conference was well attended by approximately sixty nurses and nurse practitioners.

A week following the conference, I traveled to Wellington to participate in an expert panel review as part of the process of my becoming certified as a nurse practitioner in primary health care. This process started at the beginning of the year and included Nursing Council desk audit review for completeness, educational equivalence, and reference checks. The portfolio review passed the Nursing Council board in June, who then forwarded it to the nurse practitioner review panel for examination as they formulated clinical practice and professional questions for my subsequent examination. The review panel, comprised of nurse leaders, educators, and a physician, convened for the purpose of an assessment interview, deliberation, and decision of recommendation to Nursing Council for my nurse practitioner endorsement. The panel presentation and question/examination period lasted about five hours. I learned weeks later that I passed the panel review and the Nursing Council Board of Directors accepted my certification as the twenty-seventh nurse practitioner in the country. I joined fewer than ten nurse practitioners with full prescriptive authority.

This news came late in the year after I had already made plans to return to the United States to pursue my nursing doctorate. I taught the last online cohort of pharmacology students. The course followed a similar framework as when I lived in New Zealand and included online discussion and teleconferences. Aided by an Internet Protocol phone, I held the planned two-hour teleconference every two weeks without interruption. The only difficulty was participating in the teleconferences at 3 A.M. New Zealand time.

Although the postgraduate program for nurse practitioners has closed at Otago Polytechnic, the program's legacy lives on as the program's nurses become certified nurse practitioners and begin to teach. Nurses in New Zealand, like their counterparts in other countries, are stalwart individuals who face daily challenges in health care and their profession. There are many great nurse practitioner programs across New Zealand and plenty of opportunities for nurses and nurse practitioners to practice.

The success of my professional journey to New Zealand cannot be measured in the short two years that I taught various courses. Successes for me are the nurses and former students moving forward with successful nurse practitioner portfolio audits and certifications. The first nurse practitioner conference's impact was followed by annual conferences. The success of our research and the nurse practitioner courses at Otago Polytechnic were carefully reviewed by University of Otago School of Nursing leadership, with some concepts now incorporated in postgraduate course offerings, especially those in the nurse practitioner tract. Although I talked to leaders across the country regarding access to health care and nurse practitioner job opportunities, my ongoing challenge is that change has not moved forward as quickly as I would have liked. I am optimistic that the health of New Zealanders will continue to be enhanced by more nurse practitioner clinical practices and patient health advocacy from these advance practice nurses.

PANAMA
Sandra J. Cadena

Building partnerships across international borders starts with building relationships. Only after there is true connectivity among universities, schools of nursing, and dedicated and innovative faculty is it possible to provide sustainable international exchanges that potentially impact the global nursing community. A journey started in 2005 continues to flourish, bonding programs and commitment between the University of South Florida and the Universidad de Panama nursing programs.

In March 2005, the University of South Florida Colleges of Public Health, Nursing and Medicine's faculty were invited to Panama City, Panama, in Central America to meet with Arlene Calvo, Ph.D., a new University of South Florida graduate who returned to her native Panama. Dr. Calvo's passion was to create a connection between her alma mater and her homeland's endless opportunities. This began a gradual relationship building among faculty, staff, organizations, and the peoples of Panama and Florida. Little did we know that the initial visit would blossom into a sustainable exchange of knowledge and research, and create new relationships.

Our second trip to Panama that same year brought us to the Universidad de Panama School of Nursing. Entering the institution's doors, with its faded paint and rudimentary supplies, we were welcomed with unconditional acceptance. That "coming home" experience to a place never before seen lingers today, four years later.

Carving a global program is not easy. Diligence, unconditional respect, and a passion to overcome barriers motivated faculty and staff from both institutions. This opportunity brought us together, and no one wanted to miss it. Language barriers were minimal; however, there were situations when forty-five minutes were needed to clearly explain and understand an aspect of the discussion. Invitations were given to two nursing faculty who traveled from Panama to Florida as our guests to explore agreements and understanding. How can we passionately bridge distance and culture to promote nursing together?

We accomplished those initial goals and more. Promotion of international ties flourished. Flattered by formalities ingrained in the Panamanian culture, the College of Nursing from the University of South Florida signed our first international agreement. Within the second year, we traveled to Panama with thirteen undergraduate students for a three-week immersion course in the culture and health care of Panama along with community health nursing students from the Universidad de Panama. Not only were the United States' students challenged by climate, culture, and food, they were also confronted with learning from Panamanian students in an impoverished community. Traveling to an indigenous community in Panama City's outskirts set the tone for one endless opportunity.

Las Nubes is a mountain-side community of over 200 men, women, and children residing in hand-built shacks with five to eight persons in each room. Homes were constructed from scrap metal, cardboard, mud, twine, and other material harbored for building. The terrain was rocky, muddy, and slick, and without walking paths. Mud seemed to permeate everything from floors in the homes to the water used for washing clothes and dishes.

The population's health is a matter of social concern that should be promoted through both individual and social means. Community-oriented care for Kuna Indians addresses these disparities in a collaborative effort among Panama's Ministry of Health initiatives, the University of Panama School of Nursing, and considerable community support. The Ministry of Health approves the settings in which indigenous community nursing care can be provided, the nurses determine when and how care is delivered, while the equipment and supplies are largely supported by donations from individuals and organizations. The medicines offered to the Las Nubes community were donated by various sponsors and greatly appreciated by the recipient professionals and individuals. However, the drug therapy offered to Kuna did not consider indigenous customary practices.

Cultural insensitivity, another risk factor for illness, can mean the difference between sustainability and extinction for indigenous communities that are already small in numbers. During door-to-door visits, we came upon a man who resided in a single-room home with three children under the age of four, and found his youngest child suffering from a respiratory infection. The single father acknowledged he had known about his one-year-old son's illness for some time, but did not take him to the doctor. Unbeknownst to me, Kuna believe it is the woman's responsibility to take children for medical treatment, and therefore the husband refused to walk his child to the clinic. A nurse escorted father and son to obtain medications and a referral.

During orientation provided by University of Panama nursing instructors, cultural nuances specific to Kuna were discussed and suggestions made altering those affecting health care. There was a preconceived need for aggression when performing nursing assessments. One instructor's suggestion for environmental evaluations was "do not ask if you can enter their home, just say 'we need to see your home' and walk in." Our experience was very different, in that a polite request to enter a home produced a welcoming response and no one seemed opposed to a request to assess the home.

Cultural sensitivity competence stems language barriers that also affect the indigenous population's health. The Kuna speak a language not found among the Spanish-speaking mainstream. Occasionally one would find a Spanish-speaking Kuna, but Kuna-speaking Panamanians were more rare. While the most wide-spread method of education was through pamphlet distribution, all educational materials were written in Spanish, making most Kuna hesitant to accept them. The lack of linguistic sensitivity resulted in Kuna women who had received Pap smears at the mobile clinic believing they were receiving birth control.

For all nursing students, participating in the Las Nubes Mobile Health Clinical was the highlight of the three-week, international, community health nursing experience. Indigenous community assessment, cultural competency, and health system critique were part of learning experiences that impacted all students in different ways. In sum, indigenous community health nursing involves education, cultural sensitivity, and disease prevention. It is learning to care for others in their world.

PHILIPPINES
Elvira Phelps

My country, the Philippines, is an archipelago composed of more than 7,000 islands accessible by land, water, and air transport. The village where I taught is two hours by boat from the mainland. During one trip from the mainland, we were caught in the sea by a hurricane. One passenger was a young mother in labor, a widow and accompanied by her grandmother. I assisted her in delivering a healthy baby boy amid the howling wind and massive cold rain drenching our bodies as we fought for our lives. While we worked at keeping the boat afloat, a huge wave hit us and shoved me overboard. I looked around in the heavy mist but couldn't see the boat. The young mother and her baby and the other passengers were nowhere in sight.

After less than an hour's ordeal, we were rescued by fishermen. When we reached the mainland, I saw the most horrible sight I ever saw in my life—piles of dead bodies from other boats that capsized lay on the white beach. I saw the grief-stricken mother with the lifeless body of her newly born baby in her arms. He was her first born and the first grandchild in the family. We were not acquainted, we did not know each other, but at that moment, I felt she was my family. She looked at me, tears flowing down her cheeks, not uttering a word; her eyes revealed everything and I understood. I saw the ashen frail body of her son with the umbilical cord still intact, dangling at his mother's side and I cried. I was touched, really touched. I can still see the joy on the mothers' face when she held her child for the first time, until that huge wave snatched and buried him under the water. I realized the real meaning of living and dying, of hopes and dreams, of despair and suffering.

Upon my return to the village, I organized a mothers' class with the help of the Parents and Teachers Association and the Village Council, organized a health committee, drafted a request to the Department of Public Health formally requesting that a health team visit the village monthly, and assigned a midwife to care for young pregnant mothers. The first volunteer who attended the temporary clinic was the young mother. After three years, I left that village with a heavy heart, as I was assigned in a provincial secondary school in the capital city. I know my stay made a difference in their lives and mine.

In 1987, I graduated from nursing school and practiced in a government hospital and taught part-time at the university. Before I migrated to the United States in 1993, the last position I held in my country was Director for Women's Service. I was responsible for the overall leadership, direction, coordination, and supervision of the Women's Services Department and the successful implementation of programs that provided varied women's health services. The program content primarily includes women's general health and well-being, reproductive health, family planning, planned parenthood, and women's disease prevention. In this role, I met challenges, especially regarding family planning, planned parenthood programs, and prevention of sexually communicable diseases. As a nurse, I know that my fundamental responsibility is to promote health, facilitate healing, and alleviate suffering, but where do we stand when a patient's religious beliefs or cultural values, and health care practices stand in conflict?

I created a core of health workers living within the community, enlisting them to sow "seeds" of knowledge and information, and to teach that there are some health practices that would not conflict with their conscience, religion, or beliefs. I created a community theater guild that presented dramas whose storyline depicted population education, family planning, and moral values of rearing a family. I started with a small number of women attending meetings and watching the drama plays. Gradually they persuaded their husbands to come with them.

In 1993, I migrated to the United States, worked initially in nursing homes and hospitals, and then worked as an RN in a state detention facility in 1997. The state of Colorado offered me a scholarship contract to continue my studies and in 2000, I enrolled in the MSN-NP program and became a nurse practitioner in 2002.

Barely a few months into my present job, I met a Hispanic young adult. He was soft-spoken, timid, and because of language barriers, had difficulty communicating his needs. With me, he politely requested a Tylenol tablet and when I asked the reason, he shrugged and said "for a headache." His frequent requests for Tylenol aroused my interest in discovering what was wrong. As I asked questions, he gradually withdrew and refused to answer. I invited him to the clinic to assess his symptoms further. I know how to speak functional Spanish and talk in halting Spanish. While I took his health history, he shared his involvement in a car accident, and the CAT scan revealed a brain tissue growth. The emergency department doctor advised him to consult a neurologist; he had no medical insurance and was unable to follow up.

Further physical assessment confirmed that he had a neurological problem and he was referred to a physician who recommended him for medical assistance through a court order because he is only detained in the facility. The court refused to award him Medicaid assistance. The Division of Corrections Regional Director intervened and persuaded the court to grant him medical assistance because it was a life-threatening condition. After communications with legal authorities, he had brain surgery to remove a fast-growing tumor about two centimeters in size, which would be life threatening if not removed quickly.

This young man and his family were grateful for what we did. He realized that health personnel are there to advocate for him. When his teary-eyed mother embraced me and said, "You saved my son's life," it flashed memories of the newly born child who perished years ago in the sea, and my quest for knowing my humble self and the nature of meaningful interactions with others occupied my mind.

There are a great number of experiences in my twenty-one years as a nurse, and these led to an increased awareness of myself as a person. Nursing has made me aware of life's realities that cannot be controlled or overcome, a self-awareness of life's issues that confront us, and the challenges everyone must overcome as we experience our varied life roles. As a nurse, my heart and soul has inner contentment, comfort, calm, peace, and joy.

RUSSIA
Marvel L. Williamson

In 1994, I arrived in Moscow, still unable to believe that I agreed to teach in the very country that, from birth, my father had taught me to hate and fear. Just a few short years earlier, Mikhail Gorbachev had risen to power in the Soviet Union. He began promoting an attitude of *glasnost,* or openness, by the government and revealed aspects of decision making previously hidden from the public. He granted new freedoms, loosened religious restrictions, permitted libraries to provide banned literature, gave the media access to formerly forbidden events, and allowed greater freedom of speech.

The steps that led to my participation in a project to develop curriculum for Russian nurses facing *perestroika* was merely an interesting service opportunity. My unlikely immersion began with an invitation from Carla Sunberg, a registered nurse and member of my church's denomination. She and her husband were obtaining official status for the Church of the Nazarene in Moscow to initiate a mission. The Russian bureaucracy was complex, and permits required evidence of tangible benefits for Russia. The influx of new international organizations, primarily charitable and religious groups, led to creative bartering. Providing social services became a primary way to gain legitimacy in the newly liberated former-Soviet society. Early converts began helping missionaries take meals to homebound elderly in crumbling high-rise apartment buildings that were characteristic of Moscow housing. Because the elevators were frequently broken, ill and elderly people who could not climb stairs were stranded without food.

Carla had another idea as well. Hospitals and clinics in Russian infrastructure were suddenly faced with the "freedom" to support themselves. Russian agencies that were facing new expectations to oversee inventories and to manage personnel became more open to Western help. With the blessings of Moscow Polyclinic #78 and a promise to release nurses for eight weeks of intensive education, Carla called on nurse leaders from our American churches to develop an instructional program on nursing process, professional issues, administration principles, and other topics. In 1993 a group of us gathered in Kansas City to learn about the situation, develop an action plan, and begin writing curriculum. Within three months, we were ready. Carla later asked if I would teach the first group of Moscow nurses. My husband urged me to accept, but my fear would not let me go alone. My only excuse disappeared when I received permission to bring my husband and my older teenage son. Invitations were extended from the Russian embassy, permits obtained, supplies gathered, and away we went. We took extra suitcases full of insulin, gifts, one-hundred blood pressure cuffs, stethoscopes, textbooks, toilet tissue, and other precious goods that were in short supply to give our hosts and the clinic.

We spent the next several days working with translators to prepare materials, and the initial cultural trauma gave way to joy. They had a great time laughing at my mistakes and odd American ways. "Why would a diabetic wear a Medic-Alert bracelet? That's something to keep secret!" "Telling a patient that he has a terminal disease would be cruel, especially if we have no way to treat him. Let him be happy as long as possible." Lunches were simple, usually just fruit bought at street stands. Sometimes, though, we had no lunch. Food was minimal and precious. One-third of Russians at that time had less than eight ounces of meat to eat in a typical month. On the first day of class, Svetlana (Sveta for short), my interpreter, guided me through the maze of Metro, bus, and "taxi" rides (taxis were private citizens who picked up passengers to earn money) to the Polyclinic where I taught. The Polyclinic was a large, diagnostic, outpatient facility that was not handicapped accessible. As we began the first class, I used up my entire Russian language ability by introducing myself and welcoming the nurses. I gave each one my business card, which they received with great respect, a custom common in many parts of the world. Only one nurse answered my discussion questions. I wondered if they had attended under pressure, felt intimidated, or resented an American coming to teach them how to function in the new economic system. Carla assured me that I had the best first day of any American teacher she had observed so far, so I was grateful for her encouragement.

After the first class Sveta, Carla, and I met with the Polyclinic director in his 1950s-style office. He served us bitter espresso and Russian chocolate. His demeanor clearly communicated that he expected respect and deference. He asked for more medical supplies and teachers, but refused to consider offers to provide direct services or education for the patients, citing the difficulty of obtaining needed permits. I later learned that Russia was drowning in bureaucracy and red tape. Carla said that buying a car required over thirty permits, something she had not been able to accomplish after nearly a year of trying.

In 1994, Russian nursing was one of the few things not heavily regulated. An educational pathway to the role existed with no licensure system. Russians attended basic school at six years of age until they were fifteen. Nurses were educated at a level similar to American LPNs, but they had difficulty explaining how nursing and medical care differed. Nurses who demonstrated superior intelligence were sent for medical education to become physicians, creating a situation that left nursing staffed by personnel with less motivation, acumen, or creativity. Medical students attended one of the three medical institutes in Moscow for six years. The first three years were spent studying history, philosophy, Leninism, and other general courses. The last three years were for medical studies, graduating them as young as twenty-one years of age. A one-year hospital internship followed, then a mandatory three years as a general practitioner in a clinic, split between office hours and making home visits. By the age of twenty-five, they specialized or stayed in general practice. Most male physicians specialized in narrow areas, such as pediatric neuroradiology. Because of the excess of physicians, each one saw only a few patients each day and usually worked only a six-hour shift.

Nurses were also micro-specialists and task oriented. For example, one nurse did only Pap smears, but her rate of positive findings was suspiciously low. Diagnostic rigor seemed to be lacking across the board, often because of limited resources for assessment or treatment. For example, chest x-ray films were only two inches by two inches, to save on silver needed for film developing. Many people said that Russians do not trust physicians because of their limited education, their requirement to report information to the government, and their reputation for not caring about doing a good job for patients.

At first I was impressed by how many physicians were women, outnumbering male physicians two to one. My interpretation of that statistic was completely wrong, however. Under Communism, preservation of the government and strength of the military was most important. People who drained resources, such as the ill or infirm, were viewed with impatience. Those assigned to care for the sick were to be pitied. Women, as second-class citizens, were more often directed into health care, while men received the status jobs. Physicians were paid the equivalent of $100 a month, but subway drivers were paid $300 because, as we were told, "Drivers have very important jobs transporting workers, but doctors merely take care of sick people who are not making useful contributions to the Motherland." Nurses earned about $30 per month.

Not surprisingly, I learned more than my students. They taught me about Russian public health issues, culture, and philosophical differences. They told me how much they disliked disassembling disposable syringes and counting the pieces at shift change, just as we count narcotics. They suspected the syringes were being reused, even though they were told otherwise. At that time, Moscow had a diphtheria epidemic because people feared immunizations, being distrustful of reused needles that were sometimes HIV contaminated.

Teaching the concept of caring was a challenge; the students did not respond much, except to say that an individual's needs were unimportant. Everyone conformed to the system. Differences were not accommodated, and this was an understandable attitude because Russians were afraid to be different. People who stood out were targets. Those with certain ethnic or religious backgrounds were particularly at risk. Conformity and blending were preferable. Another difference was that the nurses believed that what they said to patients was more important than what patients said to them. They were offended by noncompliant patients or patients who took extra time. I had difficulty inspiring the nurses to imagine a better future. They did not want to visualize doing more for their patients, and did not believe that Russian health care systems were changing.

These nurses did have dreams for themselves, however. When I asked what they wanted to be doing in five years, each replied that she wanted to be a better nurse (defined as more skilled), have children, and live outside the city in the country. Thousands of Moscovites resided on every city block, and crowding was an urban stress issue. Leaving Moscow required a permit, but that didn't stop most people from spending vacations in a rural area. The same need for contact with nature soon overcame me, so one afternoon my husband and I walked to the neighborhood's edge to explore a birch tree forest, which we could see in the distance; we arrived and found the ground covered with rotting trash and the campsites of homeless people.

The nurses, my students, were reflecting a type of starvation of the spirit ingrained by decades of oppression and shortages not limited to food and syringes. Contraceptives were almost nonexistent, resulting in an abortion rate nearly twice that of the birth rate. Having insufficient medical supplies led to imaginative practices using available equipment for unintended purposes, such as shining laser lights on acupuncture points, guessing at diseases by looking at the eyes, and taking aura prints of fingertips on x-ray film to aid diagnosis. Limited resources resulted in some harsh, but necessary decisions. For example, *babushkas* who fell on the winter ice and broke their hips were simply bound in stabilization wraps and sent home. Of course, they usually died in a few weeks. Medicines were difficult to find and hospitals provided few prescription drugs. Families were urged to buy on the black market and to bring medicines to the hospital for nurses to administer.

Signs of generalized economic and emotional depression were manifested in the trash strewn about and the decay apparent everywhere in Moscow. Sveta told me that before the fall of the Soviet Union, one day every spring was designated to clean the city of the dirt and garbage that accumulated under layers of snow over the winter. She sounded sad as she said that all of the old ways were being abandoned, even the good ones.

Even so, early signs of *perestroika* were around on that extraordinary day we visited the Kremlin. I could hear my father's fears resurfacing within me, as if he were there voicing them himself. I hoped he was somehow aware that Communism had crumbled and that his daughter, walking through Red Square, was asked to teach Russians about free enterprise.

We were fortunate to tour Maternity Hospital #4, a 120-bed facility that delivered approximately 4,000 babies annually. Before going to wards, we donned cloth caps, gowns, and shoe covers that came to our knees. We felt we were walking into the 1940s. Fathers were not allowed in the hospital; patients had no access to telephones or visitors during the typical five-day stay after a vaginal delivery, so one popular activity was shouting out windows to family members on the sidewalk. The cesarean delivery rooms looked well equipped, but women having vaginal deliveries were required to walk from the labor room to the delivery room. Delivering in a labor room was strictly forbidden, so we were entertained with stories of women walking down the hall holding their babies' heads between their legs with their hands. All labor, delivery, and postpartum beds were flat and nonadjustable, overlain with mattresses that were only three inches thick. Linens were stained and patched. The delivery rooms had large windows with no curtains to reduce the need for electrical lighting during the day.

This hospital was state-of-the-art for Russia. The staff was proud to show us everything and encouraged us to take pictures. Again we were reminded of the difference in philosophy toward patient care, this time by the practice of placing women whose babies had died in the same five-bed wards as women who had delivered healthy children. The nurses kept babies on strict three-hour feedings between 6 A.M. and 11 P.M., but allowed no feedings during the night. Security was not tight; babies were often left alone, and none had identification bracelets.

After many more adventures, our last day came. When I finished class, I gave Sveta a Kansas City Royals baseball cap, a portfolio notebook, and a calculator. She was thrilled with them all, but liked the cap best. The nurses presented me with three red roses and two boxes of Russian-made chocolates. I later learned that the flowers had cost 21,000 rubles, a fortune. I was so overwhelmed and surprised, that I decided to reveal more about why I came to Russia to teach in spite of my fears, and my belief that God had sent me to serve them. They then asked me take back a message to nurses in the United States: a wish for happiness for them and their families, and that we would "be friends now and enemies no more." As they completed their evaluations, I passed around the chocolates for everyone to enjoy and then dismissed them. No one moved. They had been whispering among themselves until finally Natasha, the most outspoken nurse, asked if I would tell them what being a Christian meant to me. That opportunity made the whole trip worthwhile. I shared my personal beliefs and how my life was lived based on those beliefs. We then conversed until we had to face the realization that the time had come to separate. We were forever changed, and simultaneously sad and glad to be leaving. My heart had bonded with all my Russian colleagues with whom we had worked or taught. I will never forget them. I only wish I could have done more for Russia.

ST. KITTS
Catherine Garner, Agnes Beachman, Kimberly McClane, Vicki L. Rogers, Brenda Simmons, and Cara Stone

The International University of Nursing is a U.S.-modeled, pre-licensure nursing program located on the island of St. Kitts in the West Indies. Founded in 2005, this private school is U.S.-owned and managed, with the goal of providing the first six semesters of a bachelor's degree on the island, with the final two semesters at a U.S. partner school. Graduates are eligible for U.S. licensure and Caribbean licensure. The faculty members are largely American, many of whom have lived and worked abroad. The staff is primarily residents of St. Kitts, commonly referred to as Kittitians.

There is one hospital on St. Kitts, with an average census of sixty and one on Nevis, with an average census of twenty-five. The hospital is without modern diagnostic or treatment equipment and has limited treatment capabilities. All births are without analgesia or anesthesia. For major health care, one must leave the island for Jamaica or Miami, depending upon the economic circumstances of the individual or family. There are nine community health centers located within two miles walking distance of any resident. These offer primary and secondary health care through community nurses and government-paid physicians. There are two long-term care facilities, one private, focusing primarily on the elderly, the other public, accommodating a vast majority of health issues requiring residential care. In the process of finding clinical experiences for the students, we reached out into the community to locate any opportunity for learning and, in the process, created some unique service projects.

In September of 2006, there was no traditional "blood bank" at the hospital. When a person required surgery, he/she was requested to bring in two donors of the same blood type. If this was not used, it was saved for others who may need emergency care. In true emergencies, a call for blood donations is issued on the radio. However, it is not part of the culture to give blood on a regular basis. The International University of Nursing Student Nurses Association went to the local hospital and met with the head of the laboratory to discuss the possibility of a regular blood drive to the island. The director was very receptive, and the students and laboratory staff from the hospital organized and conducted this event in the clinical skills area of the school. The first drive in 2006 netted twelve units of blood. The Student Nurses Association has continued to do this three times per year, and the most recent collection netted thirty-one units, the storage capacity of the laboratory. The drives have also generated a listing of those donors who wish to be "on call" for emergencies. In addition the publicity and the education of the general public over the last two years have resulted in a greater number of persons donating blood.

Ade's Place is a privately owned, not-for-profit organization founded by a local mother of a developmentally delayed son named Ade. It is the only organization on all of St. Kitts that provides training and educational services specifically to developmentally delayed adults. The training site is a tiny house located in a residential neighborhood near the International University of Nursing. The organization is staffed by volunteers with large hearts and much compassion, but no formal education about the specific diagnoses and special needs of this particular population. International University of Nursing students started spending time at Ade's Place as part of their community clinical experience. Each week our students assisted the trainees in learning various life skills ranging from making sandwiches to making crafts. Before long, such a significant amount of trust and mutual respect had been established that the director of Ade's Place decided to designate one day per week for our students to be solely responsible for planning and executing a health education program for the trainees. Guided by our nursing faculty, our students embraced the challenge with a high level of enthusiasm, knowledge, maturity, and ingenuity.

Empowered with relevant information from their community health lectures, our students developed, executed, and then evaluated teaching plans that specifically addressed both the educational and developmental levels of the target audience. The weekly teaching sessions quickly became the favorite day of the week for the trainees and staff, who greatly appreciated both the information and positive energy shared by our students. Topics taught included proper hygiene, proper nutrition, road safety, seeing unique qualities in oneself and others, identifying feelings and ways to help others, communication skills, self-worth, mental and emotional health, how to act as a responsible citizen, anger management, and respect of self and for others. Our students chose to wrap up their semester by planning and hosting a Field Day for the trainees with multiple activities specifically designed to increase self-esteem and build team spirit while enhancing fine and gross motor skills. Anyone who saw the smiles on the faces of our students and the trainees that day would find it difficult to determine which side of this therapeutic relationship benefited more...sacred reciprocity at work.

Project Strong is a voluntary alternative high school on St. Kitts that focuses on teaching troubled youth a trade or a skill, which will allow them to support themselves upon graduation. The school arranges apprenticeships in carpentry, fish trapping, computer support, tiling, mechanics, and even beekeeping. Students of Project Strong enter with a damaging history of crime and poverty. In fact, many of the students are sent to Project Strong as an alternative to juvenile incarceration. Nearly all of the graduates become contributing members of society. Guided by International University of Nursing faculty, mental health students organized and implemented educational group-work sessions at Project

Strong on a weekly basis. Topics of the group-work sessions included self-esteem building, therapeutic methods of managing stress, and how to become a productive member of society. International University of Nursing faculty and students also designed and shared a day during which Project Strong students, International University of Nursing students, and elderly community members positively interacted while participating in a variety of learning and social activities. Students of Project Strong expressed their gratitude for the attention, respect, and knowledge provided by our nursing students by hosting a Fish Fry event specifically for the nursing students. The event continues as an ongoing expression of thanks and is made possible by the exceptional vocational training in fish trapping provided at Project Strong.

With the desire to improve the financial support for both Ade's Place and Project Strong, one nursing student approached her community health professor to discuss ways to raise necessary funds. The professor and student met with executives of a large resort hotel on the island. A plan was made for the hotel to sell merchandise and artwork created by individuals at Ade's Place and Project Strong. The relationship resulted in a secure source of funding for two very vulnerable programs.

William Conner School is the special education program for children with a variety of disabilities on the island of St. Kitts. There are approximately 105 students and 22 teachers. The majority of the teachers have the equivalent of a United States high school education. The most common student disabilities are those involving mental retardation, fetal alcohol syndrome, and hearing- and vision-impaired students. Nursing students have the opportunity to observe and communicate with the teachers and students during their mental health clinical rotation. International University of Nursing students assist the teachers by helping provide structure and simple educational instruction in the classroom setting. Nursing students also work with the Conner School students during recess to develop social skills through redirection and role modeling of appropriate social skills.

Last semester the principal communicated concern about the high stress level the teachers were experiencing at her school. She requested assistance from International University of Nursing. Faculty discussed the principal's concern with the mental health clinical group. One student decided to make it her priority to help the teachers manage their stress. With guidance and direction from faculty, the student performed a needs assessment through observation, interviewing teachers and the principal at the school. Afterwards, the student developed an educational presentation for the teachers at the school. The presentation took place during a scheduled teachers' meeting. The student's teaching plan ensured that the stress reduction techniques presented were simple and could be incorporated into the teachers' daily work schedule. Furthermore, techniques were presented that could be used to involve teachers and students.

The presentation was met with initial success. Through much laughter and playing the teachers demonstrated relaxation techniques. Many verbally agreed they could use the measures throughout their day to help manage their stress levels. Because the presentation was at the end of the academic year, there was no time to reevaluate effectiveness. Plans are in the works to follow-up during the fall semester to reinforce the presentation and reassess the teachers' stress levels.

The Ministry of Industry, Commerce, and Consumer Affairs approached the university about doing something for the 3,000 women who comprise much of the workforce in ten factories on the island. Her interest was in reducing the incidence of heart disease, the number one killer of women in St. Kitts. The result was a year-long research program designed at improving healthy behaviors among the women. We expected only 75 to 80 participants, but had to close the enrollment at 389 women due to capacity issues. While this represents only 1% of the population, most women have children and live with extended families. Under the guidance of faculty, fundamentals students have conducted the interviews and physical screening, with the junior students doing the phlebotomy. Community health students have conducted monthly education sessions in the factories, using materials developed by the students in the nutrition classes. Students in research, epidemiology, and statistics all participated in the evaluation of the program.

Nine months into the project, nearly everyone on the island was aware of the project or knew someone who was participating. The women have come to trust and respect the International University of Nursing students, often approaching them on the streets of the community for health advice. Several private companies and the factories that did not initially participate have asked the university to conduct the program with their workforce. The government has asked International University of Nursing to submit a proposal to expand this program over the next three years, as what has resulted is a model public health intervention in the Caribbean. The preliminary results are very positive with respect to lowering blood pressure, control of blood sugar, and reduction in cholesterol and other risk factors.

Building trust around topics as sensitive as HIV/AIDS on a small island requires persistence and patience. As dean, I was invited to attend a five-year planning committee meeting. Not only did I go, but I stayed to work long after the "higher ups" disappeared. The first event was an AIDS Awareness March. I immediately volunteered our students to staff water stations and to be available for emergency assistance. This was followed with a request for our students to be available at local screenings to survey participants. The statistics professor at International University of Nursing processed these to provide outcome data to the AIDS planning team. The results showed a preference for additional local screenings, despite the fact that screening is available at all of the local clinics. Residents felt that there was more confidentiality at these local events, especially with our students. It was this increased level of trust that residents had with our students over their own nurses that prompted the HIV/AIDS coordinator to train International University of Nursing students as voluntary testing counselors. This additional manpower has allowed the Ministry to substantially increase the volume of testing. It is also working to foster trust in a very sensitive cultural area.

In the quest for creative clinical sites, opportunities present that not only provide strong challenges for the students, but also avenues to community outreach. One of our resident nursing faculty runs a food distribution each Saturday morning in the Catholic Church in the downtown area. A clinic has been set up for students to interview, screen, teach, and refer clients with varying needs. They are confronted with a variety of clients—the elderly poor, the homeless, single mothers, the developmentally and mentally disabled, the unemployed, and the chronically ill. The students see as many as twenty-five clients each Saturday, and thus learn to organize their time and practice efficiently. Many of those who practice in the "clinic" become advocates for these clients, and have voluntarily collected clothing, household items, and school supplies for them. This experience has also assisted the university in developing a Parish Nursing curriculum that focuses on the unique needs of the community.

In a little over two years, the students and faculty at International University of Nursing have firmly bonded with the people of this island nation. The rewards of approaching the community under the principle of sacred reciprocity have been many. The community members have benefited from the expertise and enthusiasm of our students and the supportive work of faculty members. The respect for our students is palpable as they engage in various activities, resulting in a greater sense of confidence and responsibility in our students. These experiences have changed all of us, too.

VIETNAM
Priscilla Limbo Sagar

The author had the experience of a lifetime while teaching Vietnamese nurse leaders in nursing practice, nursing education, and nursing administration. I saw first-hand the overwhelming effect of a series of wars and was offered a glimpse of the challenges facing nurses as they endeavored to advance nursing as a profession.

While pursuing the doctoral degree at Teachers College, Columbia University, I participated with my mentor Marie O'Toole on her project in the Socialist Republic of Vietnam. Dr. O'Toole was project director of the Nursing Education Development Project, which was part of the Vietnam National Rehabilitation Association Program. The work was supported by Health Volunteer Overseas, the United States Agency for International Development, and a Teachers College grant, the McKenna Award. Thus, Teachers College's relationships with two educational institutions in Vietnam—Hanoi Medical School and Thanh Hoa Medical College—were formalized. I have traveled twice to Vietnam with faculty and student delegations to attend the nursing congress in May of 1997 and to teach a two-week professional nursing course in July through August of 1997. While in the country, I pursued my doctoral dissertation, which was a case study of the lived experience of Vietnamese nurses.

Much-needed nursing textbooks were shipped by students, faculty, and alumni through Health Volunteer Overseas to stock the school libraries. Through Health Volunteer Overseas' donations, the nursing laboratory has models; flip charts; transparency machines; mannequins for measurement of temperature, pulse, respiration, and blood pressure; and models for dressing changes and tracheostomy care.

Friendship Bridge, a humanitarian group based in Denver, Colorado, sponsored the course and the expenses of the other two faculty members.

Twenty-seven nursing leaders in practice and administration attended the two-week workshop. Participants were nurse administrators of provincial and city hospitals including chief nurses, nurse leaders such as two vice-presidents of the Vietnamese Nurses Association, and nurse educators, including the head of school's nursing department.

The group developed and refined their definition of nursing. Group leaders appointed on the first day remained as leaders. Future course requests were for teaching methodologies, nursing management, and nursing research. The Vietnam nurses' thirst for learning and their desire to advance nursing and to be on par with international nursing colleagues were impressive. They want more power and equality in the health sector and in society.

Working directly with Vietnamese nurse leaders provided insight in assisting them to develop standards of practice and a professional code of ethics. It is imperative to upgrade the current nursing workforce of Vietnam. Upgrading primary and secondary nurses to the registered nurse level is a priority. To bridge the gap between Vietnam nursing and the rest of the world, continued collaborations, mentoring connections, and partnerships among nurses from various nations continue to be needed.

VIETNAM
Sara L. Jarrett, Faye Hummel, and Kathleen L. Whitney

The nature and focus of this vignette is about a long-term international partnership between nurses in the United States and nurses in Vietnam. The key to success was built upon relationships, trust, and collaboration to improve nursing, nursing education, and health care in an underserved country. Paramount was to draw upon the Vietnamese nurses' strength to ensure sustainability and ownership.

The Friendship Bridge nongovernmental organization was founded in 1988 by Connie and Ted Ning after they returned from a fact-finding trip to Vietnam to assess the women and children's health care needs. They began a grassroots medical relief project that grew, and in the spring of 1990, Friendship Bridge sent the largest single shipment of medical relief to Vietnam from the United States since 1975. After spending many days with a team of health professionals visiting Denver through Friendship Bridge, Sara Jarrett, a nurse educator, recommended that a nursing delegation go to Vietnam to learn about the country's current health issues and needs. In 1991, a delegation of three nurses (Sara Jarrett, Kathy Whitney, and Karen Terry) traveled to Ho Chi Minh City to assess nursing education programs and hospital nursing conditions. They found that despite poor physical conditions in hospitals and minimal educational resources, the Vietnamese nurse administrators and educators envisioned a new way of nursing and were committed to its development. Sara also had a long-term connection with the country; she and her husband supported an orphanage during the 1970s and adopted two babies from Vietnam before 1975.

Following the initial fact-finding trip, the Friendship Bridge Nurses Group was founded, with Sara Jarrett and Kathy Whitney as the initial facilitators of nursing activities. Additional Vietnam trips followed the supported development of relationships between the Friendship Bridge nurses and nurse educators, and the members of the Vietnamese Nursing Association. These relationships were foundational for collaborations that sustained all Friendship Bridge Nurses Group projects. In 1995, a Steering Committee for the Friendship Bridge Nurses Group was formalized with three members: Sara Jarrett, Kathy Whitney, and Faye Hummel. The Friendship Bridge Nurses Group sponsored several delegations of nurses to travel to Vietnam and conduct educational in-service presentations, clinical teaching, and consultation for hospitals in the Ho Chi Minh City and Dong Thap Province areas.

In 1995, the Friendship Bridge Nurses Group launched a program of certificate courses for Vietnam nurses with baccalaureate nursing degrees. It became known as the Pos–Baccalaureate Certificate Program and was taught from 1995–2005 at three university sites in Vietnam. This certificate program was composed of nine or ten nursing courses that reflect U.S. bachelor's level of nursing education. Each course was developed and implemented in partnership with Vietnamese nursing colleagues to ensure context relevance and cultural appropriateness. The purposes of these courses were to upgrade the knowledge base of Vietnamese nurse educators and nurse administrators, and to help prepare them for acceptance into graduate nursing programs.

The Friendship Bridge Nurses Group partnered with nursing faculty from eleven different U.S. universities and clinical sites to teach nursing courses and mentor nursing professionals in Vietnam. For the post-baccalaureate course years, fifty-five U.S. nurse educators volunteered (some more than once). Together they taught twenty-eight nursing courses and completed three certificate programs. Eighty-eight Vietnamese nurse educators and administrators participated in these programs. The Friendship Bridge Nurses Group's success is founded on relationship building at all levels. Course by course, student by student, and faculty by faculty, professional connections were established with key nursing leaders in hospitals and nursing schools. Friendship Bridge Nurses Group leaders maintained ongoing relationships with the Ministry of Health, the Ministry of Education, the University of Medicine and Pharmacy in Ho Chi Minh City, and the Vietnam Nurses Association. Today, Friendship Bridge Nurses Group is a well-known entity among nurses in Vietnam.

With nursing scholarships from Friendship Bridge Nurses Group, six Vietnamese graduates of the Ho Chi Minh Post-Baccalaureate Project completed their graduate education in nursing administration at Burapha University in Thailand during 2001. They were the first nurses to receive master's degrees in nursing in Vietnam. The vision of graduate nursing education in Vietnam came from our Vietnamese colleagues and nationally recognized and respected nursing leaders. In 2001, around the dining room table in a Colorado home, Friendship Bridge Nurses Group leaders and their Vietnamese partners carefully crafted a curriculum for a master's degree in nursing for Vietnam. Following countless emails, phone communications, and thousands of traveled miles, a model curriculum was completed. Friendship Bridge Nurses Group nursing leaders traveled to Vietnam to accompany their Vietnamese colleagues to seek approval from the Ministry of Education and Ministry of Health. They worked tirelessly with the leaders in the University of Medicine and Pharmacy in Ho Chi Minh City for final curriculum approval. In the fall of 2007, after seven years of collaborative development and planning, eight students began the first Vietnam Master's in Nursing Program at the University of Medicine and Pharmacy in Ho Chi Minh City. The second cohort of eighteen students began classes in the fall of 2008.

Master's nursing education today in Vietnam reflects the synergy of professional nursing colleagues with the desire and capacity to cross boundaries and barriers and to create opportunities for nursing education and development. This program was collaboratively developed by the

Vietnamese Nurses Association and the Graduate Department Faculty of the University of Medicine and Pharmacy. The graduate nursing project represents a unique partnership of a nongovernmental organization, a Vietnamese university, and the Vietnamese government.

Friendship Bridge Nurses Group has aligned development strategies with recommendations set forth by the World Health Organization, Sigma Theta Tau International, and the International Council of Nurses, specifically to build an effective system of nursing education with master's and doctoral programs as the ultimate goal. Additionally, policies and direction set forth by the government of Vietnam have guided the goals and activities of Friendship Bridge Nurses Group.

The Friendship Bridge Nurses Group recognizes that time is needed to build the critical mass of MSN nursing graduates able to pursue doctorates, but in the meantime, the Vietnamese master's in nursing graduates will make a significant contribution toward educating a growing number of highly skilled, highly educated BSN graduates by teaching in baccalaureate nursing programs. These graduates will provide the building blocks of a modern nursing profession. This is the first step in graduate nursing education. We believe that Friendship Bridge Nurses Group's major contribution was to open the door of opportunity for nurses and to make graduate nursing education acceptable in Vietnam. While we launched nursing graduate education, we continued to rely on other partners, new and old, to pursue this trajectory in nursing development. The program must graduate a sufficient number of nurses with advanced degrees to build long-term sustainability and establish an educational structure where BSN, MSN, and doctoral programs are the norm.

A core tenet of our successful collaborative relationship has always been that the Friendship Bridge Nurses Group's nurses work within the host country's educational and health systems to effect gradual, culturally appropriate change, rather than attempting to impose external values and methods. Friendship Bridge Nurses Group's visiting faculty work within the university's structure, with the support of the university faculty.

Friendship Bridge Nurses Group, in partnership with the University of Medicine and Pharmacy in Ho Chi Minh City, is directly responsible for ensuring the curriculum's academic integrity. Friendship Bridge Nurses Group will measure success by the number of graduating master's-prepared nurses. Additional evaluation measures include the effectiveness of the Friendship Bridge Nurses Group mentoring program, the roles in practice and nursing education that the new master's-prepared nurses assume after graduation, and ultimately, the number and quality of Vietnamese faculty who achieve doctoral degrees.

Currently, health care, even in the major cities, is still struggling to rebuild much of the knowledge and many resources lost in the years between 1975 and the early 1990s when Vietnam was effectively closed off from the rest of the world following reunification. Vietnam's Ministry of Health and its Ministry of Education recognize that to build an infrastructure capable of meeting the country's future health care needs, they must develop a strong professional nursing program that meets international standards. It is understood that high-quality nursing education is a vital component of a strong health care infrastructure, and that Vietnam's health care system urgently needs professional nurses. Friendship Bridge Nurses Group has been proud to work alongside Vietnamese colleagues, especially the Vietnam Nurses Association. Friendship Bridge Nurses Group has made progress—in 1991, Vietnam had no bachelor of science in nursing (BSN) programs and now there are ten. However, there are only forty nurses with a master's degree in all of Vietnam and only thirty-two of those hold degrees in nursing. To obtain their degrees, these nurses traveled to other parts of Asia.

The Friendship Bridge Nurses Group's founders frequently speak to nursing associations about their successful collaboration in Vietnam. Over the course of seventeen years, Friendship Bridge Nurses Group has sent sixty U.S. nurse educators (with master's and doctoral degrees) to Vietnam from a variety of U.S. private and public universities. To date, Friendship Bridge Nurses Group operates on a small budget with an all-volunteer staff to create an exceptionally strong program. Small private donations provided a base for educational course costs and limited support for faculty travel and per-diem expenses.

Volunteerism has been the basis for Friendship Bridge Nurses Group's success. Its nurses shared the fact that they participate because of their desire to be helpful; their willingness to develop respectful, collegial, and long-term relationships with Vietnamese colleagues; and their sharing a common goal to contribute to the improvement of Vietnam's professional nursing practice. All factors created an ongoing bond that continues to call nurses into the project and to energize them.

The last seventeen years have seen a series of new beginnings, transitions, and endings. This has not simply been a project; it has and continues to be a journey. It is an ongoing cultural immersion that has been intense with the depth and breadth of experiences, both personal and professional. We have seen the unbelievable change that occurred in a developing country and know that we have been part of nursing health care changes. When any one of us travels the familiar road to Vietnam, we know that the welcome will be as sincere and exciting for both us and our Vietnamese colleagues and friends just as it was the first time we traveled to Vietnam. This journey continues; the time is coming when our Vietnamese colleagues will sustain our collaborative activities independently.

13

Nurse Educators Working in Multiple Countries

Elissa Crocker

Faculty members at the University of Oklahoma College of Nursing are involved in a variety of global projects. These include projects in Japan, Russia, Jordan, Israel, St. Kitts, the United Arab Emirates, Saudi Arabia, Bolivia, Mexico, and other countries. Utilizing technology and the availability of online course work, two College of Nursing graduate students completed the education pathway master's program while residing in Nigeria and Germany. Ethnic diversity is also present among faculty and staff, with personnel from many countries. In addition, University of Oklahoma College of Nursing is an active partner with the Council of International Neonatal Nurses, which has representatives from more than forty countries across the globe. And in 2005, University of Oklahoma College of Nursing was named as a World Health Organization Collaborating Center Affiliate under the auspices of the University of Alabama at Birmingham.

Evelyn Acheson, PhD, RN, assistant professor and director of the WHO Collaborating Center, as well as University of Oklahoma College of Nursing's international program, is a seasoned nursing educator and mentor with many years of experience in multiple countries in Southeast Asia, Africa, and South America. In 2006, Dr. Acheson was invited to accompany family medicine faculty and residents from the University of Oklahoma College of Medicine to Santa Cruz, Bolivia. Contact was made with another American physician, Dr. Toni Mercado, who has been working with the South American Missionaries to improve the health of the Ayoré Indians, an indigenous tribe in Eastern Bolivia. "The Ayoré people are at the bottom of the socio-economic ladder," Dr. Acheson said.

With partial funding from AMB Foundation in Phoenix, Arizona, University of Oklahoma College of Nursing faculty and students and the College of Public Health students traveled to Bolivia during spring break. Their purpose was to develop and implement a basic public health education program for the Ayoré villagers. Ten villages were visited—each typically consisting of twenty to fifty family groups. Although education pertinent to all age groups is provided, the special needs of the most vulnerable population—infants, children, and pregnant women—were emphasized.

Explaining that education and training of "village health workers" is a model commonly utilized in WHO public health initiatives; Dr. Acheson also used this model in the Bolivia project. Typically, individuals selected as village health workers are intelligent and respected leaders who are motivated to advocate for their village's needs. Ayoré health care workers spoke Spanish, and methods of advocating for their needs in Bolivian clinics were discussed.

The village health workers attended two-day classes that covered basic but pertinent issues, ranging from handwashing and dental hygiene to first aid for skin wounds. Symptoms and treatment of common respiratory conditions, as well as diarrhea and parasites, were addressed; emergency situations were emphasized. "We had one three-month old baby infected with scabies in the form of boils over her body." Dr Acheson said. "I almost cried."

Linda McFall is an RN with master's degrees in education and nursing. Her motivation to attend the spring 2008 trip was twofold. In addition to her desire for international experience, she was one of the students in an advanced community health nursing class who wrote the curriculum. As such, she wanted to evaluate its implementation. And while she was grateful for the warm, caring, and dedicated attitudes of the South American Missionaries group members, Linda was surprised to feel vulnerable in a foreign country when she didn't know the language.

Adding that another nursing instructor, Megan McClintock, MSN, RN, was also a participant in the spring of 2008 trip, Linda said her "comfort zone" was teaching in groups with translators. "But I also found that it's important to keep instruction simple to ensure the translator gets to the heart of what we were teaching," she said.

An eye-opener for first-timers was Ayoré's poverty and primitive lifestyle. Homes were constructed with large tree branches held together with mud. Some huts had tin roofs, but none were equipped with any modern amenity, including running water. A central water location is present in every village where residents fill jugs and buckets and carry them to their dwellings. Obviously, hauling heavy water jugs is difficult and basic hand washing can be problematic.

Consequently, "tippy bottles"—two-liter plastic bottles with a small straw for a make-do spigot—were constructed. "Fill them with water and when you open the lid, water pours out," Dr. Acheson said. "Close it and it stops. Hang it in a tree using dental floss and presto—you have running water." Another improvisation was placing soap in panty hose that was hung next to the tippy bottles. "It was super," Dr. Acheson said, "We had soap and running water and we air dried."

Rachel Schupp, a University of Oklahoma College of Nursing Tulsa campus student also made the same trip. Explaining that her motivation was to obtain public health experience in a different culture, she admitted the trip wasn't all smooth sailing. She often felt like she stood out in the crowd with her fair skin and short hair. Rachel said village women have long hair and people often stared in curiosity. However, the young nursing student took it in stride. "I really admired how receptive Rachel was," Linda said. "She was willing to do whatever was asked of her and she helped and learned as she went." Understanding cultural norms was also a learning experience. "I saw a tribesman in the marketplace and I went to speak with him," Rachel said. "The missionaries shooed me away, and I didn't understand why. Later, they said he was respected in his tribe and the Ayoré have been so oppressed [that] if he was seen talking with a foreigner in [an urban marketplace], they might lose respect for him."

Another area of culture shock involved attitudes about illnesses. If a neonate is born with any gross abnormality, infanticide may be practiced, and often sickness is attributed to "evil spirits." However, villagers were often open to gaining education and knowledge. Rachel enjoyed observing the interaction between Dr. Acheson and the children. "They would swarm around her," she said. "Dr. Acheson had paper and pencils and would write down math problems. They would work them as fast as they could and run back to have them graded. They would not leave her alone." Perhaps the children's admiration for Dr. Acheson stemmed from this being her third trip and she had built rapport.

"They have such a desire to learn," Dr. Acheson said. Classes were taught under shade trees, and one of Rachel's assignments was teaching them how to take a blood pressure. "The younger villagers caught on quicker," Rachel said. "But I also had to use body language—such as tapping—to demonstrate what to listen for in order to measure a blood pressure accurately."

Infant mortality is also high, so a good deal of teaching focused on recognizing abnormal symptoms and taking appropriate action. Dental hygiene is also an issue. "We taught them to brush their teeth and there was lots of pointing and laughing," Dr. Acheson said. When the villagers were asked what they used to treat cuts and burns, they sent someone to pick aloe vera. Dr. Acheson's goal is to foster independence and impart knowledge to enable people to care for their own health care needs. So at some point, their work with the Ayoré tribe will end. "With the proto-type for the program successfully developed and all our material trans-lated into Spanish, we could implement similar projects in any country in South America," she said. At the end of this immersion in public health education, village health care workers were given small first aid kits with bandage materials, scissors, antibiotic ointment, baby scales with trou-sers, salt and sugar for making oral rehydration solution, and tee-shirts designating their special role.

Integrating a global perspective within University of Oklahoma College of Nursing is also accomplished through the visiting scholar pro-gram, in which practicing nurses, educators, or graduate students from abroad can study on-site with faculty mentors. The scholars establish their own learning objectives for their time in residence, and their goals are diverse—some want to broaden their knowledge in a nursing specialty, while others may desire to gain exposure in information technology and its use in distance education and curriculum development. Others are seeking mentors to plan a research study or to assist with completing research studies in progress.

Visiting scholars were assisted in obtaining a visa and finding host families and transportation. They have office space and access to univer-sity facilities and a writing lab and assistance with English. Scholars are encouraged to attend meetings, seminars, and educational opportuni-ties at state-of-the-art hospital and clinical facilities. Upon completion, they receive a continuing education certificate and a written evaluation of their study plan.

Visiting scholars have included nurses from Russia, Thailand, Taiwan, and Iraq. One of the most historic cultural exchanges with far-reaching implications occurred in 2008. In January of that year, four nurses from the University of Sulaimania, the major city in the Kurdistan region in northern Iraq, traveled to University of Oklahoma College of Nursing for an immersion in the American health care system and to participate in an unprecedented cultural exchange. Representing an array of special-ties, the nurses, three men and one woman, have undergraduate degrees from Baghdad University Nursing College. The men were working toward their master's degrees while the woman was working toward her doctorate. A two-year-long, complicated, and difficult process, the proj-ect was born in the mountains of Kurdistan in a very unique situation. For over a decade, Donna Fritz, a graduate of University of Oklahoma College of Nursing's nurse practitioner program, was a nursing profes-sor in the Middle East—primarily in Turkey and Kurdistan. As a result, she saw the campaign of genocide waged by Saddam Hussein against the Kurds, the Shias, and other ethnic groups within the country. On one occasion, as Donna sought refuge in the barren mountains, living in tents with the barest of essentials, she met the current First Lady of Iraq, Hiro Ibrahim Ahmed (al-Talabani), also a Kurd fleeing from Hussein's genocidal assaults.

After the Iraqi dictatorship was toppled, her husband, Jalal al-Talabani, was elected as the president of the new Iraq. "The case was made to the fledgling democratic government that this exchange with some of their best and brightest future leaders and educators would benefit the entire country," Dr. Acheson said. Their Oklahoma itinerary included extensive exposure to the health care system in both clinical and academic settings. Experiences were diverse and included rotating though the gamut of roles in acute care and community health where they were exposed to cutting-edge technology. In addition to attending conferences and student and faculty interactions across the state, they were on a helicopter rescue mission and visited a contaminated mining site in northeast Oklahoma. They saw infection control practices and how instruments were sterilized, and read something as mundane—but unfamiliar—as policy and procedure manuals. And as they observed interactions they were impressed by the teamwork. "Nurses are more independent in the United States," said one Kurd nurse. "They can do many things and are well respected."

In an analogy very apropos in Oklahoma, Dr. Acheson said, "Being a Kurd is like being a Cherokee; it's an ethnic origin, not a religion." The Kurd nurses made multiple presentations about the Iraqi health care sys-tem to Oklahomans. Many differences exist, some of which are stagger-ing. Formerly, all Iraqi nurses were women, while about 70% of today's nurses are men. Also about 80% of nurses in the current work force completed a "primary program" for training, entering the program after the sixth grade. Comparing this preparation as being similar to a nurse's aide in the United States, Dr. Acheson said nurses in Iraq are not permitted to take vital signs.

Knowledge and use of infection control practices are minimal, and windows are frequently open because of the heat, allowing a free flow of dust and insects. Equipment is often antiquated, and many times nurses were not taught to operate and maintain it properly. Not only are nurses paid poorly, the nursing profession is not held in esteem in Iraq. Obviously, leadership skills are desperately needed.

In light of the current political unrest and war in Iraq, the nurses were frequently asked their opinion. "They are very grateful to the United States for liberating them from Hussein's regime," Dr. Acheson said. "And they worry about the return of oppression if U.S. troops are withdrawn too soon." Even traveling to the United States for this educational and cultural exchange put these four nurses at risk. As they observed the stark differences between the two countries, they became overwhelmed by the technology, cleanliness, and efficiency of the health care system in the United States.

However as time continued, their confidence grew and they began to acquire some of the American "can-do" spirit. "They've identified ways to begin making needed changes," Dr. Acheson said. "Now, they are full of ideas and are much more optimistic about the ability to implement change and improve the system."

Susan E. Fletcher

"Look out for the rapids! Oh boy, I think we're sinking. There go all our luggage and medical supplies." These words were uttered as our canoe hit unruly rapids and capsized. We were in a dugout canoe, powered by a small motor, going from village to village in the Amazon. Luckily, there were people from two other dugouts who retrieved our luggage and aided us to shore. By the time we unpacked and discarded many ruined supplies, our canoe was dry. Then the motor burst into flames, shooting fire twenty feet into the air. Our boatmen dumped the canoe, extinguished the fire, and repaired the motor, and off we went in our dugout. This occurred after we safely navigated Camino Del Muerte, the Road of Death, purported to be the most dangerous road in the world, with an average death toll of one person per day. Within the span of a two-week period, eight nursing students and I survived the death road; saw our boat capsize and then catch fire; were invaded by squirrel monkeys; swam with dolphins while Pedro, a twelve-foot alligator, served as our lifeguard; slept on a beach only to be attacked by an over-zealous sand flea population; ate grub worms; assisted in extinguishing a jungle fire; and treated 2,500 individuals with health concerns.

My initiation into global nursing work began several years ago when I taught a multiculturalism course. Students gave presentations on cultures and engaged in community multicultural events. Following these "cultural explorations" students discussed their thoughts. My "aha" moment came when one student said, "My father and grandfather were from Germany. They told me the holocaust was made up by Jews to get sympathy. I was never sure, but now after visiting the Holocaust Museum, I know what they said was wrong. It hurts me now to think of all those people dying." I realized that if we stayed in the safe confines of academia, we limited our students' understanding and exploration of the "real world."

My first venture involved a fairly easy trek to Ojinaga, Mexico. It was a three-week immersion experience, and I took along four nursing students. We met biweekly and discussed their personal goals and objectives. Students journaled throughout the experience; it was an excellent method of reflection on their thoughts, beliefs, and instances of transformative learning. We prepared students for the sights, sounds, and smells of the countries; our sensory systems were often overloaded. Whether driving through downtown Guatemala City with its partial buildings serving as homes for thousands of people, meeting beggars at Managua Airport in Nicaragua or Bolivia, or arriving in Bangladesh to throngs of people waiting to earn a few extra coins, the cacophony of noise can be quite intimidating! Preparation of students for unfamiliar experiences is important.

On my next trip, with a nondenominational Christian group, I brought ten students to Guatemala. We held daily rural clinics providing care for several hundred people. We stayed with several families, which was crucial to the immersion experience. Students learned communication and a variety of unique cultural experiences.

The next travels were to rural villages in Nicaragua, Bangladesh, and Thailand. Bangladesh was a poor country. People lived in various levels of poverty. The lowest level is that people must work or they will die. Their daily income decides; if they are too sick to work, they will probably not survive. While in Bangladesh I taught a class on community health and critical thinking to nursing students at Kumadini Hospital and College. We also taught classes on English as a second language. Because of their limited funding they had few current nursing journals. I collected journals from my colleagues and gave them to the nursing program.

Education is key to international trips. In Bolivia we presented an educational symposium to all village health care workers in a central town, and health care workers traveled some distances to attend. We offered the educational program collaboratively with Bolivian doctors and nurses with topics like dental hygiene, tuberculosis, and nutrition. Feedback about the seminars has consistently been positive.

In our Bolivian clinic, one resident was too sick to attend so a nursing student, a translator, and I made a home visit. This area was high and mountainous and we climbed to about 14,000 feet where we were greeted by their neighbors. At first I was confused by their presence, but I soon realized that education combined with health care is a communal effort, especially in remote villages where people rely on each other for basic needs. They followed us into the two-room house. An older woman greeted us and told us about her husband. He suffered from back pain for several months. The neighbors gathered around his bed as I examined him. He hurt his back while working the field with his machete. Seeing this as a perfect educational opportunity I asked neighbors to sit down and we discussed proper body mechanics and lifting. When we finished, the entire group proceeded to instruct him.

With each adventure I gained additional insight. Each trip brings new experiences and new adventures. I gradually learned what works and what doesn't. What I also learned is that in every country, the people are incredibly grateful for anything done for them. Each trip and each village holds special memories. In Nicaragua I saw an older woman crawling up the hill to our clinic. Several of us helped her to the clinic. She didn't want us to help because she was "too dirty" for us to touch. She had an infected leg lesion that made it difficult to walk so she crawled. We treated it with dressings and antibiotics. She called us her "little birds" for bringing joy to her life.

While in Bangladesh I taught at Kumadini Hospital and visited and stayed in rural villages. I visited several sites operated by non-governmental organizations. One was a factory run by women who made men's shirts for approximately eight cents each for their labor; the shirts were then sold to U.S. corporations. The women were paid minimal money but saw it as a means to become independent. Another site was a group of homes around a small lake. The people were given homes and a small tract of land. In exchange, they were required to fish the lake and sell the fish for income. The homes, built of plywood approximately twelve feet in diameter, were minimally functional. I also visited the slums where I was greeted by throngs of people with diseases ranging from tuberculosis to lice. The people were anxious to see us and tell their stories. One family was offered the opportunity to leave the slum and live in a lake home. They refused because the extended family could not go. Another lesson learned. Family, including extended family, is very important in Bangladesh.

During one of my first trips to Bolivia we went to the Altiplano (a desolate area high in the mountains). We met with the local council who gave us a meetinghouse to hold the clinic. In the front yard of the clinic, a witch doctor killed an alpaca (an animal similar to a llama), skinned it, and prepared to cook it while our clinic was in session. Several older men of the village came to us and then went to her for a bowl of brains and intestines. This combination of care and food was what people needed for total wellness.

After several years I learned the importance of asking others for help. I wrote a few small grants to help defray student expenses and provide much needed care for Bolivian people. After several trips involving treatment of parasites, especially worms, I decided to provide education about worms and offer people flip-flops to minimize their exposure to infestation. The generosity of others was amazing! I continue to look for future opportunities to combine teaching experiences with service to humanity, always anticipating new lessons waiting to be learned.

Jeana Wilcox

I made my first trip to Jamaica in July of 2003 with the youth of my church for a week-long mission experience. During the trip my passion for mission nursing was enlivened. I made numerous mission trips to Jamaica (eight in all) and one to Cambodia over the past five years. These trips provided me the opportunity to give back to the global community with my nursing abilities.

I most frequently visit a primary care clinic in Falmouth, Jamaica, which was built 20 years ago. The goal of the clinic is to provide opportunities for medical professionals to give care to the poor and indigent of a mid-sized Jamaican city while forging lifelong relationships with global friends of another culture. The clinic is managed by women from the Falmouth United Methodist Church. It is open only when a volunteer team is present, usually 25 to 30 weeks each year. Teams consist of physicians, nurse practitioners, dentists, nurses, and lay persons who bring medications, medical equipment such as crutches and orthopedic braces, blood glucose machines and supplies, gloves, and condoms. Each patient has a docket (chart) updated with each clinic visit. The clinic charges about $3 US to be seen and receive all necessary medications, and $5 US if minor surgery is needed. The money pays for the church ladies' time to run the medical records room and clean the clinic. However, no one is turned away and team members often pay the entrance fees for needy patients.

My work with the mission began with a passing comment from a friend as our dilapidated tour bus drove through the streets of Falmouth, Jamaica. My friend said, "You should bring your students here; there is a medical clinic a few blocks away." The medical clinic is a Volunteer in Mission project of The United Methodist Church.

As I investigated the opportunity, I found that a mission group from Clinton, Missouri, was scheduled to go there in 2004. I contacted the team leader who welcomed my students and we joined their team. That year, I accompanied nine students for a transcultural nursing experience. The team could not accommodate nine students in one week so I spent two weeks in Jamaica with five students the first week, and four students the second. I fell in love with the Jamaican people. Their laid-back, happy, and generous nature captivated me. Their hope and enthusiasm in the face of extreme poverty inspired me to help. Thus, I returned annually to the same clinic and the same grateful patients. The experience has been life changing for my students and me. In fact, two original students and others from subsequent years returned to the location after graduation to work as clinic nurses and to mentor students.

My work with students in the primary care clinic enabled students to interact with members of another culture, utilize clinical skills in an alternative clinical setting, and build meaningful relationships while cultivating culturally sensitive interaction skills. Patients may walk several hours in the pre-dawn to place their name on a list to be seen (first come, first served) then patiently wait on the clinic's porch. They rarely complain and often voice blessings to the team members. It is not uncommon to hear "God bless you" when handing a patient something as simple as a small bag of vitamins. Patience, perseverance, and a positive attitude are necessary for clinic work. Clinic patients speak English with a Patwa accent. The language is a combination of African, Creole, and English, which takes extreme patience and attention to understand their words. Even though a nurse spoke English, the accent required undivided attention. Another difficulty in assessing patients' needs involved their different use of terms when describing ailments. Patients' references to their "hand" may refer to anything from their shoulder to their pinkie finger.

Each trip brings new challenges and opportunities. During the second year we introduced ourselves to local school officials. We were welcomed and engaged the All Age School students in discussions on topics such as drug/alcohol use, smoking, nursing as a profession, and hygiene. The student groups have a close relationship with the local infirmary, which is equivalent to an American nursing home. The government-run infirmary cares for the poor and indigent elderly. The nurse who runs the infirmary, Matron Allen, is a remarkable woman. Students were amazed at her quality of care. Not a single resident had pressure ulcers and all residents get up daily, dress, and engage in meals and activities in the infirmary dining area. One student was so inspired by the Matron's work she is obtaining wound care nurse certification.

I was able to instill a sense of charity in my thirteen-year-old son Paul, who accompanied me on three Jamaican trips. He worked the pharmacy counting pills, entertained children while parents were seen by medical providers, and learned how blessed he is while becoming a great observer of human behavior and circumstances. Often he'd say things such as, "That boy playing in the street does not have shoes. We need to buy him some so he doesn't hurt his feet." or "Mom, that kid is hungry. I'm going to make him a peanut butter sandwich."

One student provided me with a mentoring opportunity. She was interested in the large numbers of Jamaicans who developed intestinal worms and was amazed at the cost and limited quantity of Vermox available for treatment. She researched natural methods of treatment and found that papaya seeds can treat intestinal worms. She made contact with a European physician and obtained documentation of effective dosages of papaya for intestinal worming. She began a teaching project with the Jamaican people in Falmouth. She taught the worming technique for patients and their pets on the porch as patients waited. We have several trips planned for continued teaching, follow-up, and evaluation of outcomes. It is exciting to impact the Jamaican people through inspiration of an undergraduate nursing student.

Another mission opportunity that provided me cultural enrichment was my trip to Phnom Penh, Cambodia. As a member of Health Volunteers Overseas, I accepted an invitation to visit Cambodia in 2007 to teach nursing in the Sihanouk Hospital Center of Hope in Phnom Penh. The Sihanouk Hospital Center of Hope is a Swiss-sponsored facility providing the only available free health care in the entire country. I conducted lectures related to my expertise in psychiatric nursing and therapeutic communication, led a journal club for staff RNs, and assisted nursing administration with curriculum development of a BSN program.

I met Phalla, the nurse educator, in the hospital lobby for a tour; I saw family members feeding and bathing patients, and nurses charting at three metal desks arranged in a U-shaped configuration. The library, one floor below the educator's office, was the only air-conditioned area and contained four computers with Internet access and a variety of medical and nursing texts. I spent mornings in the library creating modules for educators to use during new nurse orientation classes. Phalla asked me to work specifically on assessment modules (skin, heart and lung sounds, abdomen, and neurologic) for newly hired RNs.

Each morning there were hundreds of patients waiting to be seen. Because the hospital was small, patients were asked to return daily for treatments, intravenous antibiotics, etc. The hospital's front yard had patients sitting in "wheelchairs"—plastic lawn chairs with wheels. Families held IV tubing or hung it on trees limbs to encourage gravity flow of medications.

Teaching nursing in a different culture provided me with a professional challenge. One afternoon, as I taught about anxiety disorders, phobias in particular, the nurses began to laugh hysterically. I was confused about their reaction to a discussion of spiders being a simple phobia of many people. When the laughter subsided, one nurse said, "We aren't afraid of spiders; we eat them." Then, I began to laugh as I realized I needed a new, more culturally appropriate example. That experience demonstrated my continued learning about the effect of culture on my teaching.

IV

Nursing Amidst Disaster

This section includes three chapters focused on nurse educators and their extraordinary efforts in disasters. Not only have these nurse educators provided direct care and immediate response to disasters in their communities and abroad, they also have used these opportunities for students to learn of the complex roles required for immediate responders. The first chapter in this section is focused on disasters in the United States. The second chapter includes responses to disasters in other parts of the world. The third chapter includes nurse educators' descriptions of how they used disaster situations to teach other nurses and students.

—*Joyce J. Fitzpatrick*

14

Nursing and Disasters: Stories From the United States

HURRICANE KATRINA
Diane Blanchard

No one could predict the devastation caused by Hurricane Katrina. The victims became evacuees within a matter of hours and everyone's lives changed forever. Nobody knew that Hurricane Katrina would reduce homes and businesses to rubble along the Gulf Coast and cut them off from the rest of the world. No one could foresee that levees would breech and flood the city of New Orleans, Louisiana.

Senior-level nursing students in the BSN program at Alcorn State University were anxiously preparing for their fall semester. Students and faculty were busy getting ready for clinical rotations, homework assignments, classroom lectures, and planning experiences to ensure that the best opportunities would be implemented. Affiliating agencies for clinical rotations were dictating their latest guidelines for the students to practice at their facilities.

The word flexibility would become very familiar to the nursing students. Flexibility would be tested as never before at Alcorn State University School of Nursing, and become a way of life in the months ahead. Implementing and redefining skills in the clinical area would take on new meaning. The hours of sleep lost and the amount of time contributed to preparation for clinical experience would greatly increase.

Hurricane Katrina arrived on August 29, 2005, with a catastrophic effect on the Mississippi and Louisiana Gulf Coast. Destruction was massive, and the devastation changed many roles and responsibilities for students and faculty at Alcorn State University. The projected clinical schedule for pediatrics at the University of Mississippi Medical Center was suddenly interrupted.

Gasoline was scarce, prices skyrocketed, and travel was restricted due to hazardous road conditions. Students were unable to travel to their scheduled pediatric rotation at the Medical Center located in Jackson, Mississippi. The 120-mile trip could not be undertaken because of many obstacles, such as lack of lodging, gas shortages, hazardous road conditions, power outages, and uncertain supplies of food and water.

Hurricane Katrina's arrival necessitated the opening of six disaster shelters in Natchez, Mississippi. Already strained health care facilities were further stressed with the new evacuees. The Alcorn students and faculty could never have planned such a real-life experience for disaster training, nor could they ever expect to repeat it in the future.

Electricity outages forced many evacuees, faculty, and students to seek temporary housing or alternative means for cooking, sleeping, and showering. Nursing students and faculty began working at Ground Zero, as the media described the shelters. Nursing students who were displaced from Gulf Coast universities joined the ranks of the regular generic baccalaureate students and adapted to new clinical and classroom experiences. Their home universities were now twelve to twenty feet underwater with irreparable damage from high winds. Many students lived with their families in various local shelters. Unable to return to their schools, they became part of the Alcorn State University student population and practiced nursing in the shelters they called home.

The student nurses' roles as caregivers to over 500 evacuees and family members became the clinical experience of a lifetime. The student ratio that had been 1:2 changed and sometimes the ratio would exceed 1:20 or even 1:50. Faculty and students became one of the stable components for many victims of Hurricane Katrina's devastation. Students and faculty came together to make the best of a devastating situation. Students assessed, planned, implemented, and evaluated each and every part of their practice. If one solution proved unsuccessful, the situation was reevaluated and corrections were made in the plan to accommodate the evacuees in the shelters. Responsibility in diverse roles and creativity characterized the morning, afternoon, and evening clinical experience.

Critical thinking, assessment, history taking, technical skills, communication, ethics, and human diversity were necessary components of disaster relief from Hurricane Katrina. Organization was problematic in the beginning due to the unavailability of medical records. A roster was formed and different areas of need were prioritized by registration through the American Red Cross. Registered clients were directed to student nurses to complete a health history in order to prioritize and validate the need for medical attention.

Student nurses and other volunteers completed health history forms, which provided valuable information on allergies; medical, surgical, and social history; medications; family history; and other areas of concern. Clients then were directed to the mobile health unit, provided by Alcorn State University, to receive care from the family nurse practitioner or physicians.

When arriving at the mobile health unit, general assessments were made on health status, and health care needs were determined. Student nurses were active in assisting with all treatment based on assessed needs. This assistance included making appointments and finding transportation for referrals, making phone calls to local providers of walking canes, wheelchairs, eye glasses, and dental work. Priority was given to children and expectant mothers when specialty care was needed. Those clients requiring emergency medical attention were directed to the local hospital emergency departments. Physicians in the area agreed to open their offices to evacuees who could not afford to pay for services. Red Cross vouchers were available to clients with no existing resources for medications, supplies, or medical care. Nursing students were recruited to work in area medical offices to assist with the increasing numbers of clients.

Confidentiality, privacy, ethics, and respect for human diversity were held to a high standard. Clients were informed regarding treatments; their right to refuse treatment was respected. Privacy was maintained. Careful consideration was used concerning the placement of personal information and documentation. Clients were respected and treated regardless of their ethnicity, background, or financial status.

Nursing students became playmates for the young children in the shelters, as well as sanitizers of toys, organizers, homework assistants, secretaries, patient advocates, architects, painters, and technical advisors. Students assisted evacuees in completing online forms for assistance and they became sources of key information. Students directed evacuees with a professional ability most nurses take years to develop. Three nursing students took corrugated boxes and made playhouses for small children while their parents completed forms and information packets from the Federal Emergency Management Agency.

Alcorn State University School of Nursing also welcomed an International Disaster Relief Team of volunteers based in San Diego,

California. The team included two doctors, one nurse practitioner, one registered nurse, and a program coordinator. Housing accommodations were provided at the Alcorn State University dormitory. The International Disaster Relief Team reported to the shelter each morning, triaged the patients, and provided medical services. The team collaborated with nursing students, faculty, and shelter staff on the Alcorn State University Mobile Unit.

Nursing students gave vaccinations to evacuees before they returned to their homes in the still-flooded areas. Tetanus toxiod, hepatitis A, and hepatitis B, if requested, were given to anyone returning to areas where contaminated water remained standing. This area included all of the Gulf Coast, lower Louisiana parishes, and New Orleans, Louisiana. Educational materials, including possible side effects of the vaccination, and follow-up schedules, were given to and discussed with each client. Many clients did not know or could not remember when they had last received a tetanus vaccination. In this case, the client received the tetanus vaccine if one was requested. Tetanus vaccine was difficult to obtain in this situation and was one of the most sought-after medicines during the disaster. The local hospitals donated approximately sixty doses, only a small number of those actually needed. Local physicians donated additional doses, but many more were needed.

Hurricane Gustav did not give warning; this hurricane hit land on September 1, 2008, at 9:00 A.M. and made all of our disaster planning obsolete. Almost three years to the day of Hurricane Katrina's arrival, Hurricane Gustav landed twenty-two miles west of Grand Isle, Louisiana, and continued on a path of destruction directly toward our School of Nursing. None of the faculty or students had prepared for the direct winds or destruction that followed, but our practice and education proved to be most valuable.

Shelters were opened and supplies were provided for those seeking relief. Faculty and students signed up for shifts at shelters and felt prepared for their role. Hurricane Gustav hit with the fury of 120- to 130-mile-per-hour winds, destroying all power lines and public services. Trees were uprooted and crashed into homes. Shelters were not accessible because trees were strewn across the roads. Some of the faculty and students were able to find transportation using four-wheel-drive vehicles and four wheelers. However, they discovered the need was not in the shelters but door to door with victims.

One faculty member, along with a student and her husband, went door to door removing tree limbs and parts of buildings to help those who were trapped. First aid, ice, food, and drinking water were the most valued commodities. Because our area was the first to be declared a disaster area, supplies from the National Guard from Mississippi and Louisiana arrived quickly. The Kentucky National Guard responded and began to open relief assistance shelters for anyone who could mobilize themselves. Everyone needed to act more independently to provide the needed services. Those with the information and training learned from the previous storm worked together to restore calm and order to a devastated area. Because individuals, faculty, and students were cut off and communication was not available, the true meaning of disaster nursing became clear. Individuals using generators were now in danger of carbon monoxide poisoning. There were reports of people being hospitalized or dying because of the poisonous gas. The general public was afraid of the unknown, and the role of the nurse was that of educator.

There was no fuel, which meant that people with serious health problems could not leave their homes for assistance. Hospital services

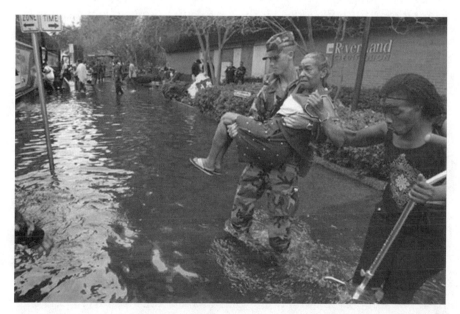

A soldier carrying a woman through a street flooded by Hurricane Katrina in New Orleans.

were not available because of shortages of personnel, gasoline, water, fuel, and utilities. The National Guard welcomed all the help that any nurse faculty or student could provide to help assess, provide care, and educate the public.

The services that we had provided in Hurricane Katrina shelters were now being offered in the streets and at relief stops. The university closed and only those students who could not evacuate to their personal residences were housed on campus. Services at the university were disabled. Students stayed in the gyms and food was distributed in the form of Meals Ready to Eat. The university did not return to full service for seven days. During that time, faculty and staff provided needed disaster nursing care to those in the community.

Because faculty and students lived in these areas, they were unable to get e-mail for online assistance or classes. Phone service was limited to working cell phones. No gas for transportation was one of the main problems and delayed classes from returning to normal schedules. Faculty and students were offered and received great hands-on experiences in the communities in place of the routine clinical. Some even helped with the delivery of a baby and the care of the new mother in the home. Students gave first injections and were happy to have those new experiences, even under those circumstances. One student reported administering over fifty injections on the first day as preventive measures for disease were put in place. Faculty and students faced the challenges with great resilience and experienced memorable and invaluable professional and life experiences.

Nursing students and faculty of Alcorn State University School of Nursing considered these disaster experiences irreplaceable. Students were able to apply the learned skills necessary to meet the needs of those affected by the disasters. These experiences afforded them the opportunity to provide immediate assistance to individuals who experienced tremendous loss, utilizing skills they developed as they matriculated through the program of study.

The aesthetic appearance of the Gulf Coast following the devastation by Hurricane Katrina has improved. The citizens have moved on with their lives. The time and the days appear to be well organized, and no damage can be detected until interviews with the people are performed. Many people report they do not enjoy the once pleasurable events of the past. Some report feelings of hopelessness and helplessness in performing everyday tasks. They often indicate that their failure to connect with others may be a direct result of the old relationships being lost. They claim something is missing in their lives and they cannot sleep and worry about the next day's problems.

Students have learned to interrupt the problems associated with hurricane survivors. These same students begin to look for the next storm and hope they are prepared because now they are the nurses in charge.

HURRICANE KATRINA
Betty Pierce Dennis

Hurricane Katrina roared ashore on August 29, 2005, making it impossible to return to New Orleans. I was serving a second year as dean of a New Orleans nursing school. The campus was completely evacuated. After using our one-night hotel reservation in Baton Rouge, attempts to stay longer were futile. The city was overwhelmed with thousands of evacuees. There were no accommodations available at any of the hotels, inns, or motels in the city or in the surrounding areas. With no living options, I returned to North Carolina where I had previously lived. New Orleans, all the newscasts said, had "dodged a bullet." Hurricane Katrina was a category 3 not 5 as originally projected. Damage was reported as minimal. With that assurance, I left for Switzerland. I was a member of Project Lead, one of the W. K. Kellogg Foundation's outstanding leadership projects.

Although the winds of Katrina were considerably weaker than expected, the true consequence was yet to come. The surge following the storm caused the topping and breaching of the protective levees and canals, dumping more than 100 billion gallons of water into the streets. New Orleans is a city surrounded by water and sits seven to ten feet below sea level. When the levees failed and the pumps were overwhelmed, 80% of the city was flooded. This necessitated the rescue of residents from rooftops and attics. Over 1,400 lives were lost, and the economic upheaval and disruption was unlike any seen before in the United States.

I attempted to contact colleagues in Louisiana. Initially, no cell or land lines in the New Orleans area code were operative. Even though I was finally able to get through, I learned the meaning and frustration of "dropped calls." Connections were sporadic at best. At last, I was able to get an update on the university and decided that instead of continuing on to England with my colleagues, I would join a small group of university faculty, administrators, and staff that our provost had assembled in Atlanta to initiate recovery efforts.

From our hotel, we traveled daily several blocks to donated office space. We reached out to our university family by contacting evacuated students, answering inquiries from families, and reaching other faculty and staff. We always worked with the hope that they and their families had managed to transit this event safely. What we found was that our community was widely disbursed in the state or temporarily relocated in other states both far and near. We were pleased and relieved to learn that our students were faring well. Over sixty colleges and universities throughout the United States had responded by opening their doors to our students so they could complete the semester started in New Orleans. Our campus, Dillard University, known for its aesthetic qualities, was a lovely spot with wide green areas and stately, graceful old oaks. After the devastation, it had the unenviable distinction of having sustained more damage than any of the other educational institutions in New Orleans.

Senior nursing students either evacuated to the Baton Rouge area or to the Houston area. They only needed the final two semesters in their baccalaureate nursing program and, therefore, had not enrolled in any other institutions to take courses, as many other students had. This class was small in number, with only twelve students. The question was should they simply sit out the semester or could the semester be organized and offered in a way that was consistent with the nursing program? In attempting to reach each member of my faculty and staff, I learned that three nursing faculty were also in the same vicinity as the students. Widespread dislocation of people, institutions, organizations, and infrastructure presented formidable challenges. The transportation system was almost nonexistent, so students would have to be able to live in close proximity. If living quarters were established, it would be necessary to ensure their safety. What about resources to maintain student support such as daily meals and laundry facilities? Where would we hold classes? We had no access to computers or to textbooks. Having evacuated with the thought that they would be returning in a couple of days, no one had brought textbooks. Clinical placements for students would be needed— was that even a remote possibility?

Our university has, for many years, received support and funding from The United Methodist Church. Among the many calls into our temporary center in Atlanta inquiring about needs, identifying available resources, and offering assistance was one from The United Methodist Church. I was referred to a minister who was director of one of the recreation centers located in Baton Rouge.

The goal was to create an environment that was not only comfortable and safe for the students, but also conducive to learning. The assistant dean, who was one of three on-site faculty, was an effective monitor of the on-site development of the project. We kept our communication channels open to anticipate and address problems and ensure that needs were identified and addressed in a timely manner. The recreation center was promising; it had a kitchen and restrooms, but no showers. There were no bedrooms, only a large, open area. And there were no computers. Assistance was obtained from several sources to make the facility ready for students. Mattresses were donated by the church. The university paid for bed frames, bedside tables, and dividers to provide privacy for each student. Dinners were prepared by members of the church. Through the minister's contacts and persistence, several computers were donated and three Federal Emergency Management Agency (FEMA) showers were installed adjacent to the center. An appeal to our most frequently used publisher brought DVDs containing all of the course textbooks. During this period, hotel space remained unavailable, so my visits to Baton Rouge had to begin and end on the same day.

Fortunately, the facility was located across the street from the Southern University campus, which had a nursing school with requisite laboratories and classrooms. I contacted the dean at the School of Nursing, and she expressed a willingness to collaborate with us. A course in nursing research was required by our curriculum for seniors. It was also offered by Southern University during the fall semester. Our students were welcomed into the course, and I engaged our financial aid personnel to work out tuition payment.

Two other senior courses were planned and offered by the on-site faculty. For the first time, learning to assess and care for patients after a disaster required no speculation; it was real and immediate. The clinical experiences focused on the health care needs of the numerous evacuees in shelters and in the newly established FEMA trailer parks. The students gained insight into some of the outcomes of disaster that directly affected all segments of the population. The ability of evacuees to cope was apparent. How state and national systems functioned in emergencies was unfolding daily, providing an exceptional learning experience.

An important concern was the safety of the students during night shifts. We developed a position description for a resident advisor, collaborated with the minister, and successfully recruited several very competent women from his congregation to provide night-time security for the students. As the relationship among the students, faculty, minister, and church developed, the caring for each other also deepened. Later, the students selected the minister as their Pinning Ceremony speaker. Both state approval and national accrediting bodies were informed of the arrangements to continue the education of senior nursing students. They communicated their encouragement and support. Students and faculty completed the fall 2005 semester, and the nursing program had successfully established its first temporary site.

Once the fall 2005 semester was completed, discussions about the reopening of the university, and most importantly, the location for reopening, were in process. We knew that the campus would not be ready for occupancy for several months. The provost led efforts to consider and visit several alternative sites—some were in Louisiana, and others in Georgia. Eventually, it was decided that the university would return to New Orleans, in part, to support the recovery of the city. The site was to be a hotel in downtown New Orleans.

Just as we had converted the recreation center into a dormitory/study hall/dining area, the hotel would have to undergo similar modifications. Over one thousand returning students along with faculty and staff occupied the hotel beginning early January of 2006. Our presence made it one of only a few fully operative hotels in a city almost at a complete standstill. The hotel's exhibit hall was divided into classrooms. All university units could not be accommodated in the hotel. For example, the computer laboratory, nursing classrooms, and music practice areas had to be installed next door in the World Trade Center building. The problem of finding clinical experiences was even more acute in this city that had gone from over 2,000 hospital beds to under 500. Again, innovation was the order of the day and students were guided to survey and assess the state of health care in New Orleans by touring sites and interviewing residents to develop reports assessing health care post-disaster. It was an exceptional learning experience, one that could not be duplicated.

For the second time, nursing would have to create an educational program in a noneducational site. Access to audio-visual and skills laboratory equipment, as well as software was necessary. When it was apparent that an early return would not happen, furniture in all offices, classrooms, and laboratories, as well as books and other equipment were packed, boxed, and stored. Arrangements were made to retrieve the mannequins, beds, pumps, models, kits, disposables, and the like. A small kitchen area was the only place with running water and became useful for teaching hand washing and aseptic techniques. With space at a premium, we shared with other units of the university such as the Offices of the Chaplin, Study Abroad, and Campus Life. Now we "lived" together. Also, because most faculty and staff had suffered total loss or damage to their homes, we were like one family "living" together in the hotel. Without the dormitories and off-campus housing, we also "lived" with our students at the hotel. These experiences were instrumental in developing a oneness of purpose, an understanding and appreciation of each other, and a deepened level of comfort. Also, in no small measure, we were in awe of the parents that entrusted their sons and daughters to our nontraditional recovery university location. To ensure that students were able to complete a full academic year, two thirteen-week semesters were developed. Graduation, usually held early in May, was held early in July.

In September of 2006, the university returned to campus. Although we are more than three years post-hurricanes Katrina and Rita and the breached levees, the campus and New Orleans recovery are far from complete. Recovery continues in areas such as housing, the secondary school system, businesses large and small, health care facilities, health care personnel, and commerce. More than 100,000 houses either sustained damage or were completely destroyed. Today, many neighborhoods include empty lots, boarded up, and unoccupied houses.

An important aspect of recovery is the psychological response of the population to a catastrophic event of these proportions. For example, depression, anxiety, and the multiple effects of stress were and are apparent in many returning evacuees. This fact is exacerbated by a severe reduction in psychiatric beds and caregivers. Some secondary school students have begun to manifest negative behaviors such as fighting, nightmares, flashbacks, or panic attacks during rainy days.

Accepting the constancy of the shifting and evolving nature of situations requires leadership that influences and supports new directions, promotes the power to create, and is informed by ideas top-down, bottom-up, and laterally. While this journey is not finished, the leadership aspect has shown how adaptability and persistence can achieve desired ends. In disaster, leaders who are open to innovation have a greater likelihood of achieving the needed outcomes because in disasters, the only certainty is uncertainty. The tenor of leadership in a disaster must be calm and unwavering, with a presence that is inclusive, able to listen, respond, care, and seek solutions. It is important to recognize that one's role is not fixed, but amenable to unpredictable circumstances. What must remain constant is commitment to purpose and understanding of our shared humanity. This event had no comparable occurrence in the United States, in the state of Louisiana, and in the 138-year history of the university. Through this experience comes clarity about the interconnectedness of all people and the breadth and depth of community.

HURRICANE KATRINA
Andrew J. Mahoney and Ecoee Rooney

Coming home to New Orleans after Hurricane Katrina and the levee breaks was not easy, but no one thought it would be. We slowly realized that what we had thought would be a long weekend visiting friends during a perfunctory evacuation to North Louisiana was the beginning of a long and arduous road home. Nothing could have prepared us for the turns and twists, the amazement at those who helped, and the level of commitment of so many lifelong friends and family members and citizens who came forward with money, supplies, and all we needed to survive those first months after leaving all we knew of our lives behind.

No amount of sensationalized media coverage could have prepared us for what we saw and smelled as we drove into the city after the hurricane, even though the mayor still banned entrance to many parts of the city. The vastness of the devastation began to truly sink in as we quietly drove down the interstate past a gray, abandoned landscape. Occasionally, houses that appeared to have been blown apart by some violent force, their guts dangling out, damaged, sat waiting to be discovered by their owners.

It is hard to imagine if we remembered to breathe as we drove into our neighborhoods. No words were exchanged as we passed through the city, tears streaming down our faces. This was truly ugly; ugly beyond what we had even imagined. The desolation was shocking, the gray, cracked patina on everything, and the inescapable black or brown line clearly marking the levels to which the water had risen. Flooded cars and abandoned boats were scattered about the caked mud and debris. The acrid scent of mold and putrid smell of decay penetrated the masks we had been advised to wear upon initial reentry. The orange lifejackets swinging in the breeze from a neighbor's front railing sent a shudder through us as we imagined their terror at the rising waters.

Returning to the city and finding a place to stay was a challenge. Many of us settled into friends' guest rooms. After we settled in, we arrived to set up our new work environment and what would become our new Education/Staff Development office in a raised building that stood unflooded and ready to be occupied across from Big Charity. Four flights of stairs up (no elevators), we met the human resources director outside of the room that was to become our new home. We peered in to see a small room, with two street-facing windows piled with eighty boxes, desks, and chairs jumbled on top of each other, and began to work to find order in this mess. This was in contrast to our large work area of several weeks before—each with our own office, eight staff members, and three large classrooms behind the locked doors of our department. Occasionally we paused to look out the window, where in front of us, Charity Hospital stood, abandoned, purposeless, patientless, and sad. Charity Hospital was one of our main campuses, the more famous of the two, and the storm and floodwaters had delivered the coups de gras that brought down this grande dame of architecture and history. Weeks after evacuation, our hospital, the Medical Center of Louisiana, had started providing care for patients in military tents in the parking lot of the flooded University Hospital campus, and then the hospital operations were moved to military tents in the Convention Center.

We made a list of things we would need to start re-creating our educational efforts from our former offices and department. List in hand, we walked to the back side of Charity and saw signs in the windows and some billowing on sheets outside that staff had made while still awaiting rescue in the days following the storm. Some were pleading "Save Us," while others showed gratitude and inspiration ("Thank you" and "9th Floor Has Heart"), and yet others expressed the ways in which their faith had been tested ("Son of Abraham—where are you?"). We ascended past the black, greasy line that showed us how high the water had risen and

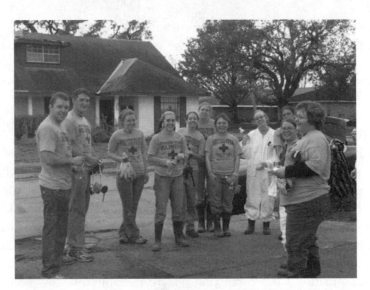

Harding University nursing faculty and students volunteering in New Orleans in the aftermath of Hurricane Katrina. Nursing faculty Karen Kellery and Elizabeth Lee (far right) aid in the disaster cleanup.

entered the hospital where weary and hot armed police stood guard. We signed in and were handed flashlights to navigate the dark corridor in the center of the building, through to the center stairwell. The dank, mildew stench was sickening.

We began the climb up the slippery steps in the dark, slowly making our way to the ninth floor. We emerged from the stairwell and found our department unlocked, the doors flung wide open. Our eyes settled onto the disorder as we began to survey the property damage, loss, and abandoned encampments of staff that had used our large classrooms as sleeping quarters in the days after the storm. Windows had been broken out either by wind or overheated staff hungry for ventilation in the sweltering heat. Pallets had been created on the floor and on chairs pushed together, with colorful quilts and pillows from home lined up in rows throughout the classrooms. As we surveyed, we began to look for the many long classroom tables that filled each classroom and could not find them. Then we saw the tangled heap of metal table legs piled in the corner of classroom 3, our largest room, and realized that the legs had been removed from the tables and the table tops used as spine boards to carry patients from the Intensive Care Units down the twelve flights of stairs to safety and evacuation.

We sighed and looked at each other as if we were both thinking "Where do we begin?" There was so much to do. We reviewed our pre-Katrina "to do" lists for any relevance to life now. Strange how so many projects lost meaning after a disaster of this magnitude. We collected Basic Life Support mannequins, several reference texts, and a few other items, including a personal item or two from our desks, and headed back down the hot, slippery nine-floor descent carrying as much as we could, and slowly crossed the street back to our new office, not noticing that we saw no cars on this usually busy downtown street.

We agreed that we would begin with a learning needs assessment and did so less than one month after the disaster. The immediate needs we identified were maintenance of currency in BLS and other required certifications, as certifications had lapsed, cards were lost in flood waters, or personnel files were unavailable; identification of depression among caregivers; anger/hostility and hostile work environments and the effects on teamwork; products of horizontal violence; burnout, stress, compassion, and fatigue; addressing post-traumatic stress disorder in our staff and patients; and providing trauma-informed care. Additionally, community partners identified that domestic violence survivor identification would be a need. Law enforcement personnel notified our forensic nursing services that there had been a 94% increase in domestic violence in the region since the disaster.

Based on these learning needs assessments, our early educational interventions focused on helping staff maintain current certifications and reorienting staff to this new environment of tents and Meals Ready to Eat, of seeing armed National Guard soldiers wearing camouflage patrolling the streets of the city in humvees, and knowing that nothing about this was normal or was going to be normal any time soon. Additionally, we recognized above all, the staff we were serving was also personally traumatized due to the staggering loss of the community we lived in and all we expected from daily life (our own grocery store, our homes, our churches, and our family near by) and secondarily by hearing all the traumatic stories of the people they served. Continued reassessment of learning needs revealed an increased interest in education regarding provision of care to traumatized patients by traumatized staff, recognizing as well that our staff are a part of that returning population.

We focused our efforts on partnering with agencies that were offering mental health services and made these services available through debriefing sessions with mental health counselors and therapists from the community, as well as volunteer psychologists and therapists from around the country and world, who provided complementary therapies in the forms of support groups and individual counseling. All of these interventions were extremely well received.

As a result of employee dispersion and layoffs, and the very limited services the hospital was providing, the hospital's Sexual Assault Nurse Examiner (SANE) services had not resumed care for people who had been sexually assaulted. We were both SANE-trained registered nurses and began taking 24-hour calls. We performed this duty over and above our usual educational roles, frequently leaving the office, or staying up all night to care for these patients. We performed these examinations in a special military tent we set up at the emergency services unit at the convention center.

Initially, a small number of employees (approximately 230 of the 5,000 pre-storm staff) were working in the emergency services unit and in ancillary services. As services returned and grew, more and more employees were called back to work. At first, we informally re-oriented people in small numbers in our tiny office, often while staff was completing human resources paperwork. It quickly became evident that we needed to provide a formal re-orientation for returning employees. We created information guides, forms, handouts, and poster presentations to support staff in their re-assimilation. As the groups got larger we had to move our orientation to a large white tent in the convention center. The tent sat on raised wooden floors and had minimal lighting and was reminiscent of a square dance hall, so we affectionately named it the "hoedown tent." In addition to the usual orientation materials (such as safety and parking), staff needed information required for working in these unusual conditions: providing care on raised wooden floors, tents, portable sinks, and loud environmental noises from generators. A formal Nurse Orientation resumed in November of 2006 when the hospital had relocated the emergency services unit and education space to a vacant building that had formerly been an upscale department store. Patient education was distributed from sources such as FEMA on post-disaster safety, water potability, and protection from environmental dangers (such as mold and chemicals). These orientation classes became the setting for many emotional reunions with former co-workers, some of them family members. Many had not seen each other since before the storm.

We also learned another facet of "staff development" when we recognized the importance of supporting a person in meeting their personal needs before they could ever meet professional goals. Employees frequently called on the phone to get information, and would begin to tell their "Katrina Stories." We learned very quickly that they were hoping to talk to someone who would listen and take their concerns seriously, even if there was not much we could do for them. We often provided on-the-spot, informal counseling. It was tremendously painful to hear the voice of a former employee, displaced and requesting educational records, barely able to articulate her request because of the severity of her stuttering, a result of the horrific trauma she had experienced. One of us ended up housing three employees and their children consecutively over the next several years because these employees had nowhere to go and needed a place to stay in order to work.

We continuously sought out mental health and material support services for employees who were experiencing symptoms of post-traumatic stress disorder (PTSD) and depression before hospital employee assistance personnel were called back. We created and presented continuing nursing education classes about PTSD and Horizontal Violence, which were very well received. We now view supporting the emotional well-being of our employees as a critical component of staff development; if people feel comfortable, safe, supported, and knowledgeable, they will be better able to provide excellent care and services.

Human Resources offered positions to people with the necessary qualifications. We were frequently consulted regarding qualification criteria for certain jobs. Employees called from all over the country requesting education records so they could obtain work. We worked to support them, and placed calls to the American Heart Association (AHA) and Emergency Nurses Association (ENA) to obtain records that were not immediately retrievable.

Our role also included serving as a de facto Employee Health Department. We administered and read PPD tests, obtained immunization records, managed blood and body fluid exposures, and provided minor first aid services in our office until a full-time Employee Health nurse was hired to manage this aspect of human resources.

We carried out other human resources-related functions such as assisting with the hiring process, attempting to locate employees using very large phone number logs, and writing and helping to disseminate critical information letters for all employees. We realized how scattered we truly were as we watched these letters leave our hands and go out to nearly every state.

Three years later, we were 2,500 employees strong and were providing services in one of our renovated campuses while we await the building of a brand new hospital. Our clinics were still in an old department store building, attached to a still-vacant shopping mall. Satellite clinics were scattered around our community and services were provided from trailers. Our team of educators became a close-knit group of people, and we admired each other for the hard work, tenacity, and dedication. We have learned a great deal about staff education in the past several years, but mostly we have seen how it can be to heal ourselves through reaching out to help others heal. We have learned that we cannot help staff learn or develop personally or professionally unless we intentionally listen to people, and work to meet their basic needs. We have learned and understand that there are other competencies that educators must possess besides the ability to write curricula and teach an in-service or course. These competencies include the ability to listen and learn from the people we serve.

HURRICANE KATRINA
Carrie B. Elkins and Deborah L. Curry

One month after Hurricane Katrina on September 29, 2005, a baccalaureate nursing program from a regional university in northeast Alabama assembled a voluntary team of six nursing faculty and fifteen senior nursing students to travel to New Orleans. The charge given to this team was to "reset" approximately 139 nursing home residents back into their residence. These patients had been evacuated pre-Katrina and had been maintained on air mattresses on floors of shelters for four weeks.

Three weeks of planning resulted in students and faculty receiving donations of a church bus, private vehicles, money from the community, and food and water. The facility had no way of providing bedding, so each volunteer brought their sleeping bag and prepared to sleep on the floor of the facility. Enough food and water were gathered to sustain the team for the three-day work schedule. Preparation is essential to improving the delivery of health care in the aftermath of disaster, and primary to the skills required to respond to a disaster is an understanding of the basic principles surrounding disaster preparedness and response.

No amount of emotional preparation could have prepared the team for what they encountered upon entering the Crescent City. The Five Mile Bridge over Lake Ponchatrain at 10:00 P.M. had only three vehicles—those belonging to the team. A surreal feeling fell upon the team, as inside the city, police officers checked credentials and provided a warning not to be outside the facility after 6 P.M. A sparkling clear autumn sky was now the only familiar aspect of New Orleans. Roads appeared toppled like dominoes, buildings were marked with flood water residue, and businesses were in shambles from flood waters, wreckage, and looting.

After settling into the facility the students and faculty determined objectives, a plan, and a time period for execution of the plan. Discussions entailed division into teams according to the facility layout, receiving of the patients, initial assessment, and triage. Each student on Day 1 was required to perform a complete head-to-toe examination, weight, and vital signs on residents in their sector. Patients with wounds, unstable vital signs, or suffering from dehydration or other illnesses were reported to the nurse in charge at the facility.

One particular nurse who became a hero to students and faculty had worked 193 hours in a two-week period. She was optimistic, cheerful, and supportive of the work the team was doing. Never did she complain. Later the team learned that she had lost her home and was living at the facility. This was only one sad story of many sad stories we encountered. The residents were worried about their children and grandchildren. Emotional stress was palatable.

After twelve hours of non-stop work that first day, the objective for Day 1 had been achieved. Many students continued working with the residents into the night singing to them and "tucking" them into bed. The perseverance and faith of the residents energized the team. The objective of Day 2 was to give each patient a bath, shampoo, and check for fecal impaction. Again, this was another twelve-hour day of pure unadulterated joy for the team. Never had basic nursing care seemed so important! Faculty were working alongside students and no one complained. Work was interrupted only by the need to eat and to toilet. Occasional bursts of laughter would emerge from students, faculty, and residents. How could this happen amid such a catastrophe? At night, crying could be heard from the same people who eight hours previously had enjoyed the gift of laughter.

Prior to September 29, assessment, planning, and implementation had appeared to be only a process from which to begin a nursing assignment for the nursing students. Now it was a lived experience that will never be forgotten. By October 1, 2005, the mission was accomplished, the convalescent center had been indeed "reset," as had the team's hearts.

OKLAHOMA CITY
Elissa Crocker

It was a beautiful spring morning in Oklahoma City. The sun was shining, and the characteristically fierce winds were calm. As winter reluctantly relinquished its hold on nature, flora throughout the city reflected the onset of a new season. Lavender blossoms of red-bud trees contrasted vividly with snow-white flowers adorning Bradford pears and the lime-green buds of elm trees.

Identified in old photographs, one such elm was more than 100 years old. Neglected and drooping in a parking lot across the street from the Alfred P. Murrah Federal Building in Oklahoma City, this elm tree had definitely seen better days. But on April 19, 1995, it saw its worst. A tribute to the untold acts of courage, sacrifice, and resiliency, this elm has been dubbed the "Survivor Tree." Why? This aged and untended tree withstood the force of a bomb equal to 5,000 pounds of TNT. Seismometers in the area recorded the explosion as measuring 3.0 on the Richter scale, and the shock and noise were felt and heard fifty-five miles away.

At 9:01 A.M. on that infamous morning, it was business as usual. At 9:02, almost the entire front of the Murrah Federal Building was decimated. Shards of glass were propelled like hand-held rocket-launchers, and all nine stories pancaked, crushing people, furniture, and the hodgepodge of items frequently seen in office buildings—family pictures, memorabilia adorning walls and desks, wallets and purses, pens, and lipsticks.

But this building also housed a daycare center. Located at the front of the building on the second floor, it received a direct hit with maximum force. In seconds, the children's daycare was compressed by the immeasurable weight of seven floors of rebar and concrete. The truck carrying the explosives created a thirty-foot-wide, eight-foot-deep crater in the recessed driveway at the front of the building.

In a sixteen-block radius, 324 buildings were damaged or destroyed, and streets were littered with glass, concrete, and rubble. Fire from eighty-six burning cars filled the air with smoke, combining to form a choking cloud of dust and debris. Weeks later, the official death toll was 168, and an extra leg is still a mystery. Nineteen of the casualties were children, and more than 800 people were injured.

And yet across the street, the 100-year-old elm tree beat the odds.

Within minutes, first responders were at the scene, and reporters from local media outlets were not far behind. Area hospitals called a Code Black—a term used at the time to signify any disaster. Health care personnel with split positions—those who worked part-time in emergency rooms (ERs) or operating rooms (ORs), as well as part-time in other departments—were sent to their respective ERs and ORs. Off-duty personnel were called in to fill the vacated positions.

The University of Oklahoma College of Nursing is located about seven blocks east and four blocks south of the former federal building. Deborah Booton-Hiser, PhD, RN, ARNP, professor and director of University of Oklahoma College of Nursing 's nurse practitioner program, said their first class of the day had just begun. "We were teleconferencing with a class in Tulsa when we heard and felt the blast," she said. "The Tulsa students couldn't hear or feel anything, but they could see us—and they knew something had just happened."

Shortly thereafter they were told that an explosion had occurred in downtown Oklahoma City and health care professionals were being asked to report to Saint Anthony Hospital—an urban hospital located about two blocks west and four blocks north of the blast. "We didn't know what caused the explosion," Dr. Booton-Hiser said. "But a bombing in Oklahoma City was never even considered."

Joined by another faculty member, Barbara McEndree, MS, RN, ARNP, Dr. Booton-Hiser began driving toward the hospital. Listening to a local radio station, they learned the site in question was the Murrah Federal Building. But the cause remained a mystery. The two instructors parked at Saint Anthony but quickly realized the hospital was overflowing with help. So they began walking south toward the federal building. Scheduled for a promotional interview that afternoon to discuss University of Oklahoma College of Nursing's nurse practitioner program, Dr. Booton-Hiser had dressed for the occasion. Wearing a kelly-green suit and matching green high heels, she was hard to miss in the crowd. A senior BSN student, Kim Allen, recognized her as a University of Oklahoma College of Nursing professor and joined them. Hindered by the growing congestion and rubble, Dr. Booton-Hiser had no choice but to continue navigating in the ungainly high heels. "We were walking down the middle of streets because glass was everywhere and debris was still falling," she said.

Rumors that another bomb was set to detonate traveled through the crowd like wildfire. Consequently, several blocks north of the building, the group made a detour to the east. Shortly thereafter, Dr. Booton-Hiser recognized the chief medical officer at the Oklahoma State Department of Health. They joined forces and a larger group began to form in a parking lot several blocks east of the site. As the dust settled and the smoke cleared, they could see the front of the building was a gaping hole of indescribable destruction.

Readily admitting that a scenario of this magnitude had never been covered in anyone's education and experience, Dr. Booton-Hiser said the group invisibly transitioned into a new dimension. "We decided to divide up into two groups and provide first and second line triage," she said. "By that time, home health nurses were dropping off car stock—blue pads, 4x4s, and an assortment of wound care supplies. Medical equipment companies started dropping off IV supplies and poles."

As they set up their triage station, police and security personnel began to cordon off the area. Several asked the health care personnel if they had seen anything suspicious. "This was unprecedented," Dr. Booton-Hiser said. "What was suspicious?"

Leaving the detective work up to the authorities, the group concentrated on establishing a rescue area. Hours passed, but no one came. "Word started trickling down that all the survivors had probably been rescued," she said. "We felt an overwhelming sense of sadness and futility." Similar to the responders on site, personnel in ERs and ORs across the city were poised to act at a moment's notice. Watching and waiting, they soon realized that their feverish preparations were also for naught.

A paradox, time had been suspended in a flurry of reflexive action. At about 2:00 P.M., gray clouds began to move in with the stealth of a thief. Rescuers had not noticed as the clouds became thick and heavy, nor were they aware that the clear-blue sky at dawn's light was now dark and foreboding. At about 2:30 P.M., a light rain began to fall, as if to weep with a city in shock and mourning. Dr. Booton-Hiser said, "It was truly remarkable that so many people came together to contribute to saving lives when we didn't even know what happened."

By the next morning, "Ground Zero" was cordoned off and centers of care were being established. However, care was now directed toward the rescue workers and displaced families—many of whom resided in the Regency Towers Apartments. An urban apartment complex with over 20 stories and about 275 units, the Regency was located a block west of the federal building.

Shortly after the explosion, the entire complex was evacuated and residents were not allowed to return home due to the instability of the high-rise. Many of the residents were elderly people with chronic illnesses. Diabetics had no access to their diabetic supplies and medications, and life-sustaining heart and blood pressure medicine were also left behind.

Consequently, care centers typically offered different services. Some provided aid and comfort to families who had no proof their loved one had escaped. Some provided shoulders to families that knew their loved ones did not. Others assisted displaced families without shelter, food, and medications. Others cared for the needs of rescue workers.

For the next three weeks, Booton-Hiser and her students and health care professionals from across the city worked day and night at Ground Zero as recovery efforts continued. Nurses gave rescue workers tetanus shots and over-the-counter medicine. Due to the high level of stress and fatigue, they also monitored vital signs and physical status as needed.

During this unexpected interlude, Dr. Booton-Hiser's nurse practitioner students—a month away from graduation—began manning sites almost 24/7. "They hadn't taken comprehensive exams," she said. "But they were so distraught, their education was secondary to reality." Despite their exhaustion, their commitment never wavered.

Of note, a completely unanticipated type of caregiving emerged. "Some of the rescue dogs actually became depressed," she said. "They had seen and smelled so much death."

Adding to the dogs' distress was that huge concrete blocks became unstable mini-mountains that were difficult to navigate and couldn't be moved. So while a rescue dog might detect a victim, rescue workers might not be able to access the area due to safety concerns. In addition, many of the dogs' feet became sore and tender from traversing the sharp stones and concrete rubble. "Their owners would ask us to play ball with them," Dr. Booton-Hiser said. "And we'd also make special trips to make sure they had doggie biscuits and other treats to reward them for their work."

And while the bombing was a grotesque and unnecessary tragedy, it did lead to some positive changes. "Before the bombing, we really hadn't concentrated on disaster training and emergency preparedness," she said. "Safety protocols hadn't been established and a more cohesive collaborative effort was needed." As a result, a tremendous body of work has been directed toward emergency preparedness. State and public health departments have developed public health protocols for a variety of scenarios, and drills are now conducted to test and fine-tune relief efforts. In addition, a body of research has emerged that addresses multiple aspects of the bombing as it relates to multiple factors. Notably, a form of shatter-proof glass similar to vehicles' windshields was used in constructing Oklahoma City's new federal building.

And even Dr. Booton-Hiser's kelly green suit and matching high heels had long-term benefits. Kim Allen, the nursing student who was able to pick the NP program director out of the crowd, took note of the instructor's actions and knowledge. The experience shaped her career path. Kim not only became a nurse practitioner; she's now an instructor in the nurse practitioner program at University of Oklahoma College of Nursing .

As for the Survivor Tree, it occupies a position of honor at the Oklahoma City National Memorial and Museum. Now the object of scientific tender loving care, the tree represents strength in times of doubt and loss. Many seedlings have been cultivated from the Survivor Tree and are now available through American Forests' Famous and Historic Trees Collection. And someday, Dr. Booton-Hiser and her husband plan to plant one of these special trees on their property located east of the Oklahoma City limits. "We'll die here," she said. "But the Survivor Trees will live on."

15

Nursing and Disasters: Stories From Around the World

CHINA
Changrong Yuan

At 14:28 Beijing time, May 12, 2008, when nurses throughout the world were celebrating their International Nurses' Day, an earthquake measuring 8.0 on the Richter scale struck Wenchuan County in the Sichuan Province of China. More than 60,000 people died in the disaster, with as many as 30,000 more injured and another nearly 20,000 declared missing. After the earthquake, about 40,000 medical staff from all over the country immediately headed for the front line of relief work. Their relentless efforts saved countless lives and lit the lamp of hope for the people afflicted by the disaster. Their work exemplified the sacred responsibility of the humanitarian creed: Heal the wounded and rescue the dying. As a nursing teacher, I am proud because so many of my students have showed so much courage and love by helping in the disaster relief. The following are stories from my courageous students.

Hong, one of my students, has worked in Sichuan Province since her graduation. She called me after the earthquake and related her experience:

> "I have never encountered any earthquake and I was really scared at the time, but I didn't let you down. On one side, I am well prepared for the situation as a result of frequent trainings of emergency aid; on the other, I am the head nurse, so I must be responsible for our department. At the time, there were 130 inpatients and all of them were elderly, at an average age of 85. The oldest was 102, while the youngest was 70.

We could not use the elevator, so it was difficult to transfer them. Some attendants put their patients on their backs and moved them downstairs. However, for most patients, whose female attendants were too weak to move them, they had to be moved by one another. The nurses and attendants moved the patients to the stair exit and together they took the patients downstairs with a wheelchair. In approximately half an hour, most patients were transferred to safe areas.

There were still twenty more patients whose conditions were too serious to be transferred. They were suffering from cerebral infarction, heart failure, and respiratory failure. Among them four patients were using ventilators and it was dangerous to move them. I decided to stay alone with them. I checked them and consoled them one by one. I told them I would accompany them all the time. The earthquake seemed endless and the inpatient building continued shaking. I was afraid that I would not be able go back to my family again. When I looked in my patients' eyes, I knew they trusted me, and I had no right to be afraid. I would not abandon any of them."

Huang, a head nurse of the surgical room of a hospital in Sichuan, would never forget the miserable scene on that Nurses' Day. Many doctors and nurses were operating when the earthquake occurred. When the earth shook suddenly, everyone was at a loss at first. Because of the sudden shaking, the operating equipment was not functioning correctly, the ceilings were falling down, and the building was collapsing. At that moment, three operations hadn't been completed, two patients were just being "closed," and another three operations were about to begin. An operating lamp shook so much that it was about to crash to the floor. Without any hesitation, Huang ran to protect the patient under the lamp. Just when the situation became stable, Huang and her colleagues promptly tried their best to transfer the patients to the first floor. It was really hard to move the patients, but the staff devised various ways to move them. After the patients were moved, the staff rushed into the dangerous building to salvage important medical equipment and drugs. First-aid boxes, stethoscopes, saline, mannitol, and other things needed to care for the patients were retrieved. Huang divided the patients into several groups according to their conditions. The staff stuck to their duties until they were taken over by the nationwide medical team that came on the morning of May 15.

During this period, Huang learned that she had lost twenty family members in the earthquake, including her mother. Her sister hoped that she could go back home as soon as possible. She refused, however, and stayed because of her responsibilities in the hospital. Huang didn't mention a word about her misfortune. It was not until May 15 that she had an opportunity to mourn her relatives who had passed away.

Lan was a head nurse of the orthopedic department in a hospital. She was attending a conference about Nurses' Day in a hotel five kilometers away from her hospital when she felt the earth shake violently. She had no choice but to walk a long distance back to the hospital because of the devastation caused by the quake. Two hours later, she reached the department, exhausted and anxious. Despite painful feet, she began inspecting the patients. She made a promise to them that she wouldn't give up on any of them. During the next few days, she always kept that belief, however difficult it was. After the earthquake, many wounded people were sent to the hospital from different areas, 90% of whom were in need of orthopedic medical treatment. So many wounded people gathered that the beds in the ward were insufficient. With colleagues, Lan made room for treatment in neighboring departments. Finally, there were 600 beds in total, three times the normal number. By taking some effective measures, Lan managed to bring order to the department's work. First, she divided the patients into several groups and then she appointed experienced nurses to be responsible for each group. Second, with the nursing department of the hospital, she trained some nursing staff from other hospitals to assist them. The workload exhausted Lan completely. She fainted at a nurse's station. Not until then did anyone else know that Lan had been suffering from acute enteritis for three days. She had kept it a secret in order not to interrupt relief work.

Carefully, Min took out a white piece of paper. She cut the paper, unfolded it, and then made it into a beautiful white flower. "It was really a nightmare," she whispered to herself, followed by long silence. Nurse Yang sat in front of her, making paper flowers with Min. Every day, at 2:28 P.M., Min would go to the primary school where she had worked as a teacher for ten years. But where was the school? Nothing stood there but building ruins. Min put the flowers on the ruins and then stood there quietly, her eyes staring at the ruins for a long time. On May 12th, suddenly and without warning, the destructive earthquake caused the school to collapse. One hundred students and their teachers were buried under the ruins. She happened to take part in a meeting outside of the school, and fortunately avoided being trapped. When she went back to school, Min could not believe her eyes. She had had breakfast with all of them that morning. For a couple of days, Min kept repeating the same words in a low voice. She was not able to accept the reality. During the following relief work, children's bodies were carried out of the ruins, covered with dust and blood. Some little hands were even holding pencils and books.

During the whole process of relief work, Yang encountered so many clients with serious depression just like Min. The big earthquake caused severe psychological trauma to our people. Yang and her fellow workers' main task was to treat them with psychological interventions. Yang hoped that with their help, people in the disaster area could step out of the shadow and begin a new life. Facing the catastrophe, nurses attached more importance to a new professional demand—psychological guidance.

Nurses' Day of 2008 appeared to be much more somber because of the Wenchuan earthquake. People will never forget this Nurses' Day. During that unforgettable time, nurses in China learned how to appreciate others, how to cherish what they have, and how to strive for their sacred mission.

MEXICO
Cheryl Herrmann and Rita Knobloch

On a Friday evening in the small village of Ixtlan, located in the state of Michocan, Mexico, we had just completed a week of training for the Cruz Roja (Red Cross Ambulance) and the local police. The elected government had changed, which meant that all the policemen in town were new. They were chosen by the new president and had little training. Because the police are typically the first on scene, we worked with them on First Responder skills—controlling bleeding, burn treatment, splinting a fracture, and scene size-up and safety. To assist with learning the skills, they set up a safe accident scene with toy cars.

As our grand finale, we simulated an earthquake scenario. The scene was a local school that already did earthquake drills. At 10 A.M. the drill started. Twenty students were assigned to stay in the building, acting as the injured with cards around their necks indicating their injuries. The school director called the Cruz Roja and the police, who responded quickly and began to triage. The Cruz Roja and police worked well together to get all of the injured students to the treatment area. When the drill was over, we had a debriefing about the assessments and areas for improvement, and were pleased with how well the simulation went. We thought our week was ended; however, Carlos, the Cruz Roja Director, received word about the need for the ambulance to transport a patient on a ventilator. Four American team members left with him and headed to Guadalajara Hospital, two and one-half hours away.

"Rosie and I volunteered to go with Carlos to transport a patient on a ventilator to Guadalajara. When we arrived in Zamora, we learned that there was a baby on a ventilator that had to be transported. Alberto, an Ixtlan EMT, told us the baby we were to transport weighed one kilogram—2.2 pounds. Carlos, the Cruz Roja Director and physician, told us we were not taking the baby because the ventilator was not working. Alberto gave Rosie and me Cruz Roja vests to put on and we went into the hospital to the pediatric ward. The baby was in an isolette in the hallway with doctors and nurses around it fixing the ventilator, changing tubes, and bagging the baby.

"In the back of the ambulance were the baby's parents, Rosie, and myself. Rosie and I visited with the mom and learned that the baby girl's name was Maria del Rosario. She was only eight days old and had problems with her lungs. Her endotracheal tube was very tiny and she also had an oral gastric tube taped together with the ET tube. A temperature probe was on her chest. She had an IV to her right foot with a glucose solution dripping with a mini drip of buratrol. There were no monitors. The IV was dripping too fast and was a constant challenge to adjust and readjust.

"The alarms for the vent started going off.... There was no pressure. We had to bag the baby. Then the oxygen attached to the vent tank ran out. Carlos and Alberto tried, but were unable to get it attached to the other tank. Meanwhile, I continued bagging. The ambulance turned back and raced toward the hospital because the baby looked bad. We took Maria into the pediatric ward and into a room. The team fixed the ventilator and put in two new oxygen tanks. Then we headed back to the Red Cross ambulance. The parents did not go with us. We drove off and went only about twenty feet when the vent alarms went off. Carlos

stopped the vehicle and the back doors opened. The man who had fixed
the vent before was there and proceeded to fix it again. The baby was
pink and resting. Carlos went into the hospital and came out twenty minutes later with the news that now instead of one preemie to transport,
there were two preemies to transport. The Ixtlan police were contacted
to locate Dr. Bruce, the pediatric intensivist on the team. The other
preemie was taken by another ambulance.

"At 6:25 P.M. we arrived at the Urgencias Pediatria (the Pediatric
Emergency Room) in Guadalajara. The hospital was only expecting one
baby but received two preemies. We were so relieved to hand over the
care of baby Maria Del Rosari. We arrived back in Ixtlan twelve hours
after our experience had begun...."

As I listened to Rita's story, I reflected on the educational opportunities of the past five years for the Ixtlan Cruz Roja that made it possible
for this local ambulance and crew to transport a critically ill neonate. For
several years we had considered taking medical teams to Ixtlan. Initial
assessments indicated a small community with several physicians where
medical care was available. It would be unwise to do a medical clinic
campaign in Ixtlan as we did in Juarez, as we would take business away
from the local doctors. We prayed that when the doors opened for medical missions in Ixtlan, we would be ready and able.

Early in 2003, my fifteen-year-old niece, Brittany, said she really
wanted to go to Ixtlan to visit Rosa and Claudia and learn more about
their culture. These two young Mexican ladies from the Ixtlan Apostolic
Christian Church spent time in our home to experience our culture and
practice their English. The door was open, so we started planning our
trip, which at first was planned as "just a visit."

We had recently completed teaching a fire-medical training mission
in Imuris, Mexico, and I wondered if there was a need for training in
Ixtlan. Sandy, an American physician assistant, was living in Ixtlan and
working with a local physician. I e-mailed an offer to do some CPR/med-
ical training for the community. Sandy met Carlos—a local who is just
finishing his medical degree. He is the director of the Ixtlan Cruz Roja.
Carlos had a vision; his vision was to provide emergency medical care
to his community and a critical care ambulance transport service. This
was a lofty vision, especially when one only has a pathetic looking old
ambulance with no equipment. Sandy was invited to be part of the local
volunteer women's group that was helping the Cruz Roja raise money to
get a new ambulance for the town. At this point, our understanding was

that this group would be the first responders to a call. They did not know CPR, so I was scheduled to teach CPR and some basic first aid.

Carlos, the Cruz Roja Director, brought a new ambulance to the church for everyone to see. The ambulance was very bare with little equipment. When some of the medical team members learned of the need for equipment, especially a defibrillator, donations came in to purchase equipment.

Through an Internet search, I found a defibrillator with a monitor to purchase. Carlos needed a defibrillator with a monitor to meet the critical care ambulance government criteria. Meanwhile, other things were happening in Ixtlan. They recruited ten volunteers to be the ambulance squad. Carlos taught a four-month EMT class. Now, instead of untrained personnel responding to calls, they had a professional squad. And, then a bigger miracle—the squad attended the Mexico National Red Cross meeting and *won* an ambulance! God was working…the time was right for medical missions in Ixtlan.

Besides the defibrillator training, they also wanted information on how to prepare for a community disaster. At this point Don, a fireman, volunteered to go with us and do a disaster drill as he did in Imuris.

On our arrival day, we flew to Guadalajara. Carlos, his wife, and one ambulance crew member drove two and one-half hours to the airport to pick us up. The next evening we thought we were meeting to discuss the plans for the week. However, the whole squad arrived—ready to learn! We couldn't turn them away so I taught them how to use the defibrillator. The next day, Carlos brought the ambulance to the church parking lot; it was bare. We worked with Carlos to stock his ambulance with the supplies we brought. The government had an extensive list of supplies needed for a critical care ambulance—various sized ET tubes, a nasal cannula, laryngoscopes, and dressings. We were able to stock it with everything except a large oxygen tank and ventilator. Before we left Ixtlan, money was given to supply the oxygen tank. It was exciting to see the ambulance turn into a fully equipped vehicle. Carlos was the most excited of all of us, yet overwhelmed by the generosity.

Another aspect of our training was trauma education. We did a trauma scenario with Brittany as our patient who fell from a fifteen-foot tree—well, they laughed at our scenario as there are no fifteen-foot trees in Ixtlan. Her "injuries" included a broken leg, massive cuts on her arm and head, and a spinal injury. We demonstrated how to use splints, c-collars, and a spine board. They strapped Brittany to the spine board and transported her to the ambulance. This team had an impact on Brittany as she changed her career from teaching to nursing. She has participated in two other Mexico medical missions and spent six weeks volunteering at a children's home in Magdalena.

The last day was the day of the anticipated simulation to practice what they learned. The scene was staged: A drunk driver in a pick-up truck was headed toward a van with passengers. The van swerved to attempt to miss the truck and hit a boy on his bike. Several victims were thrown from the van, and the boy on the bike was under the front of the van. Each victim had a tag indicating his injuries and was instructed to act the part of their injuries. Everyone was ready and waiting for the sirens indicating the ambulance was coming. Ten minutes later, the ambulance had not arrived. Don was perplexed and concerned at the slow response. Then he realized that in all of the excitement and translation, the police commander forgot to call in the accident. The call was placed and the sirens started in town. Two ambulances and two police cars quickly responded to the call. The crew started immediately triaging the victims and transporting them to the treatment area. It went remarkably well for the little experience the squad had.

Carlos was appreciative that his squad now had more training and that the police were willing to work with them—it was great publicity for the new ambulance and Cruz Roja. Besides providing training and supplies, we felt the biggest benefit was that we taught Carlos and the police commander how to train their crews by using scenarios and drills. Tears came to Carlos's eyes as he gave us certificates and Cruz Roja badges in appreciation for our efforts. They wanted to know when we would come back. We thanked God for opening the doors in this community for medical missions and looked forward to continuing this work.

A year later, we did another medical mission in Ixtlan. Upon our arrival, we found that just as it is in the United States, it is hard for volunteers to stay committed, and many of the crew we taught a year ago were no longer with the squad. Most of the new crew were fourteen and eighteen year olds. The youngest crew member was eleven years old and had a Barbie doll in her backpack. We quickly learned that our "Barbie doll" Cruz Roja member was motivated and a fast learner. We hoped to return again the next year to continue our work. Prior to that time, we wanted to get more supplies to make the ambulance ready for inspection. The one big item still missing was a portable ventilator. We struggled with the wisdom of having this type of critical care equipment on the ambulance when the crew was just beginners.

It was eighteen months later when we returned for our next training session. Carlos asked again for a portable ventilator because it was the only thing missing that he needed to pass inspection for the Critical Care Ambulance Certification. I called International Aid to ask if they had any portable ventilators that could be used on an ambulance. I had been in contact with them other times and they did not have any, so I was not expecting a positive response. However, they told me they had an LP10 ventilator for $450. It was small, had a battery, was easy to run, and was a reasonable price. And, another miracle, a pediatric intensivist was scheduled to be on the team. Not only were we able to provide them with a ventilator, but had a physician to teach them. Some of the crew, such as Lupeta, had taken three classes from us and was an excellent asset to Carlos. Three local physicians came for training during their lunch break, making a total of five physicians counting Carlos and his father. This was the first time we had local physicians in our class. Dr. Bruce gave a lecture on intubation and then had a skills practice session.

In summary, this project shows how nurse educators can make a difference. It also illustrates the basic mission rule and Chinese proverb: "If you give a man a fish, he will eat for a day. If you teach him to fish, he will eat for a lifetime." By giving them the equipment and the training they need, the Ixtlan Cruz Roja provides a critical care transportation service for an area that encompasses a driving area of two hours in diameter. And little baby Maria was able to be safely transported to a higher level of care.

ZAMBIA
Sarah J. Williams

As the people of Zambia struggle with the high death rate, a major challenge imposed on the family structure is the increasing number of orphans. Adults and children suffer from emotional disturbances rooted in their lack of coping skills to effectively grieve as they witness the death of friends, family members, and acquaintances due to AIDS. A team of nursing professionals at a Texas university responded to professional and educational needs in a rural Zambian village. Through the development and implementation of two cross-cultural distance education training programs on coping with grief and loss, Zambian teachers, caregivers, and guardians of orphans were given coping tools and shown how to help others.

In fall of 2002, a nonprofit charitable organization at a private, faith-based university in Texas implemented a Virtual Learning Center designed to promote learning and leadership of Christian women around the world. The organization is a collaborative network fostering personal and social transformation through community education and research. A major emphasis of this organization is working with economically disadvantaged women. The center provides a space on the Web for women working locally to create peaceful and sustainable global communities to share their experiences, wisdom, and personal values.

Within a year of implementing the interactive website, an idea grew from the interaction among the diverse population of women. The team's mission was to explore outreach initiatives that would enhance the potential of the Web-based virtual community and promote collaboration in addressing the reality of women in developing areas of the world.

The initiative was named Reach-Out-Africa and two sites were selected: Mongu, Zambia and Bukoba, Tanzania. From both locations, immediate interest in collaboration with the charitable organization was expressed by the women. A volunteer team composed of faculty from the Texas university selected Africa as the continent to begin implementation of global initiatives because of its vast poverty and high mortality rate resulting from the HIV/AIDS epidemic. Four specific initiatives were identified: develop cross-cultural leadership programs, offer teacher and caregiver onsite workshops, create virtual learning centers, and promote women's economic development.

By summer of 2003, it was clear that the two teams were needed to support development of outreach activities in both sites. The Zambia team focused on teacher and caregiver on-site workshops, and the Tanzania team focused on developing cross-cultural leadership training for women. In the spring of 2004, the Zambia team traveled to Mongu, Zambia, to present the first training workshop, and again in spring 2006 to present the second workshop.

The first step in developing and implementing the grief and loss training workshops was for the program developer to understand the specific problems and needs of teachers, caregivers, and guardians of orphans in Mongu and surrounding villages. A rapid needs assessment using in-depth dialogue via the Virtual Learning Center was conducted by the Zambia team with local community leaders, community ministries of the province, and home-based volunteers. The major themes that emerged from the needs assessment described Zambian society under pressure from the burden of HIV/AIDS. Home-based care volunteers reported that adults and children have overwhelming sadness and stress. The feelings of loss do not dissipate over time, but continue to impede the individual's ability to lead a healthy, productive life. The volunteers realize that supporting physical needs—nutrition, health, and education—is not enough. Addressing emotional needs is also essential. Programs are needed to help children, adolescents, and adults to move effectively through the grieving process. Teachers, caregivers, family members, and guardians of orphans need support and assistance to cope with death. To be effective, these efforts need to be rooted in the community.

A pre-assessment of specific learning needs relative to working with grieving children occurred on-the-ground, with the administration of a survey during the first hour of each workshop. The survey assessed participants' opinions about who should explain death to children, and their attitudes and perceptions about how children respond to death. Items assessed participants' comfort in discussing death with children, answering children's questions about death, belief about children's involvement in funerals or memorial services, understanding how children think about death, religious and spiritual beliefs, and comfort in discussing their own death with others. Additionally, participants were asked whether they had experienced the death of a friend, relative, or significant other within the past year.

While a majority of the participants in both workshops had a positive attitude toward assisting children with questions about death, many were not comfortable talking to children about death and grieving. The pre-assessment revealed that religion and spirituality were important factors in determining how Zambians cope with bereavement, and that 100% of the participants in both workshops had experienced the death of a loved one within the past year. These on-the-ground assessment results assisted the program developer/facilitator to alter or refocus the content to better suit the participants' immediate needs.

Learning objectives aimed at increasing the knowledge and changing the attitudes of the Zambian leaders were identified. Distance complicated the development of content. Teaching with visible images and oral traditions has been shown to be effective in disseminating didactic information in the Zambian culture. The overall key to developing the content for both workshops was to provide culturally appropriate, constructive information that would improve the coping strategies for adults and children, and to present activities that would accommodate the unique customs and practices of the Zambian people. Participants freely offered examples based on cultural practices. Program sponsors who were of the local Catholic ministries located in the Mongu and surrounding provinces selected the participants who were to attend the workshops.

The charitable organization, along with local leaders and program sponsors in Mongu and surrounding communities, planned for a five-day workshop, eight hours daily with two twenty-minute breaks and a one-hour lunch period. Energizing activities were added throughout the long days, which included song, dance, readings, and prayer.

Analysis of the workshops revealed that the majority of participants felt the need for presentations in grief and loss, and that more opportunities should be available for more of the community's population. Participant responses in reference to what was liked best about Workshop 1 revolved around common themes such as facilitator's openness, topics surrounding how to help children grieve, motivating and stimulating course materials, good interaction and participation, and the songs and dances. Participants would have liked more time allotted for the training.

Implementing an outreach program to developing countries using distance education methods presents a number of anticipated and unanticipated challenges relating to language barriers both in presentations and on written forms. The biggest challenge was ensuring effective communication while planning from a distance with a group with limited technological access. This was compounded by the language barrier and scarce resources in the host community to support training.

Internet access and e-mail were the primary methods of communication. These methods posed challenges for consistent communication with the host program sponsors. The communication infrastructure lacks capabilities to support a strong telecommunications system. This is due in part to prohibitive costs for this region. In the western region of Zambia, the basic tools needed for Internet access—a computer and a telephone line—are luxuries and unaffordable by most Zambians. As a growing country, some progress is these areas is evident; however, these challenges will likely continue. Persistent, careful, and timely preplanning is essential for distance program planning. Consistent dialogue with the on-site program sponsors was necessary as much as possible, given the limited access of the charitable organization to the host community. Designation of specific time frames for synchronous online web discussions proved to be successful. Identification of "best times" for accessing the Internet for discussions and chats worked well; however, international time differences posed difficulties for some in gaining access during the designated time frames. Despite limited access during various periods, it is recommended that communication via e-mail be continued as one of the quickest and consistent modes of communication if distance planning is to be used for future programming.

Even though English is spoken as a second language, there were language barriers that required additional effort to ensure maximum participant understanding of content during workshop presentation. Utilization of an interpreter was key to the success. Limited availability of basic educational resources, such as pencils, paper, and notebooks, posed another challenge for ensuring that maximum learning occurred.

Finally, the issue of cultural differences requires continued attention. Preparing trainers through dialogue with onsite native Zambians about the range of learning styles, issues of interpersonal communication such as eye contact, touch, distance, and social and economic differences in daily life should be done prior to travel and training. Researching the culture, values, mores, and ways of the people is helpful and recommended prior to traveling to the country. Emphasis must be placed on the culture shock experienced by trainers when first entering a country with very diverse cultural differences and overwhelming poverty. Prior knowledge allows trainers the ability and time to reflect on their own values.

The ultimate goal for the workshops was to begin an empowering process to assist the Mongu and surrounding communities to meet the needs of grieving adults and children. Working along with the program sponsors from both communities, a team of three Zambian women are now trained and fully capable of providing training totally independently. The program sponsors and the Texas university's team have worked together to build a structure within the Zambian community that ensures follow-up, maintenance, and consistency, which will exist for future training workshops. The positive outcomes of this project are proof that the distance education approach is an effective means for assessing, planning, implementing, and evaluating an outreach program in Zambia.

In concert with the mission of the university, the Reach-Out-Africa Project continues to work toward achieving social justice in a world of poor and underserved populations. This success story attests to the university's mission of social justice and cross-cultural diversity, and of promoting global health and preventing disease.

16

Disaster Preparedness

Cheryl K. Schmidt, Joy Jennings, Shannon Finley,
Susan Ritchie, and Jan Rooker

Since September 11, 2001, nursing faculty throughout the United States have been compelled to develop strategies to prepare for disasters. This includes preparing themselves, their students, and their nursing programs, as well as developing the knowledge and skills to provide education and care to clients before, during, and after disasters. Professional and accrediting organizations have included expectations for disaster preparedness in their guidelines for nursing education.

More than just pragmatic reasons have driven the inclusion of disaster preparedness in nursing curricula. Nurses are drawn to community service activities in order to extend their caring beyond institutional walls. This service-oriented spirit is one of the factors that draws students to the profession. Nurse educators serve as role models by participating in community activities outside of their scheduled classes, and they nurture their students' interests by involving them in a wide variety of service activities.

In June of 1999, Dr. Cheryl Schmidt served in an American Red Cross canteen/first aid tent a few hundred yards from American Airlines Flight 1420 after it crashed in Little Rock, Arkansas. She joined the American Red Cross Disaster Services Human Resources system and took every disaster training course she could find. When tornados hit downtown Little Rock in 2000, she took her Community Health Nursing students to help the Seventh Day Adventists set up a Federal Emergency Management Administration (FEMA) warehouse to collect and distribute emergency supplies to the tornado victims. That event, however, was one of the few disaster-related experiences our students had, and we did not provide any specific classes about how nurses can serve in the American Red Cross.

Everything changed after September 11, 2001, for both faculty and nursing students. In December of 2001, Dr. Schmidt taught a lecture in the Community Health Theory course called Bioterrorism: Recognition and Response, and she has since expanded that content to include Biological, Chemical, and Nuclear/Radiological Terrorism: Recognition and Response, Pandemic Influenza: Are We Ready?, and Preparing Yourself Personally and Professionally for Disasters. During spring semester 2002, Dr. Schmidt certified her own clinical group in the American Red Cross Community First Aid course, which is a prerequisite for enrollment in other American Red Cross disaster courses. When students in other clinical groups heard about the training, they asked to be included. We now certify all traditional and RN/BSN students enrolled in our Community Health Nursing course in the following American Red Cross Disaster Courses: Introduction to Disasters, Community First Aid, Shelter Operations, and Disaster Health Response. These four American Red Cross courses provide the primary information nurses need to become American Red Cross volunteers, and they are presented in two eight-hour clinical days. The first morning is spent in the Introduction to Disasters course, which includes a video about the American Red Cross, plus many examples of the wide variety of roles nurses play. The day-long Community First Aid course takes only a half day because the students are already certified in CPR and automated external defibrillator use. The second day includes the Shelter Operations and Disaster Health Response courses, which overlap because the nursing roles and required paperwork are similar in both. All students receive four certification cards that they can show to future employers and American Red Cross chapters as they move to other states.

Our nursing students are also required to take three of the National Incident Management System (NIMS) courses offered free through the Internet by FEMA. These courses introduce learners to the Incident Command System, the National Incident Management System, and the policies and procedures required of all agencies participating in disaster response. Health care facilities and other agencies that receive federal funding for disaster preparedness are now required to ensure NIMS-compliance for any employees who partici-

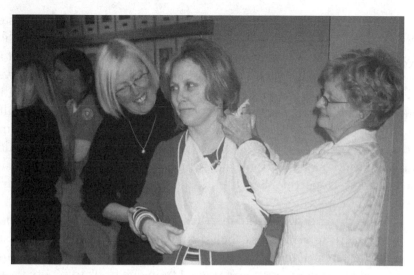

Alice Martin-Watson, Sue Ragsdale, and Sarah Mobley, doing a first aid class "check off" at the American Red Cross of Greater Arkansas in Little Rock, AR, in 2009. The class was part of the Accelerated Disaster Training Model that Cheryl Schmidt developed for the University of Arkansas for Medical Sciences College of Nursing in Little Rock. The model won the American Red Cross Susan Hassmiller Award in May 2009, and a process is being developed to disseminate it throughout the United States. Photo by Cheryl Schmidt.

pate in disaster response. Our graduates are a step ahead when they interview for their first nursing position.

The American Red Cross and NIMS courses provide our students with a strong theoretical base for disaster response, but the most valuable learning occurs through service during actual disasters and community disaster drills. Actual disasters are often unpredictable, and they vary with geographic location. Arkansas faces frequent tornados, floods, ice storms, heat emergencies, and tanker and railroad accidents. The New Madrid earthquake fault crosses northeastern Arkansas, forcing citizens to plan for either the direct effects of a massive earthquake or the subsequent evacuation of thousands of people. During hurricane season, Arkansas is a primary host for thousands of evacuees from the coast. For example, after Hurricanes Katrina and Rita, over 70,000 evacuees spent several weeks in Arkansas shelters. All states face the potential of pandemic influenza, as well as terrorist attacks. Finally, fires destroy hundreds of homes each year.

Our students are encouraged to participate as individuals in disaster response through their churches, for example, by collecting and distributing donations. They can list such activities on their learning contract in an independent study course, which awards academic credit for involvement in the National Student Nurses' Association and participation in leadership and service activities. Whenever possible, nursing faculty identify opportunities for students to practice the nursing role during a disaster. After Hurricane Katrina in 2005, all Community Health Nursing faculty members took their clinical groups to shelters to assist the Arkansas Department of Health nurses in doing assessments and providing immunizations.

During Hurricane Gustav in 2008, several nursing faculty helped staff an American Red Cross shelter in a local church. Undergraduate students were invited to work in the shelter under faculty supervision, and they cared for clients whose ages ranged from one week to ninety years, with a wide variety of acute and chronic health care problems. Several graduate students interviewed shelter residents to meet a requirement for an Advanced Health Assessment course, and they ended up staying to help with individual needs. For example, local police had delivered one client to the shelter who was wearing only a patient gown, pajama bottoms, and no shoes. He had been getting daily dressing changes for severe leg and foot burns from a work-related accident prior to the storm. One of the graduate students completed a sterile dressing change and created a "shoe" from a diaper and plastic bag, then sent the client to the local burn center. Another graduate student accompanied a faculty member to another shelter in town to help Arkansas Department of Health nurses do health assessments on hurricane evacuees. A part of the learning process for graduate students in our program includes expanding the database, validating the information gathered, and identifying and using community resources to meet a variety of needs. By working in the disaster shelters, the graduate students are positioned to call upon their education and experiences as registered nurses, expand their learning process, and serve the community. This is the ideal setting for case management practices as well.

Every fall semester, the Arkansas Department of Health provides thousands of flu vaccinations throughout the state in order to practice the state's emergency mass vaccination/dispensing plan. Staff and volunteer nurses provide hundreds of vaccines in one day at the state fairgrounds, and they invite nursing students from local nursing programs to administer the vaccines under faculty supervision. Besides practicing their injection technique and providing a priceless community service, the students have first-hand experience in one of Arkansas's strategies to respond to a bioterrorism event or pandemic influenza.

Each summer, the American Red Cross of Greater Arkansas hosts high school students throughout Arkansas at a Rapid Response Team Leadership Training Camp. The high school students leave the camp certified in Community First Aid and the Incident Command System, and with leadership skills to guide them as they return to their schools to lead school-based Rapid Response Teams. With the guidance of faculty sponsors and American Red Cross volunteers, these high school students develop emergency plans to respond to disasters such as school shootings, tornados, fires, and other disasters. They learn to respond quickly during such events, providing leadership and first aid while waiting for other emergency responders to arrive. Arkansas is a rural state, so the delayed arrival of responders is often significant. Nursing faculty serve as nurses for the Rapid Response camp, and nursing students volunteer to play "victims" during a disaster drill to test the campers' first aid skills. The erupting chaos, realistic sounds, complex wounds, and high casualty counts witnessed by the high school students during the mock disaster reinforces the need for disaster preparedness education.

Students can also choose the American Red Cross of Greater Arkansas as a clinical site and spend time learning about the wide variety of roles nurses play in the American Red Cross, including health and safety education, blood donation services, and disaster response. The students are given the opportunity to take the beginning safety and disaster courses; if a crisis or disaster arises, they are encouraged to participate as volunteers. This is a highly beneficial experience for both the RN students and the American Red Cross, because the students are able to use their years of nursing experience and their newly acquired knowledge to help with relief efforts. The goal is to motivate the students who choose this experience to enroll as official American Red Cross volunteers.

Nationwide, there is a serious shortage of American Red Cross nurses, and this is compounded by the general nursing shortage. Fewer than ten of our sixty nurse educators are currently certified as American Red Cross nurses. American Red Cross policies require that shelters have at least one health care provider on site or at least on call at all times while the shelter is open. If only a small percentage of the 100 to 120 nursing students we educate each year become American Red Cross volunteers after graduation, future shortages will be less severe. If we can also certify additional nurse educators as American Red Cross volunteers, we will increase the number willing to provide disaster response experience as part of their clinical courses. Nursing students who volunteer for ten or more hours for the American Red Cross earn a special American Red Cross pin; nurses earn a pin after volunteering for twenty or more hours. We will present pins to those who have earned them during their recent work in hurricane shelters, in hopes of motivating others to become involved in this vital community service.

In summary, nursing programs are encouraged to replicate the model our nursing program has developed, which prepares nursing students to respond to the many types of disasters in our country.

Florence Keane and Elicia Egozcue

Having being a victim of a disaster, I know from first-hand experience the initial response is panic and pandemonium. At first there is anger and disbelief that this has happened; next there is panic. Will anyone know that disaster has struck? Will there be aid in a timely manner? Then one starts to focus on the loss. There is loss of life, loss of belongings, loss of jobs, maybe even loss of everything. My first experience of a disaster was Hurricane Andrew on August 24, 1992. Man-made or natural disasters are occurring more frequently in the United States and all over the world. This increases the need for nurses at all levels to be trained in disaster nursing.

Once a disaster is declared, the needs assessment begins. Nurses are in a unique situation to participate. They provide education, advocacy, treatment, and prevention at all levels. Nurses are instrumental in developing educational materials for health care workers to use in catastrophic events. Nurses and other health care workers must be able to rapidly and to effectively assess, treat, lead, and communicate during events that may result in mass casualties.

After Hurricane Andrew, the nursing schools in South Florida sent students, without any prior training or preparation, to Homestead to help victims of the hurricane. There was the problem of transporting the students to and from the hurricane sites, and also the fact that the students had no preparation in disaster nursing. Classes were suspended. Every nursing student was taught first aid, infection control, and assessment during their first year in nursing school, but the concern for safety was a major consideration, and so the senior students who were learning community health nursing were the ones who went to help. This, however, brought about a new awareness that there was a need for preparation for disaster nursing. The ailments that the students and their instructors cared for ranged from minor lacerations, eye irritations, and sprains, to fractures and cardiac and respiratory conditions.

Students on the Gulf Coast should be trained in all types of disasters. South Florida, in particular, sits at the mouth of the Caribbean and lies in the path of many hurricanes. In 2004, the area had four hurricanes and accompanying tornadoes that caused great damage to the land and people. The following year, neighboring states, Louisiana and Texas, suffered from extensive flooding after Hurricane Katrina. The neighboring islands surrounding South Florida have all suffered from the after effects of hurricanes, volcanoes, and earthquakes, and South Florida has always come to the rescue. In 2008, Cuba and Haiti suffered extensive damage, and once again South Florida provided medical, nursing, and economic aid.

After September 11, 2001, Florida International University , began teaching disaster nursing to the beginning nursing students. The basic training consisted of mock disaster drills geared for man-made disasters and triaging after a disaster. This provided great preparation for a man-made disaster but did not address training for a natural disaster. The neighboring hospitals also provided disaster training, but again the training was focused on military disaster fueled by the aftermath of the September 11, 2001, attacks.

The Center for Hurricane Disaster is housed on the campus at Florida International University, and the university is the designated hurricane relief shelter for residents from the Florida Keys. In 2004 the community nursing students were very instrumental in caring for the hurricane victims at the shelter. As a part of their course they were taught disaster nursing, so they were able to provide assessment and treatment for those residents in the shelter. Again most of the hurricane victims had minor respiratory distress and minor lacerations from securing their homes in a hurry. The majority of the hurricane victims were stressed and they needed therapeutic communication and stress management, which the students who were primarily from our Foreign Physician Program were more than capable of providing.

In the aftermath of September 11, there was the postal worker anthrax scare. While the IMSURT team was screening and treating many postal workers with antibiotics, a South Florida Hospital in 2001 admitted a patient who developed a respiratory infection after an anthrax exposure. This patient was not a postal worker but an office manager.

Even though anthrax had been around for a while, when this patient was admitted to a local Miami hospital and his diagnosis was anthrax, there was panic in the hospital. None of the nurses had been trained in caring for an anthrax patient, so safety was the main concern. No one wanted to care for the patient for fear of contracting the "anthrax infection." Nursing ethics would not support this attitude so it was decided that in an attempt to lessen the exposure, a different nurse would care for the patient each shift.

Then, there was the matter of the press. There was a leak that the patient with anthrax was in this hospital, so every day numerous reporters would show up at the hospital hoping to speak with the nurses who were caring for this patient. Of course the CDC and IMSURT were contacted, and the local nurses and other medical staff were educated on safety measures. Fortunately, the patient recovered and returned home, and none of the nurses who cared for him contracted the anthrax disease.

In 2004, I traveled to Mbarara, Uganda, to visit the university there and to learn about their nursing program. Because I was planning to start my own disaster training at Florida International University, I asked about their role in the Ebola outbreak. I learned that safety was the key. A physician and several nurses lost their lives while caring for some victims who had contracted the Ebola virus because they did not follow the standard precautionary measures. The Ebola is a bloodborne virus; when one of the nurses became delirious with fever one night, several others rushed to the rescue and broke the quarantine and contact isolation precautions. It was determined that the most important principle I could impart to my students and fellow nurses was safety first, especially when caring for individuals from different cultures.

On August 15, 2007, at 18:40 hours local time, a magnitude 8.0 earthquake struck near the town of Chincha Alta, ninety-five miles south-southeast of Lima along the Pacific coast, according to the U.S. Geological Survey. A total of 519 were killed, and 1,844 were injured; 52,891 houses were destroyed, and 22,939 houses were damaged. Lives were turned upside down in a matter of seconds, and families were devastated not knowing what the future had in store for them. The cities of Chincha, Pisco, and Ica were affected the most.

Thousands were convinced that this was the end of the world as powerful tremors forced families to spill into the streets. Many mud-brick houses crumbled, residents placed the bodies of relatives and neighbors on street corners, and hospitals were overwhelmed with injured in Chincha and the nearby city of Pisco. Organizations such as the Red Cross, UNICEF, and USAID rushed to bring much needed help to those most affected, offering temporary shelters created from sheets of plastic, food, supplies, and water.

In 2001, Dr. Orlando Silva founded what is known as the Emmaus Medical Mission, which seeks to meet the medical needs of the poor who have no other means of receiving any medical attention due to socioeconomic circumstances. This medical mission now travels to Guatemala biannually, as well as Ecuador and Peru. After hearing of the devastation brought upon Peru as a result of the earthquake, we realized that this was a great opportunity to provide much needed relief to the people of Chincha and surrounding areas. Upon arrival, the team of forty-five doctors, nurses, and volunteers set up what was going to be the "clinic" for the next three days, which in all actuality was a school. Over 100 bags of medications, each weighing fifty pounds, were collected months prior, categorized, labeled, and now sent to the cubicle of the corresponding medical specialties.

The working conditions were not the most comfortable. The sun was beating down on volunteers as they guided locals through the triage area and attempted to maintain order among a sea of thousands in need. Meanwhile, doctors and nurses were working in a school with temperatures reaching over a hundred in a desert land that does not see one drop of rain on any given year. Although locals may be accustomed to such temperatures and extreme conditions, it can be quite a trying time for others. Some of the volunteers suffered from dehydration yet continued to successfully complete the mission.

The Florida International University nursing team had many roles to fill within this large group of health care providers. Among her many duties, Elicia, an undergraduate nursing student, was the leader of the triage team. She trained the nonmedical volunteers to triage and screen for psychological stress, especially among the children, in addition to taking blood pressures, monitoring blood sugars, and screening for other disease processes. The pediatric nurse practitioner student, Sue Hellen, worked along side the pediatrician as she treated approximately 150 children during the three days of the mission. Both students spoke Spanish and Sue Hellen was born in Peru, so they were able to provide culturally competent care and teaching to the earthquake victims.

Hygiene was a big problem in this region. Most of the residents were now living in tents and they had no running water or electricity. After assessing the needs of the residents of Chincha, Dr. Keane realized that they needed teaching on infection control. Many of the residents, including children, were suffering from stress and needed psychological teaching on stress relief. The school-aged children were no longer in school, as the schools were destroyed. Many were in need of psychological help as well as medical help. The Florida International University trio spent a great deal of time educating the residents on hand hygiene. There were many skin infections, respiratory ailments, and gastrointestinal problems. The residents were taught to boil their water before drinking, to ensure they did not eat food that had been sitting outside for too long, and to make sure that their foods were cooked and heated properly before consuming.

There is a need for more culturally appropriate disaster training in nursing programs. The faculty must first be knowledgeable of disasters and find new ways to involve students in helping. Nursing students need to learn more than triaging and must have more than military-type disaster trainings. As disasters continue to strike, it is important to prepare future nurses to assist in disasters while keeping themselves safe.

Joanne C. Langan

Who would have thought that a global tragedy could result in something positive and make our world a better place? Following the tragic events of September 11, 2001, the dean of our School of Nursing asked the faculty to form a task force to develop disaster preparedness content and programs for our nursing students. We had very little disaster preparedness content in our program at the time. In October 2003, a group of us traveled to Jerusalem, Israel, to study disaster education with nurses at the Henrietta Szold Hadassah Hebrew University School of Nursing and Hadassah hospitals. The group consisted of four nurses and a faculty member from the St. Louis University Institute of Biosecurity in the School of Public Health.

The education we received included such topics as trauma care, ideology of terrorists, bereavement, identifying loved ones, and psychological support for victims, families, and first responders, as well as nurse and nursing student roles in disaster management. The experience included approximately eight days of intense classroom and field learning. Our teachers were experts in their fields. They had frequent and recent experience with man-made disasters in the form of suicide bombers and the aftermath of other terrorist-related activities. The nurse faculty member who was instrumental in planning the curriculum also serves as a health educator volunteer worldwide.

Upon return to the United States, we immediately began concurrent work on both a textbook and an online disaster preparedness certificate program for nurses. The textbook includes some of the very powerful stories we heard from both nurses as professionals and as parents, and from the parents of a teenage girl, a victim of a suicide bombing in a pizza restaurant. The purpose of the textbook is to prepare nurses in a variety of settings to assist in planning for, and responding to, both man-made and natural disasters. The online distance learning disaster preparedness certificate program consists of six mandatory modules and the learner's choice of four of the twelve elective modules offered. We also have a module recorded by a nurse who participated in disaster relief efforts in many countries. Through these recorded modules, registered nurse students can access additional nurse and disaster preparedness experts' experiences that can broaden their ability to help others in times of tragedy. Without this format, many would not be able to receive this content or hear the stories of nurses who have had experience with assisting victims of disasters that have occurred in the United States and abroad.

Originally the online program was offered only to registered nurses through the continuing education program; however, undergraduate students voiced an interest in disaster preparedness. Disaster nursing content continues to be taught in our on-site Public Health Nursing course. The author/faculty member delivers the content in both the traditional and accelerated options of the baccalaureate nursing program. To enhance the on-site lecture, the material is peppered with real life disaster experiences involving earthquakes, hurricanes, tornadoes, snow storms, and power outages. Mitigation of disaster effects, disaster response efforts, and lessons learned are described in the lecture presentations.

For example, while living on the Gulf Coast of Mississippi, we evacuated twice during the threat and hit of Hurricane Elena. We heeded the first evacuation order and drove to Northern Mississippi on the Friday before Labor Day in 1985. Within twenty-four hours, the "all clear" was given and most returned home. The hurricane moved back to sea. As we have learned, a hurricane can strengthen over water. The power of the storm does not break up until it hits land. On Sunday of the same weekend, the hurricane headed straight to land and another evacuation order was issued. Some of our neighbors chose to stay behind, as they did not believe the hurricane would hit our area with anything more than heavy rains. They were wrong. Homes along the bayou were flooded, trees were downed and crashed through roofs. Mud was strewn so hard against homes that it stuck like concrete and cracked any non-shuttered windows.

Two of our neighbors with young children chose not to evacuate. The four-year-old child of one of our neighbors was so traumatized by the sound of the gale force winds that he subsequently fled to his closet at the sound of large trucks going down the street. Another neighbor's sixth-grade son was so frightened during the onslaught of nature's fury, that he chewed ulcers inside his mouth.

Because of the request of undergraduate students to have access to the online program for credit, an online disaster preparedness course was created for them as an elective. The two-credit course is distance learning only with no direct face-to-face contact with classmates or the faculty member. The three-credit course requires the student to attend two disaster preparedness or related meetings, actively participate at the meetings, and share the experience through the on-line format provided. Additionally, those taking the course for three credits are required to actively participate in one disaster drill in the community. They are prepared to play a variety of roles in the disaster drills.

In the spring of 2008, students attended the drill planning meetings at a nearby children's hospital. They learned about the myriad of details involved in planning a successful field drill, as well as the importance of collaboration with community partners such as police, fire, rescue, agency security, and state and local emergency management agencies. The purpose of this drill was to determine if our School of Nursing building could serve as an alternate care site for the hospital. Students participated as victims, family members, nurses caring for victims at the disaster site, transporters, and nurses receiving patients at the alternate care site.

Following the drill, the nursing students shared perceptions of the drill at the "hot wash" or debriefing session. A great deal was learned through this exercise by hospital personnel, students, faculty, and community leaders. Students had the opportunity to see the application of concepts learned in real-time practice. Again, students who participated in the drill shared the experience with classmates on the discussion board and fielded questions. Some of the questions prompted the students to do further research and interview disaster preparedness content experts for clarification and answers. While the drill was considered a success by all, it was decided that evacuation of patients to an alternate care site should only be implemented in the case of extreme circumstances when the hospital building could no longer offer refuge or shelter to any degree. It was also recommended that a table-top drill follow the drill planning phase before a live field drill was held in the future.

Students also participate in community flu shot clinics and learn how to set up mass prophylaxis sites. Students are welcomed at university-wide meetings of the Pandemic Response Planning Committee and the university's Emergency Preparedness Committee. Their active participation at these meetings keeps committee members aware of the needs and concerns of one of our key stakeholders in the academic setting. In the immediate aftermath of Hurricane Katrina, one of the physicians at St. Louis University organized physicians, nurses, and students to assist evacuees in a homeless shelter clinic in St. Louis. We were able to volunteer short periods of time in the clinic to assess the needs of the evacuees. At times, the evacuees simply needed to be heard and seemed to find the sharing of their experiences through the displacement of their families to be cathartic.

Through involvement with community disaster planning agencies, the nursing students receive a great learning experience. In return, the community and future employers receive an RN workforce prepared to participate in disaster preparedness prevention, planning, mitigation, and response activities. It is reassuring that a tragedy such as September 11, 2001, can be seen as the end of an era of not knowing and not believing that atrocities can occur at any time, anywhere in the world. It is the beginning of an era of knowing and believing that we can prepare ourselves and future nurse leaders in disaster preparedness. These future leaders will be the new nurse educators who will continue to change the world.

17

A Time to Give Back
Personal Philanthropy

Diane M. Breckenridge

As a nurse who has been supported by others, I wanted to give back in recognition of those that supported my career progression in nursing from the early 1970s. In recognition of excellent academic educators and the socio-cultural support I received, in 1977, I began to fundraise for those in need financially, and also to be a mentor and advisor both academically and personally.

My philanthropic mission began when I was twenty-three. I raised scholarship funds for those who wanted to become nurses. These funds were raised through the District Nurses Association of Montgomery County of the Pennsylvania State Nurses Association of the American Nurses Association, where I continue to be an active legislative liaison member, co-chair of PA State Government Relations Committee, and a past president of the County Nurses Association.

My philanthropic efforts continued annually and were increased in the 1980s when I became very active in fundraising for student nurses at the Abington Memorial Hospital School of Nursing (now known as the Dixon School of Nursing), where I have continued employment for thirty-four years. I continue to fundraise for the Dixon School of Nursing today. In 2007, the Diane Breckenridge Scholarship Award was given to three nurses to bridge from the Dixon School RN-Diploma program to pursue their BSN and one student with a non-BSN baccalaureate degree to pursue the MSN. From 1981 to 2007, I raised approximately $250,000 in personal and private gifts and grants for those wanting to pursue nursing careers.

In 1992, while a doctoral student at the University of Maryland, I learned of the New Access Student program for high school students and students in second careers attending or returning to community colleges to gain access to a college education. I was intrigued with the term "New Access Student" and adopted its use for nursing students who had the same characteristics of being from under-represented, diverse populations.

Characteristics of the "New Access Student" led me to do qualitative field work during my doctoral education in the 1990s. I studied recruitment of students who wanted to attend nursing school. There was a major decrease in the number of traditional students attending nursing schools at that time. Also, many nursing schools in the United States closed or decreased in size. Thus, students recruited for nursing programs tended to be the nontraditional, second career, older students predominately at the community college associate degree and diploma school levels, especially in the Philadelphia region of the country. Risk factors that were identified included attending colleges and schools of nursing from under-represented, diverse populations, including speaking English as a second language; first-generation high school students entering college; entering nursing at an older age, as a second career; working part-time or full-time to finance their undergraduate and graduate education toward an RN, BSN, and/or MSN; and those with family responsibilities.

Beginning in 2002, I developed the Career Ladder Program for New Access Students for the Nursing Education, Training and Skills (NETS) Program. Hospital employees, nursing assistants, licensed practical nurses, high school students, and second career student/employees and their family members were eligible for the program. The first phase was initiated to identify resources for students during preadmission and remediation into an RN-Diploma hospital nursing program, and to identify strategies to overcome risk factors to assist students to complete the RN-Diploma program and pass the NCLEX-RN.

The second phase of the Career Ladder Program was initiated in the fall of 2004. This phase was focused on the RN to BSN and to MSN Bridge for RNs who have non-nursing baccalaureate degrees. Both groups of RNs graduate from associate or diploma programs and pursue upper division nursing courses, including the advanced skills and knowledge of research, genetics, safety, and leadership. I coordinated an undergraduate research course for hospital nurses to engage in evidence-based practice and to carry out research as our hospital sought Magnet designation. In 2008, the hospital received Magnet designation for the second time. The nurses were engaged in evidence-based practice, with fifty-one completing the program. Presently, five nurses are pursuing doctoral degrees.

In 2006, I assumed a joint appointment position as Associate Research Director at the hospital where I have worked for thirty-four years. I also am in a tenured position as Associate Professor at La Salle University. In the undergraduate part-time evening program at this university, 53% of the students are from under-represented, diverse groups. I developed a program titled "ACHIEVE a BSN" to assist students from under-represented, diverse groups that presently have a 72% first-time NCLEX RN pass rate. The goal is to raise this first-time pass rate to the national average of approximately 82–84% in the first year of the program, and then to incrementally raise the rates over the next three years and sustain this level of success. The challenge I now face is to bring strategies for success to this inner-city university at-risk student population. It is also important to continue to fundraise for stipends and scholarships for students to have the resources necessary for success.

INDEX

Abdellah, Faye, 15
Acheson, Evelyn L., 124–132, 313
"ACHIEVE a BSN" program, 381
Ade's Place, 301–302
Africa, nurse educators in, 97
  Burundi, 97–100
  Cameroon, 100–103
  Eritrea, 104–109
  Ghana, 109–113
  Kenya, 113–121
  Southern Africa, 121–124
  Swaziland, 124–132
  Uganda, 132–154
  Zambia, 359–364
  Zimbabwe, 160–166
African Refuge Family and Youth
  Center, 48
Africa Program, The, 140
AHA. *See* American Heart Association
  (AHA)
Ahern, Kathleen, 48–49
Ahmed, Hiro Ibrahim, 317
Aiken, Linda, 233
Akaragian, Salpy, 231–234
Albright, Angela V., 104–109
Alcorn State University School of
  Nursing, 327, 329–330, 332
Alex's Lemonade Stand, fundraising
  event, 56
Alfred P. Murrah Federal Building,
  346–350
Al Gasseer, Naeema, 22–23
Allen, Kim, 347, 350
Allen, Matron, 323
Allen, Patricia, 59–61
al-Talabani, Jalal, 317
American Assembly of Men in Nursing, 16
American Board of Commissioners for
  Foreign Missions, 12
American Heart Association (AHA), 343
American Red Cross, 3, 4, 366, 367, 369
Anthrax, 372
Argentina, 167–173
Arkansas Department of Health, 369
Arkansas State Board of Nursing, 68
Armenia, 231–234
Armenian Nurses Association, 232

Ashton, Kathleen C., 218–222
Ayoré Indians, 313, 314–315

Bailey, Brooke, 152–153
Bangladesh, 320, 321
Bankert, Esther G., 173–177
Barrett, C., 232
Barton, Clara, 3–4
Beachman, Agnes, 300–306
Bell, Deborah, 188–194
Bell-Scriber, Marietta, 234–239
Bessent, Hattie, 16
Bethel University, 132–140
Billings, Lynda, 59–61
Bingham, Janice, 63–67, 70
Bittner, Nancy Phoenix, 222–226
Black infant health program, San
  Francisco, 44–45
Blesch, Pam, 97–100
Bobonich, Margaret, 192
Bolivia, 313–316, 320, 321
Booton-Hiser, Deborah, 347, 348, 349
Botswana, 128–129
Bourke, Mary P., 57 58
Brazil, 173–177
Breckinridge, Mary, 5–6
Brice, Linda M., 41–44
Brown, Mary Ann, 190, 191
Bumpers, Betty, 65
Burt, Jeanie, 66
Burundi, 97–100

Cadena, Sandra J., 289–292
Calvo, Arlene, 289
Cambodia, 234–246, 324
Cameroon, 100–103
Canada, 25–26
Carnegie, Mary Elizabeth, 10
Carnegie Foundation for the
  Advancement of Teaching, 195
Cash, Jamie, 153–154
CBNC. *See* The Chicago Bilingual Nurse
  Consortium (CBNC)
CCID. *See* Community Colleges for
  International Development (CCID)

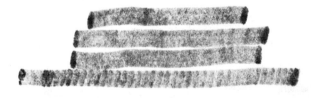